Color Atlas of
Canine and Feline Ophthalmology

Color Atlas of
Canine and Feline Ophthalmology

JOAN DZIEZYC, DVM, Diplomate ACVO
Texas A&M University
Department of Small Animal Medicine and Surgery
College of Veterinary Medicine
College Station, Texas

NICHOLAS J. MILLICHAMP, BVetMed, PhD, DVOphthal, DECVO, MRCVS, Diplomate ACVO
Texas A&M University
Department of Small Animal Medicine and Surgery
College of Veterinary Medicine
College Station, Texas

ELSEVIER
SAUNDERS

ELSEVIER
SAUNDERS

11830 Westline Industrial Drive
St. Louis, Missouri 63146

COLOR ATLAS OF CANINE AND FELINE OPHTHALMOLOGY
ISBN-13: 978-0-7216-8239-6
ISBN-10: 0-7216-8239-1

NOTICE

Veterinary medicine is an ever-changing field. Standard safety precautions must be followed, but as new research and clinical experience broaden our knowledge, changes in treatment and drug therapy may become necessary or appropriate. Readers are advised to check the most current product information provided by the manufacturer of each drug to be administered to verify the recommended dose, the method and duration of administration, and contraindications. It is the responsibility of the treating veterinarian, relying on experience, and knowledge of the patient, to determine dosages and the best treatment for each individual patient. Neither the Publisher nor the editor assumes any liability for any injury and/or damage to animals or property arising from this publication.

The Publisher

ISBN-13: 978-0-7216-8239-6
ISBN-10: 0-7216-8239-1

Publishing Director: Linda Duncan
Acquisitions Editor: Anthony J. Winkel
Developmental Editor: Shelly N. Dixon
Publishing Services Manager: Patricia Tannian
Project Manager: Sarah Wunderly
Design Manager: Gail Morey Hudson

Printed in China

Last digit is the print number: 9 8 7 6 5 4 3

Preface

When initially approached by Saunders to produce an atlas of canine and feline eye diseases, we hesitated. However, over the years we had accumulated many photographs that we knew would be a great source of material for the atlas. "How difficult can it be to produce an atlas?" we asked ourselves. Well... the daunting task soon became readily apparent! Sorting through more than 20 years' worth of photographs, selecting 10,000 of *those* images to scan electronically, and then distilling that number down to the 1000 or so we felt best represented the conditions we would be presenting was more difficult than we could have imagined. With this final set of images, we now have developed a new atlas that depicts normal and diseased eyes as they might be seen during an ocular examination by any general practitioner. We have also included some material that would be of benefit to those veterinarians with a more specialized interest in ophthalmology and to residents in ophthalmology. Furthermore, there are many fundus photographs, representing both normal and abnormal views, which are not available in most other atlases.

The aim of this atlas is simply to illustrate the canine and feline eye and its lesions. There are excellent ophthalmology references and textbooks available, and we do not intend to duplicate what is written elsewhere. In fact, the text in this atlas is intentionally limited to a brief introduction at the beginning of each section and legends that describe simply the structure or condition presented. We do not provide detailed information on etiology, diagnosis, and treatment.

In ophthalmology, more than any other specialty, the clinician relies heavily on what he or she can actually see. Visual recognition of structures and lesions is key to making a proper diagnosis. We believe the strength of this atlas lies in its comprehensive depiction of the many normal and abnormal features of the eye that will be encountered during an ocular examination. Proper identification of what is seen by the clinician's own eye is the most critical step of the process when treating an ocular problem. The goal of this atlas is to provide as much assistance as possible toward that end. For more thorough understanding of the anatomy and pathophysiology of the eye, we refer the reader to a more general ophthalmology textbook. Following the conventional format of most of those books, the chapters and illustrations in this book are arranged from anterior to posterior, and include the orbit. Throughout the atlas there are numerous images of normal ocular features as well as lesions commonly seen in practice. We have also included a number of illustrations of conditions that less frequently occur.

For those readers who would like to begin photographing eyes in their practice: Most of the photographs were initially (over many years) taken with either a Nikon 35mm SLR/105mm macro lens and ring flash combination using Ektrachrome 64-100 ASA film or a Kowa II fundus camera with 25 ASA Kodachrome. More recently we have abandoned film photography altogether for the anterior segment and use a Fuji S2-Pro SLR camera (Fuji Photo Film, Inc, Greenwood, SC)/105mm Micro Nikkor macro lens and ring flash (Nikon Inc, Melville, NY). Most of our digital photographs were taken with manual focusing (faster than using the auto-focus mode for macro photographs), at a shutter speed of about 1/60 second at f22 to maximize the depth of field. There is still no *handheld* digital camera (as of December 2003) that comes close to the quality achieved with Kodachrome 25 ASA for the posterior segment, although it is hoped that this will soon be possible.

Joan Dziezyc
Nicholas J. Millichamp

Acknowledgements

This book is dedicated to our families who have provided support and tolerance over many years. We probably should thank each other since it is really amazing that we managed to finish this project without killing each other. It is difficult to single out particular colleagues for acknowledgement because so many have provided us with support, advice, material help and friendship over the past twenty years and to these folk we say thank you. We would like to acknowledge the opportunities given to us by two outstanding ophthalmologists without whose help and guidance we would not be where we are today. Keith Barnett gave Nick the opportunity to get involved in ophthalmic research at a time when few openings existed in the UK. Kirk Gelatt provided the environment and encouragement for both of us to become clinical ophthalmologists. Both Keith and Kirk have advanced the careers of many of us involved in ophthalmology today and for their support we are profoundly grateful.

We have included several photographs contributed by colleagues and have acknowledged this in the text. We would like to thank Larry Wadsworth at the College of Veterinary Medicine, Texas A&M University who contributed digital photographs and was an invaluable source of information on photographic technique.

The publishing staff of W.B. Saunders and now Elsevier has been very patient with us, especially since they were warned early on that we have a tendency to procrastinate. Shelly Dixon, who inherited the project at a late stage, has been especially helpful and managed to coax us to complete the book at a time when we had doubts that it would ever happen.

Contents

1 **Eyelid,** 1

2 **Conjunctiva,** 17

3 **Third Eyelid,** 24

4 **Lacrimal System,** 28

5 **Cornea,** 34

6 **Sclera,** 62

7 **Uvea,** 65

8 **Lens,** 96

9 **Glaucoma,** 117

10 **Vitreous,** 126

11 **Retina, Choroid, Sclera,** 129

12 **Optic Nerve,** 214

13 **Orbit,** 220

Chapter 1

Eyelid

INTRODUCTION

The eyelids are composed of skin, eyelid muscles, eyelid glands (particularly the meibomian glands), and the palpebral conjunctiva, which lines the inner surface of the eyelids. The eyelids are affected by conditions that affect skin elsewhere on the body and a variety of anatomic abnormalities, as well as conditions that involve the conjunctiva and eyeball. Many eyelid abnormalities seen in dogs are breed related (e.g., distichia, entropion, and ectropion). Inflammatory diseases (e.g., blepharitis) may be associated with more widespread dermatitis. Various tumors may affect the eyelids in older animals and are illustrated in this chapter. Because the integrity of the eye may be affected by eyelid disease, careful observation and accurate diagnosis are important.

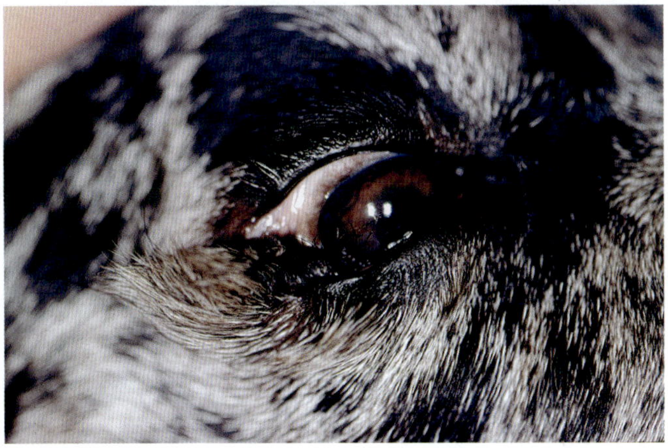

Figure 1-1
An Australian shepherd with a dermoid and eyelid agenesis of the lateral lower eyelid and conjunctiva. A dermoid is an occurrence of normal, haired skin in an abnormal location. Dermoids can be found on eyelid margins, conjunctiva, and corneas. Eyelid agenesis is the absence of normal eyelid in part of the palpebral fissure.

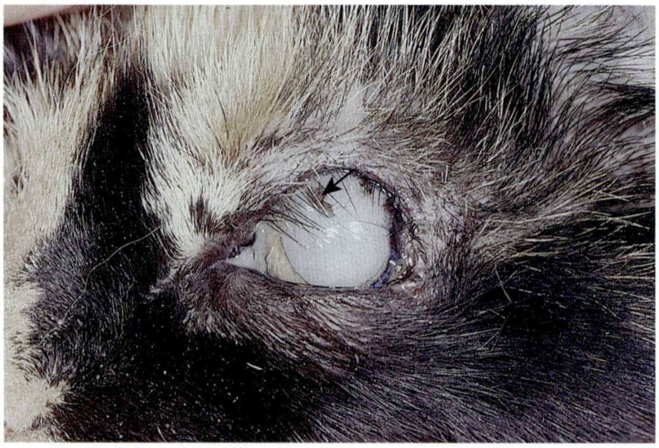

Figure 1-2
Left eye of an older domestic shorthair cat with bilateral eyelid agenesis. The upper eyelid agenesis involves most of the eyelid and lateral canthus. Pigment is present on the cornea *(arrow)* as a result of chronic exposure and hair contact. A mature cataract is present and is an unrelated problem.

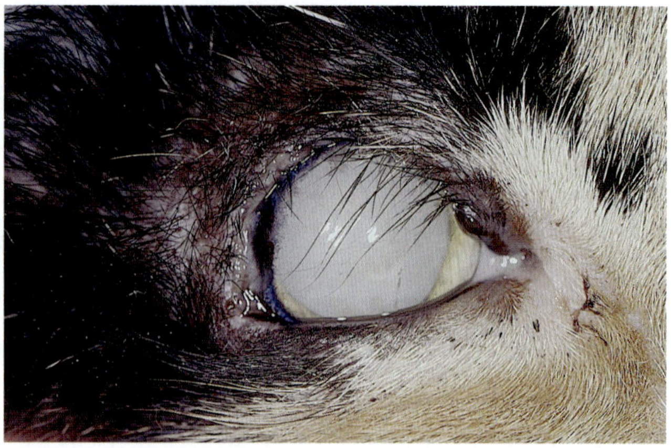

Figure 1-3
Right eye of cat in Figure 1-2. The upper eyelid agenesis involves most of the eyelid and lateral canthus—the most common location for eyelid agenesis in cats. Pigment is present on the cornea as a result of chronic exposure and because hair has come in contact with the cornea. The defect is corrected by the grafting of skin and conjunctiva to fill the defect. A mature cataract is present and is an unrelated problem.

A

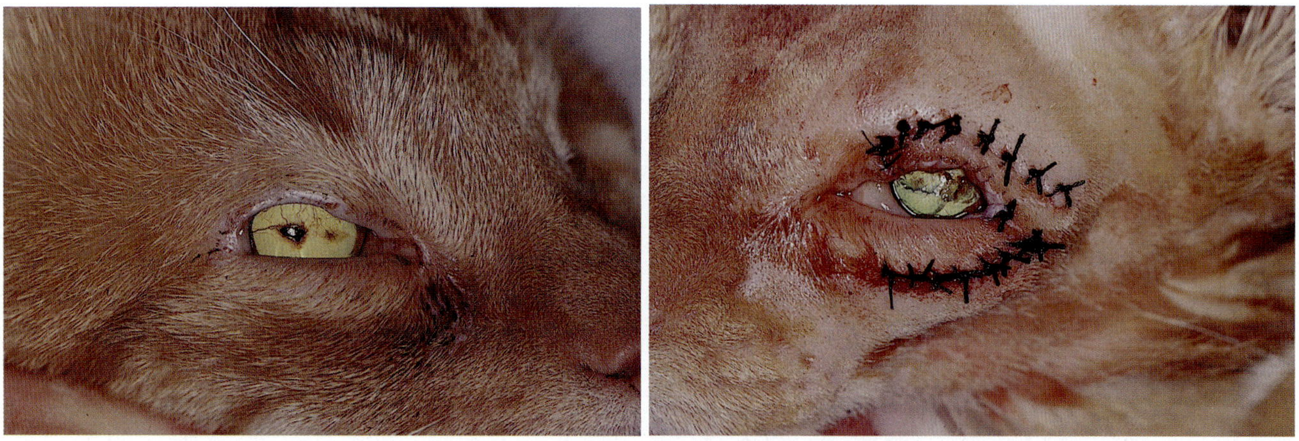

B

Figure 1-4 A-B
A, Right eye of a cat with bilateral upper eyelid agenesis. Most of the upper eyelid is involved. **B,** Postoperative view. Skin from the lower eyelid has been rotated into the defect on the upper eyelid and lined with conjunctiva from the nictitans.

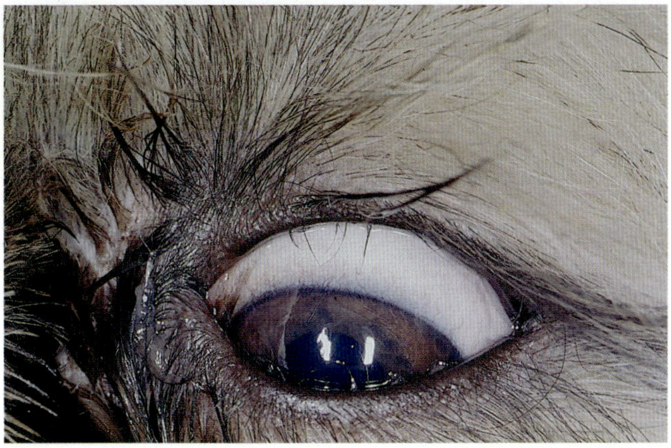

Figure 1-5
Distichiasis in a Pekingese. Distichia are cilia that exit from the openings of the meibomian glands at the eyelid margin. This dog has fine, delicate distichia in both the lower and the upper eyelids. Such hairs often cause a dog no problems. Excess tearing occasionally results from distichia. In rare cases distichia causes corneal ulcers. If treatment is necessary, electroepilation or cryosurgery can be used to remove the hairs permanently.

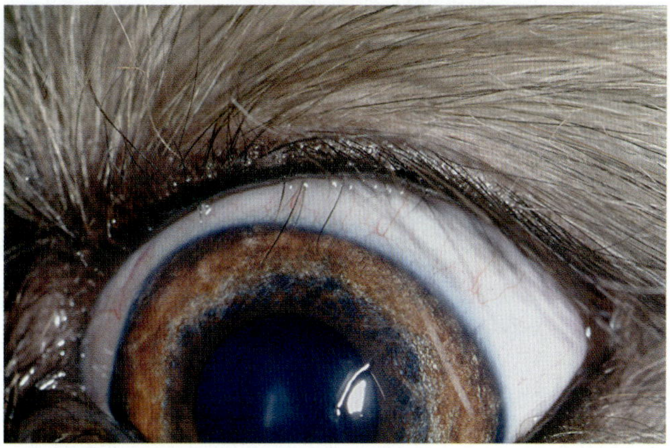

Figure 1-6
Fine distichia arising from the eyelid margins in a dog. No corneal pathologic problems are present because the distichia are fine and tangential to the corneal surface.

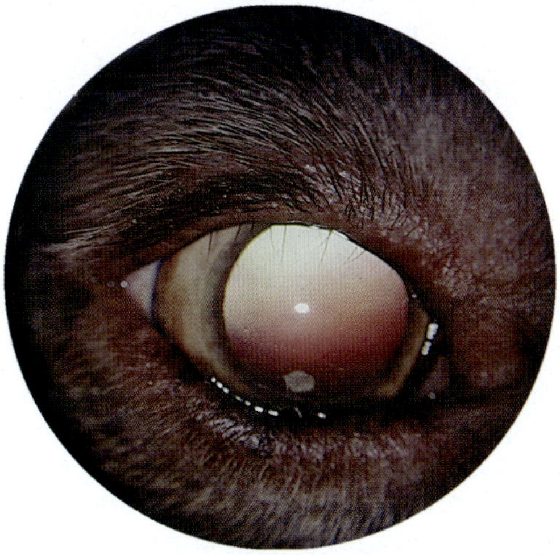

Figure 1-7
Distichia on the upper eyelid of a dog. A focal lipid deposit unrelated to the distichia (possibly a corneal dystrophy) is present in the ventral corneal stroma.

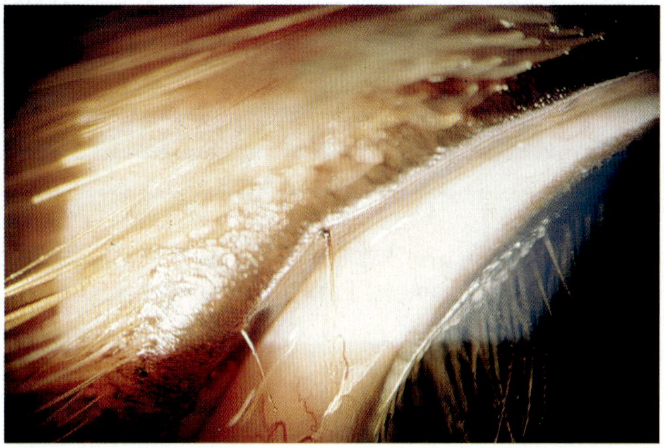

Figure 1-8
Distichia in a dog. The more central cilium is quite stout.

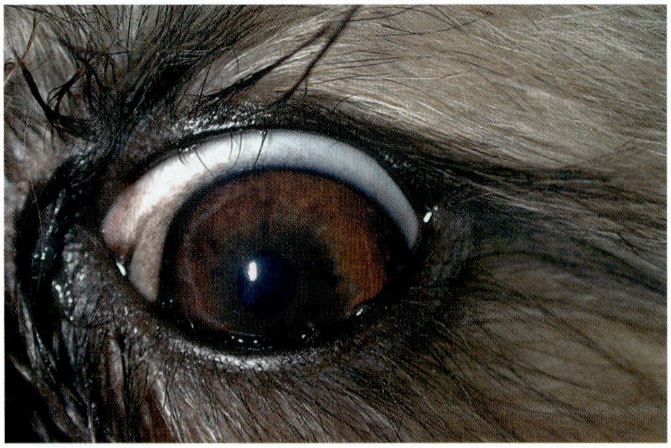

Figure 1-9
Fine distichia arising from the upper and lower eyelids and causing serous lacrimation.

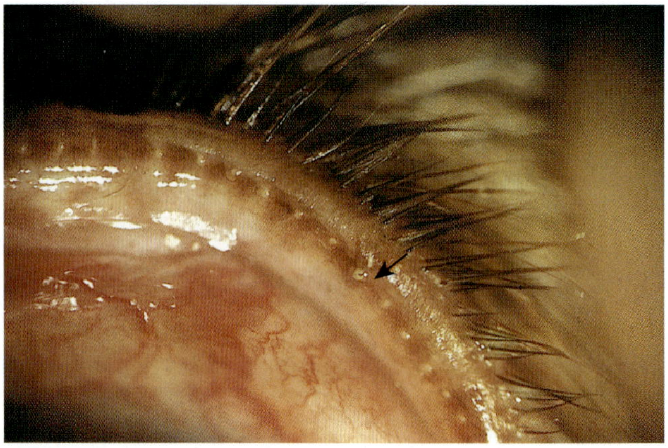

Figure 1-10
Tip of a solitary distichium emerging from the meibomian gland opening in a dog.

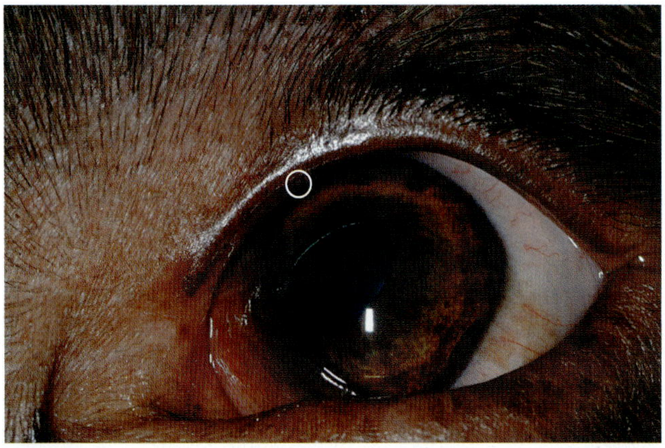

Figure 1-11
Single, stout upper eyelid distichium in the upper eyelid of a 7-year-old Labrador retriever.

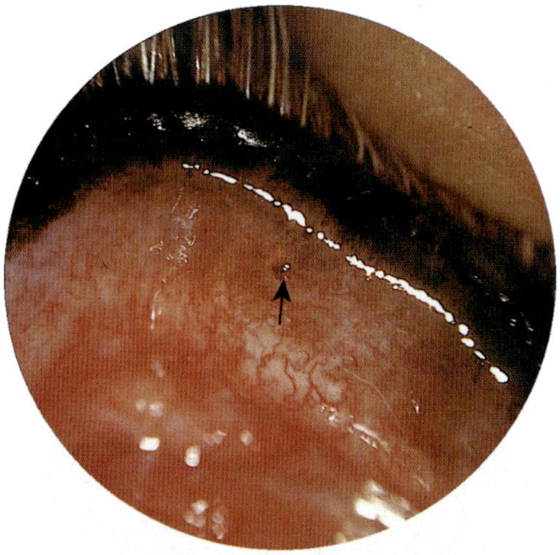

Figure 1-12
Small pigmented papilla on the conjunctival surface of the upper eyelid of a 10-year-old golden retriever. The dog had a history of a very painful eye and a nonhealing ulcer. The tip of an ectopic cilium was present in this papilla and protruded through the conjunctiva at the time of surgical removal. Ectopic cilia are abnormally positioned eyelid hairs that exit the conjunctival surface of the eyelid. They cause great discomfort and corneal ulcers that do not heal. Usually these cilia are found in young dogs but, as this case illustrates, can occur in dogs of all ages.

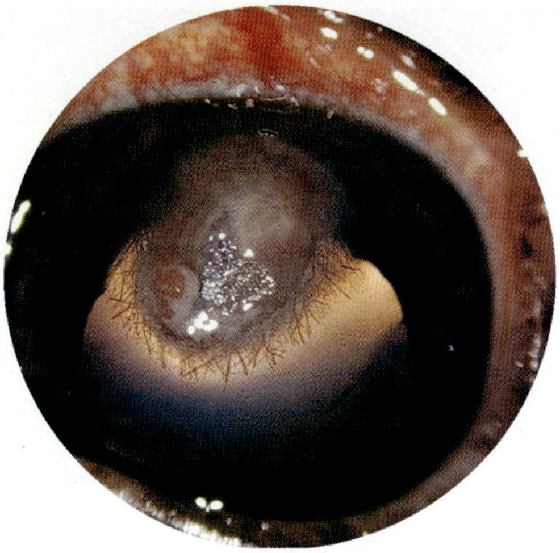

Figure 1-13
Chronic corneal ulcer with neovascularization and granulation caused by to an ectopic cilium, which is not shown in this photo.

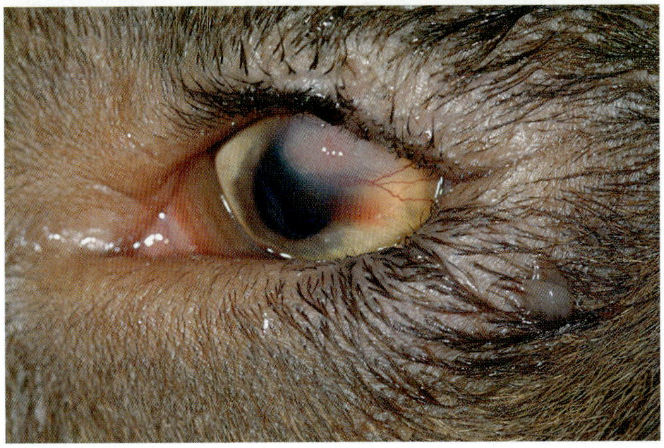

Figure 1-14
Lateral entropion of upper and lower eyelids in a German shorthaired pointer. Entropion is the rolling in of an eyelid. Haired skin then comes in contact with the corneal surface, which leads to chronic corneal ulcers and scarring. In this dog the eyelid disease has caused corneal ulceration, neovascularization, and granulation.

A

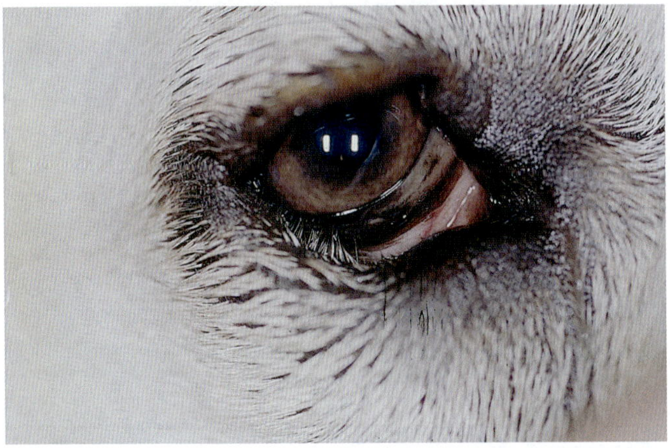

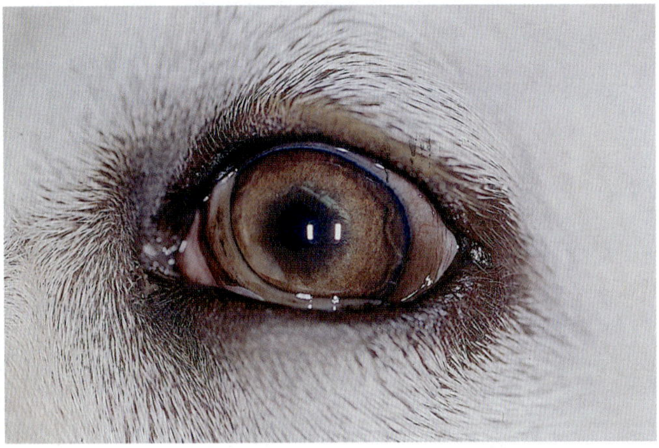

B

Figure 1-15 A-B
A, Left and **B,** right eyes of a dog with entropion of the right eye. The entire length of the eyelid margin is seen in the left eye, but in the right eye the lateral part of the eyelid is not seen. Lateral eyelid hairs contact the cornea, causing ocular irritation, retraction of the globe, and protrusion of the third eyelid.

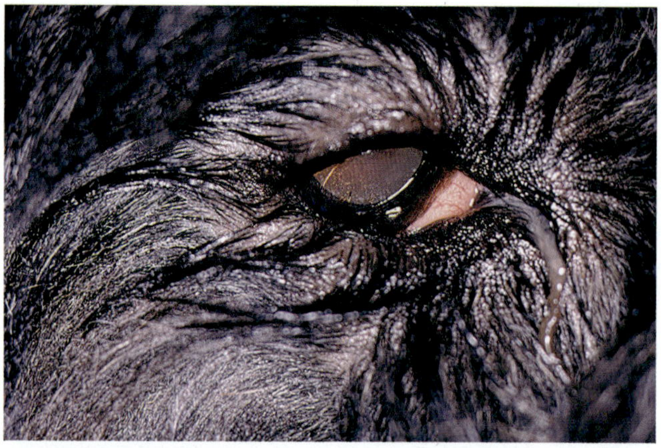

Figure 1-16
Entropion of the lower eyelid. The eyelid margin cannot be seen, and hairs from the lower eyelid are in contact with the cornea.

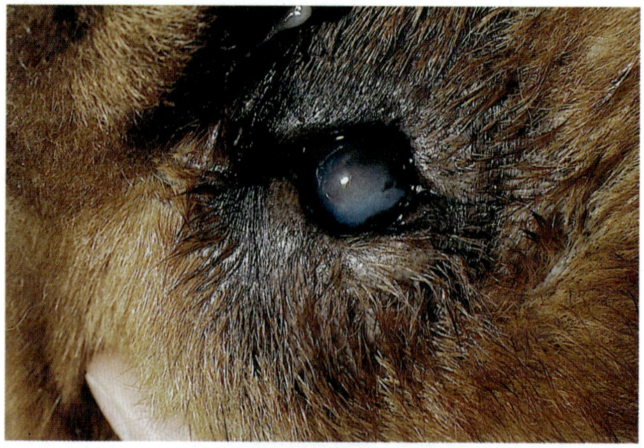

Figure 1-17
Upper and lower eyelid entropion with secondary pigmentary keratitis in a chow chow.
(Courtesy Dr. Robert Playter.)

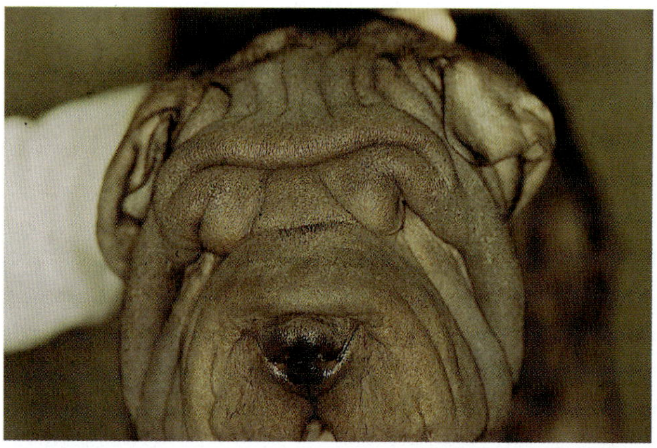

Figure 1-18
Bilateral severe entropion in a Shar-Pei.

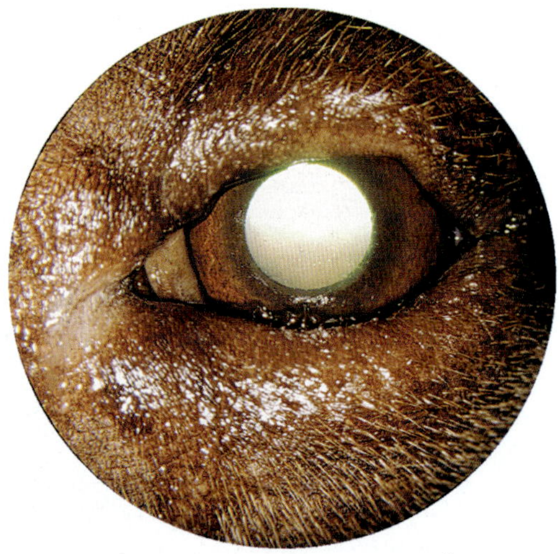

Figure 1-19
Lower eyelid entropion occurring laterally in a dog. The dog also has a V-shaped upper eyelid, indicating poor conformation of the upper lid.

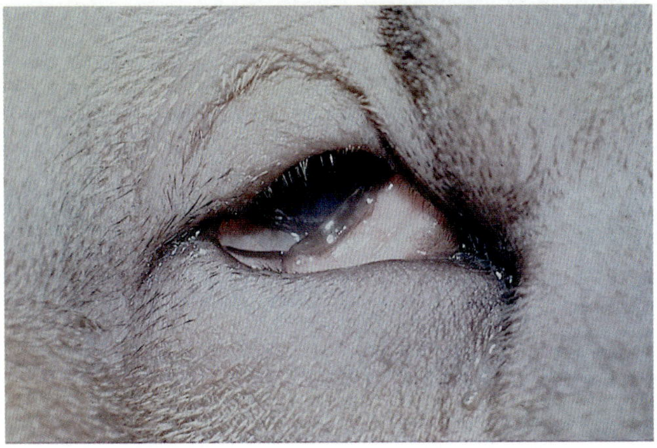

Figure 1-20
Upper and lower eyelid entropion in a shar-pei.

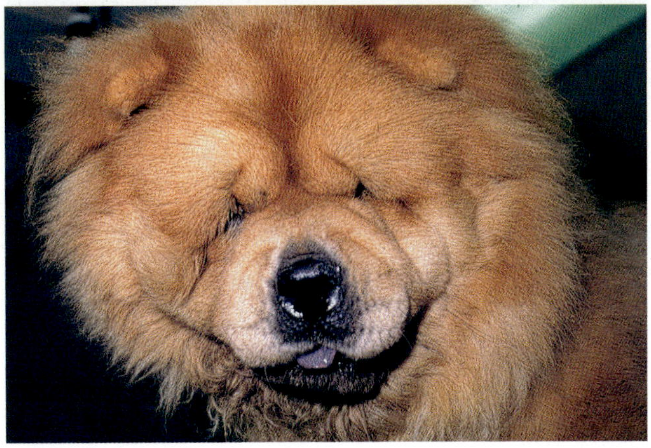

Figure 1-21
Bilateral upper and lower eyelid entropion in a chow chow.

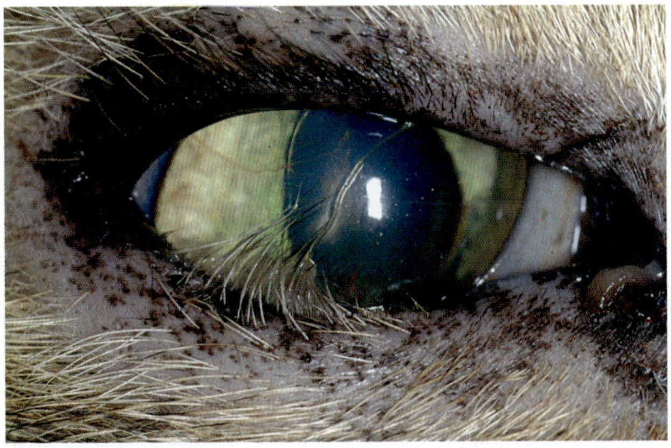

Figure 1-22
Entropion and trichiasis of the lower eyelid in a cat, which have caused chronic keratitis.

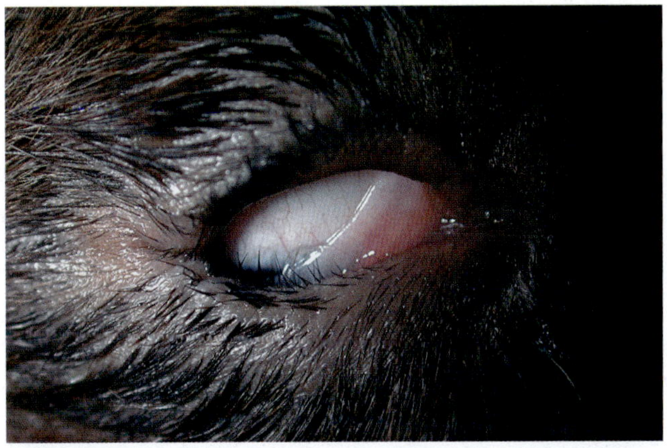

Figure 1-23
Lower eyelid entropion in a dog.

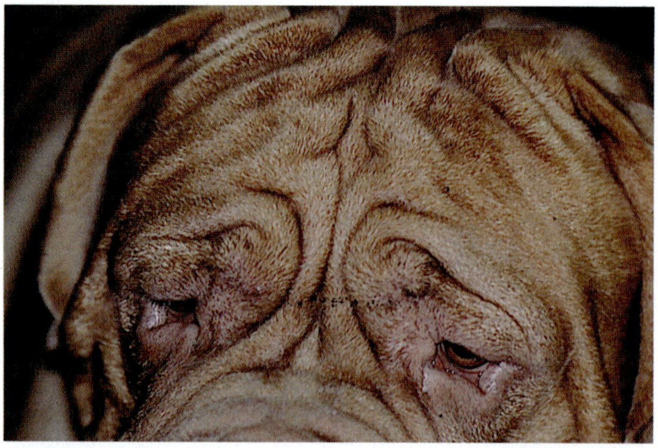

Figure 1-24
Bilateral lower eyelid ectropion occurring centrally, and entropion laterally, in a Dogue de Bordeaux. Ectropion is the outward rolling of an eyelid (usually the lower eyelid).

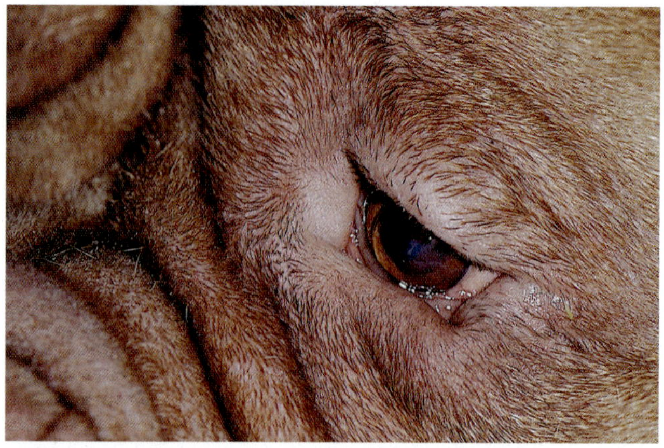

Figure 1-25
Close-up of the dog in Figure 1-24. Bilateral lower eyelid ectropion is occurring centrally and entropion laterally. Corneal neovascularization is present secondary to the eyelid malformations.

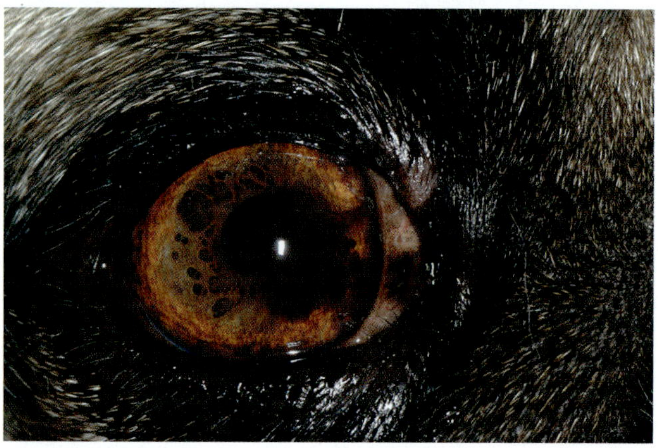

Figure 1-26
Medial entropion and trichiasis in a pug, with resulting nasal keratitis and pigmentation.

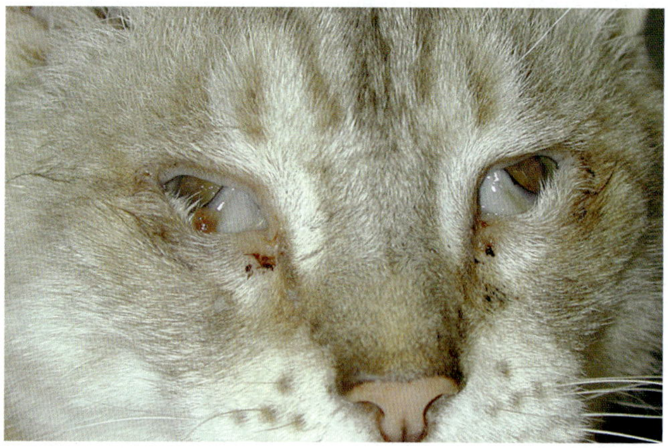

Figure 1-27
Cat with bilateral combined eyelid agenesis, entropion, and trichiasis, which have caused keratitis. Trichiasis is a condition in which normal eyelid hair is in contact with the cornea despite the absence of entropion on that eyelid.

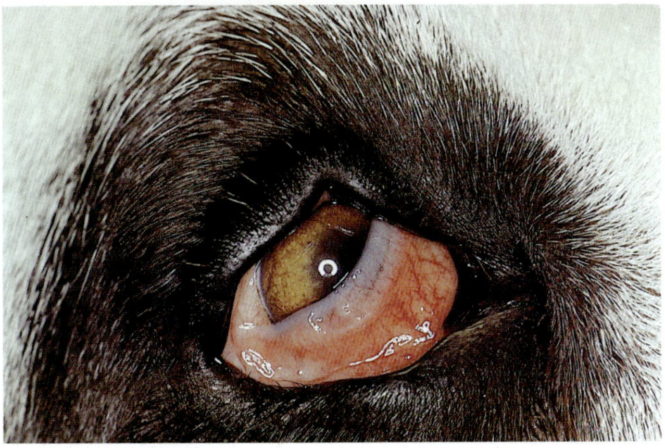

Figure 1-28
V-shaped upper eyelid, indicating conformational abnormality, and distichia of the lower eyelid in a Great Dane.

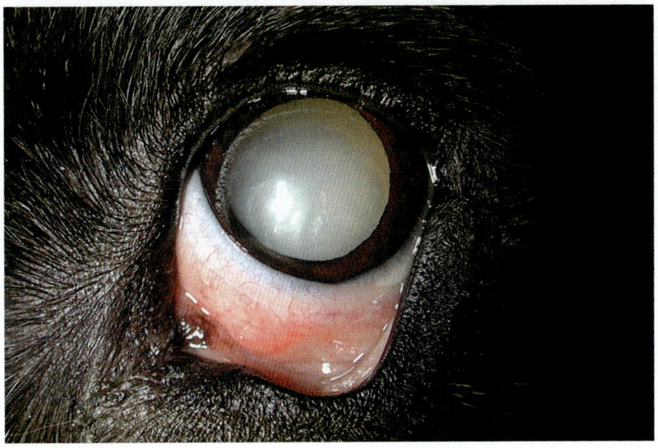

Figure 1-29
Ectropion of the lower eyelid (and unrelated immature cataract) in an 8-year-old Saint Bernard.

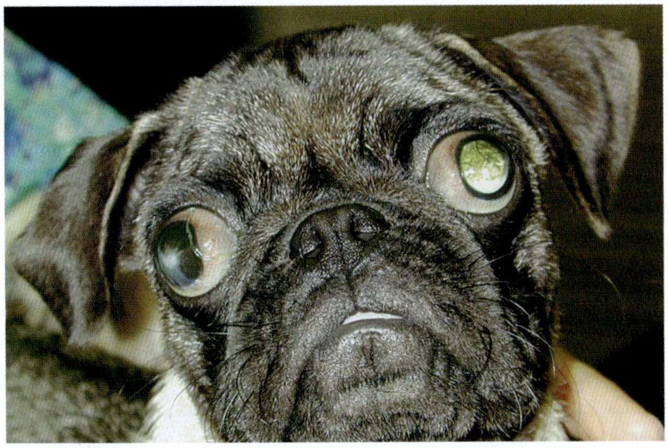

Figure 1-30
Bilateral macropalpebral fissure and a shallow orbit in a pug. Exposure and poor blinking have resulted in keratitis and pigmentation.

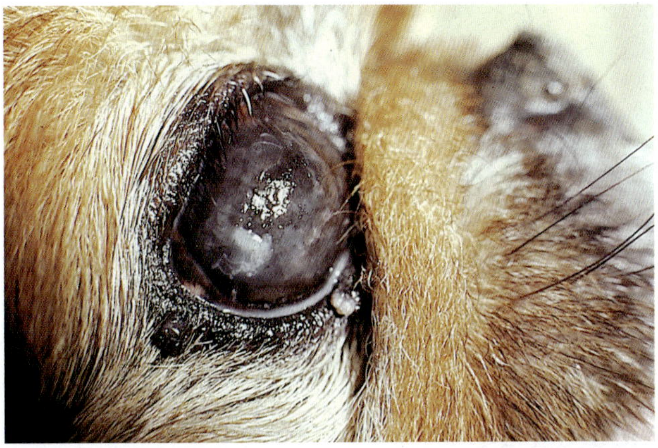

Figure 1-31
Facial folds are rubbing the cornea in this Pekingese. Upper eyelid trichiasis is present. Pigmentary keratitis has resulted from the rubbing of these hairs. Facial folds are found in most brachycephalic breeds; if the hairs touch the cornea and cause pathologic problems, the facial folds can be removed surgically.
(Courtesy Dr. Robert Playter.)

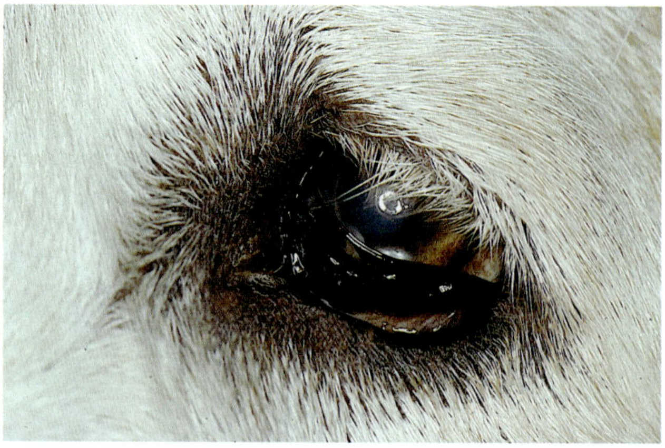

Figure 1-32
Trichiasis of the upper eyelid in an 11-year-old golden retriever. Trichiasis is often seen in older dogs when eyelid muscles have become lax with age.

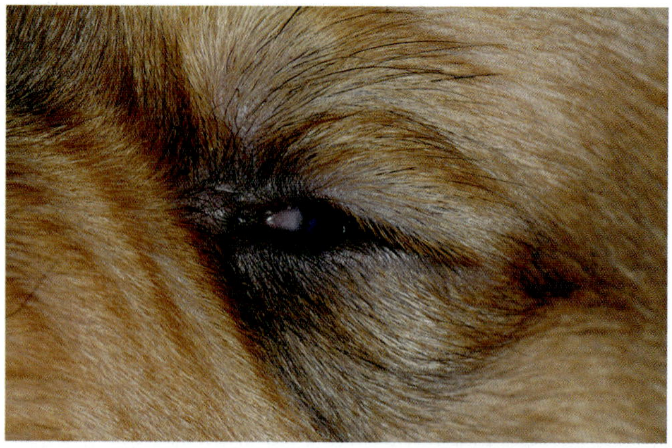

Figure 1-33
Ankyloblepharon (the physiologic fusion of eyelids in newborn pups and kittens). The upper and lower eyelids of this 10-day-old puppy are still partially fused together laterally. The eyelids open in dogs and cats at approximately 14 days of age.

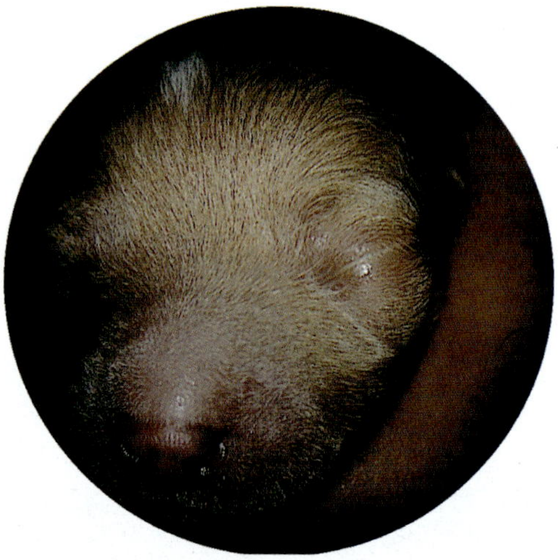

Figure 1-34
Ankyloblepharon with bacterial infection beneath the closed eyelids of a week-old puppy. This condition is also known as *ophthalmia neonatorum.*

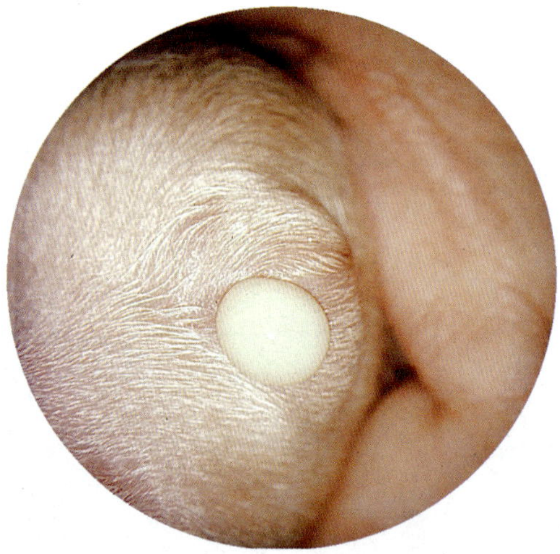

Figure 1-35
Same puppy as shown in Figure 1-34. Purulent material is expressed during gentle separation of the upper and lower eyelids, allowing drainage of pus and application of antibiotic to the eye.

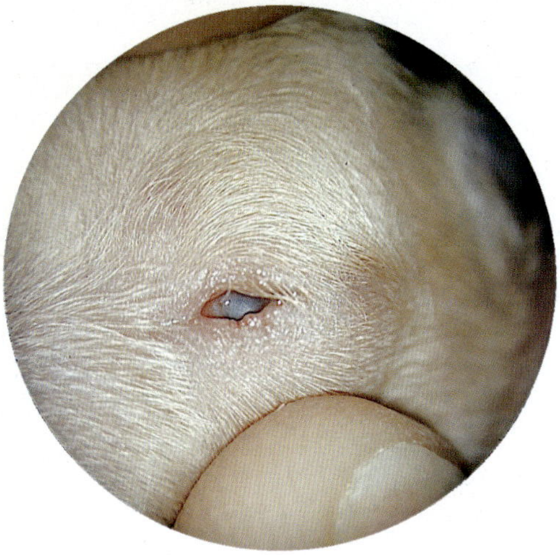

Figure 1-36
Same puppy as shown in Figures 1-34 and 1-35 after the eyelids have been opened.

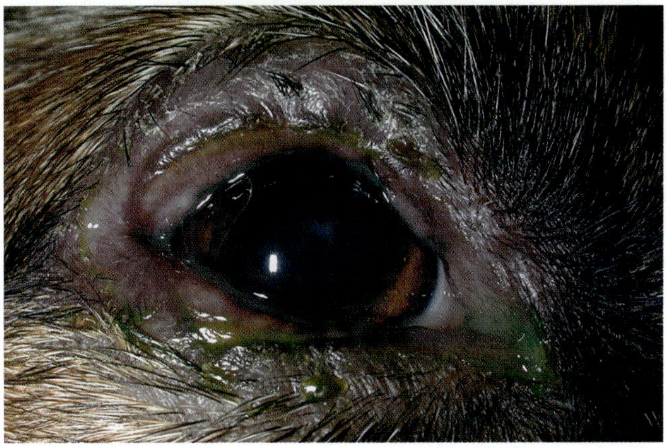

Figure 1-37
Bacterial blepharitis in a dog. Mucoid discharge, thickening, erythema, and erosion of the mucocutaneous junction of the eyelids are present. Bacteria cultured from eyelids in dogs with blepharitis are often common commensals. These dogs possibly have impaired immunity, which allows the commensals to become pathogenic. Systemic antibacterial drugs are needed to treat affected dogs.

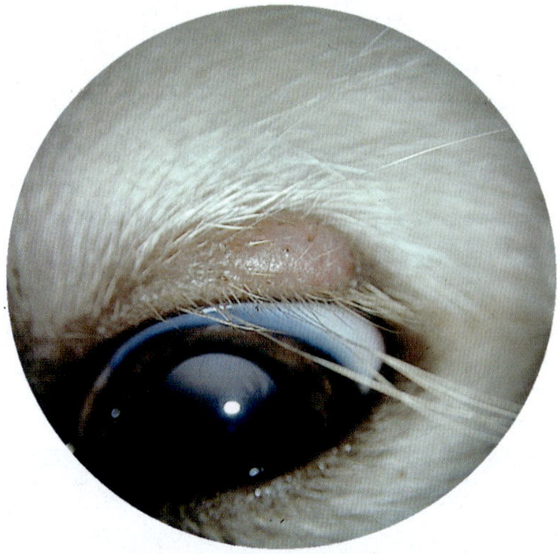

Figure 1-38
Focal area of blepharitis on the upper eyelid of a puppy. Such blepharitis represents a small abscess in the eyelid margin. Redness, swelling, and some discomfort are present.
(Courtesy Dr. Robert Playter.)

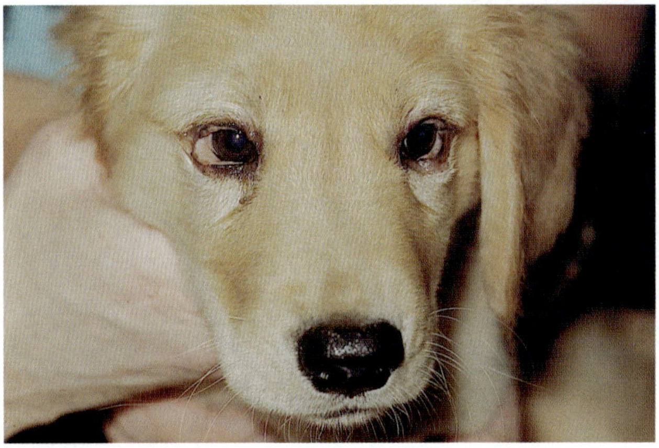

Figure 1-39
Bilateral blepharitis in a golden retriever puppy. Thickening and swelling of eyelids and increased lacrimation are present.

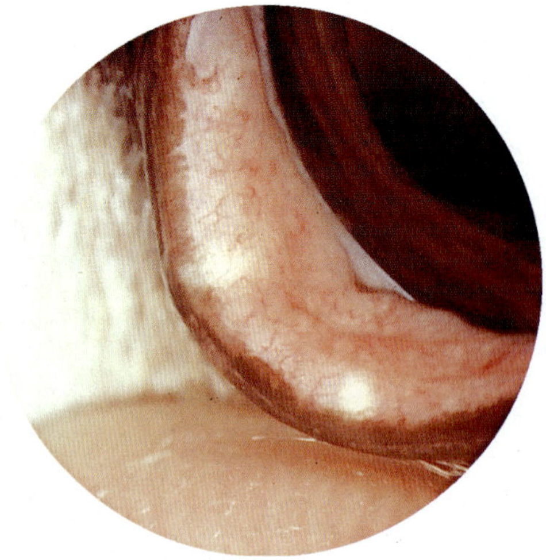

Figure 1-40
Meibomianitis (view from conjunctival surface)—blepharitis in which the meibomian glands are affected.

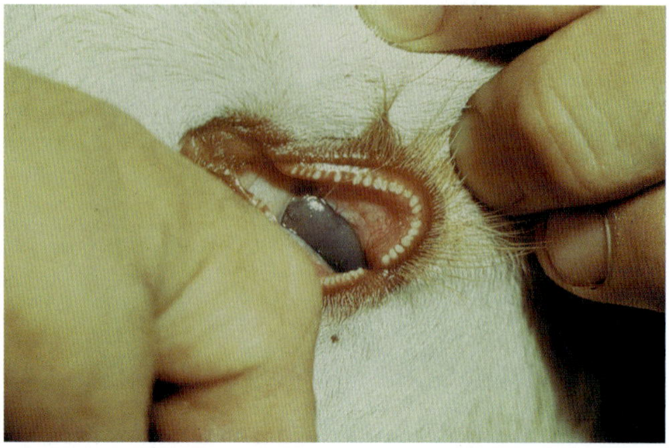

Figure 1-41
Meibomianitis.
(Courtesy Dr. Robert Playter.)

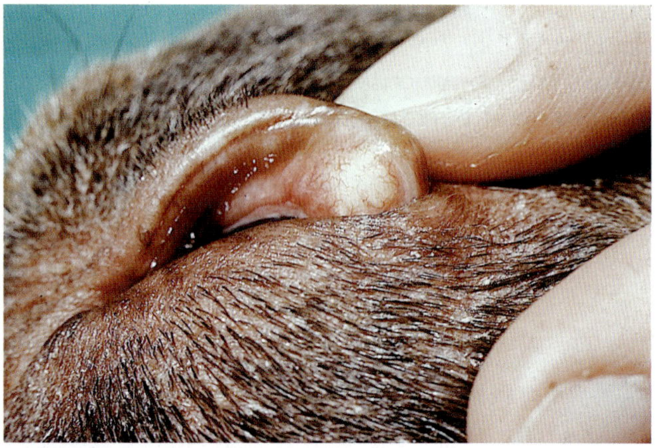

Figure 1-42
Abscessed meibomian gland.
(Courtesy Dr. Robert Playter.)

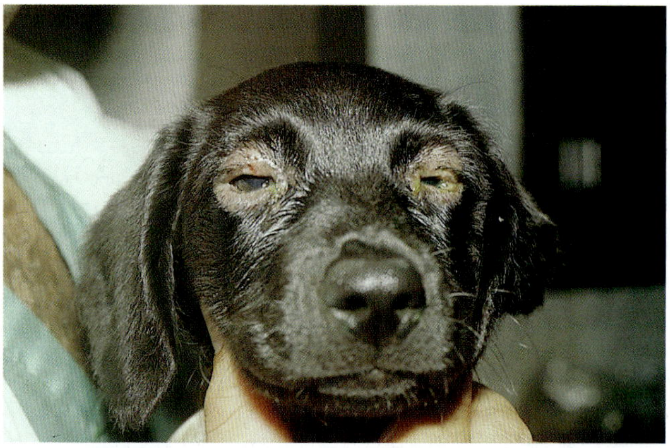

Figure 1-43
Bilateral blepharitis with redness, swelling, and excoriation in a 3-month-old puppy. Treatment consisted of oral cephalexin and prednisone.

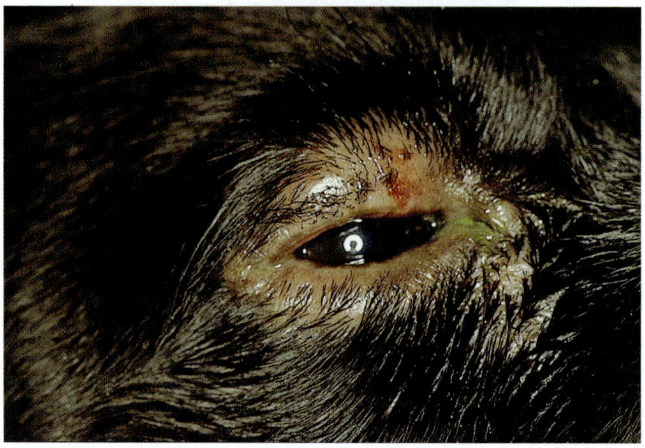

Figure 1-44
Close-up of the dog in Figure 1-43 showing redness, swelling, and excoriation from the blepharitis.

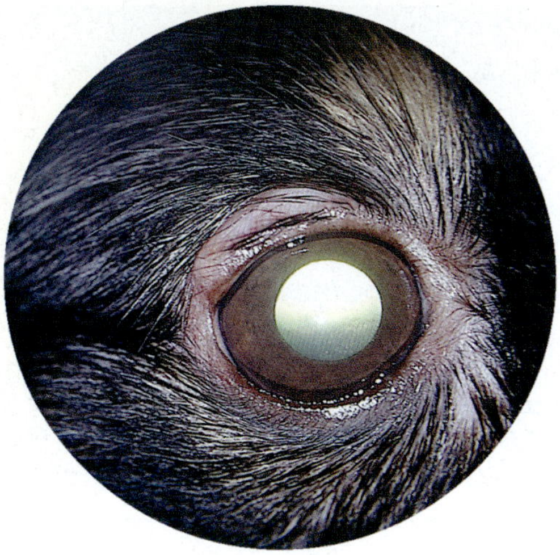

Figure 1-45
Blepharitis in a dog, with redness, swelling, and hair loss.

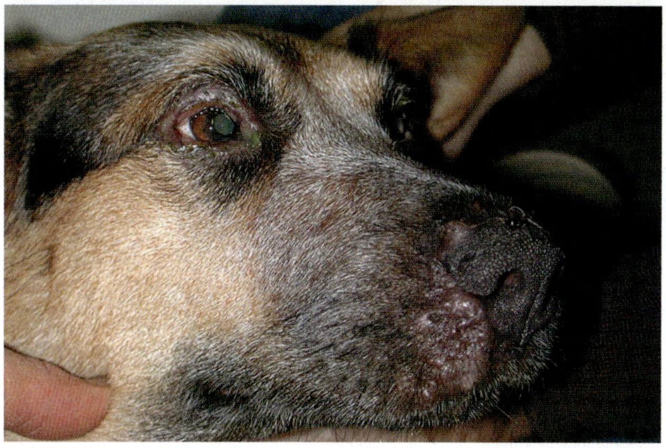

Figure 1-46
German shepherd crossbreed with staphylococcal blepharitis and dermatitis around the muzzle.

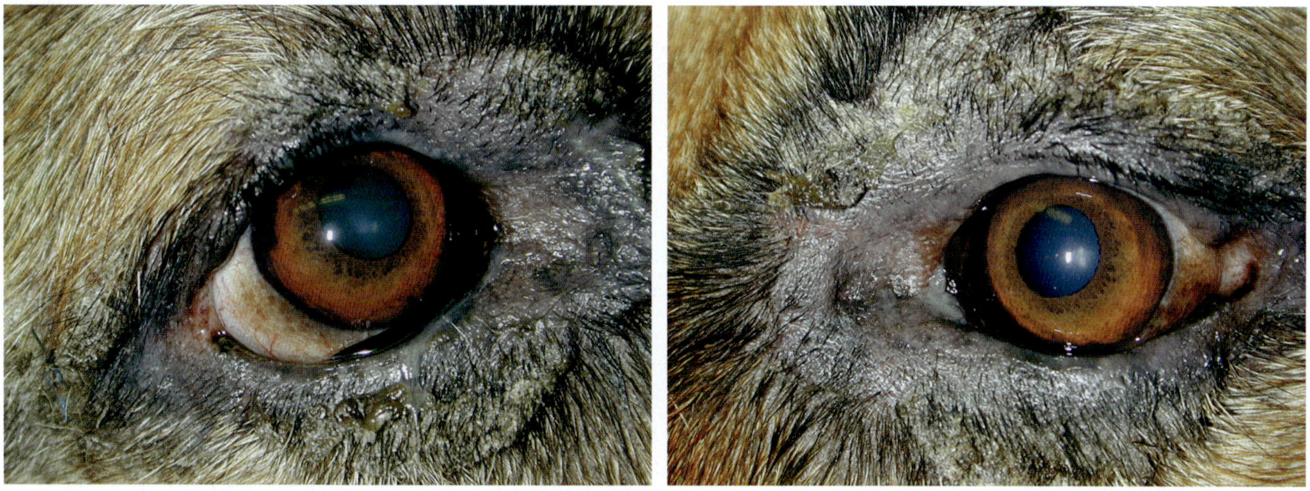

Figure 1-47
Bilateral blepharitis in a dog. The disorder was suspected to have an autoimmune cause.

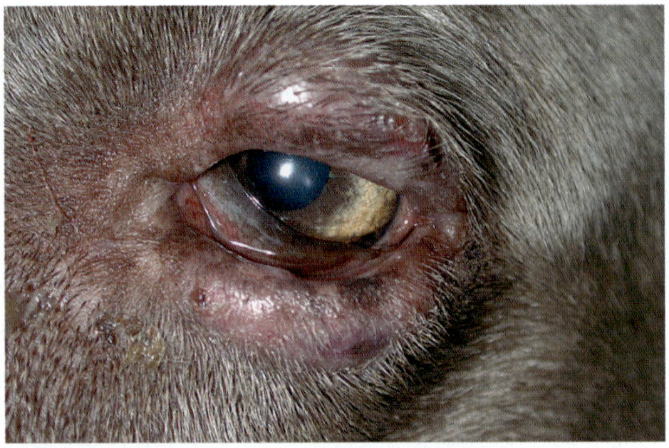

Figure 1-48
Staphylococcal blepharitis in a 5-year-old mixed-breed dog, which responded to treatment with cephalexin and low-dose prednisone.

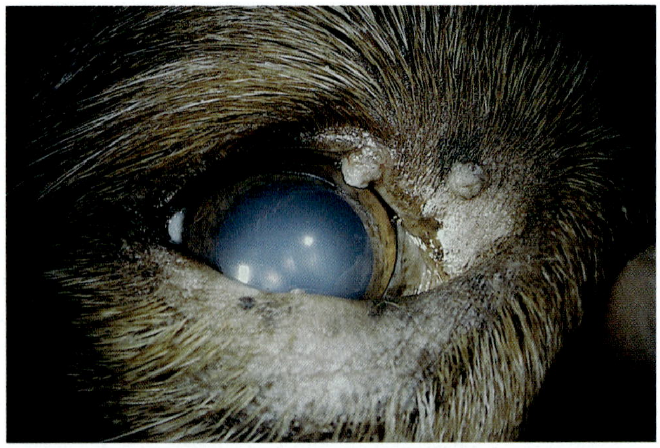

Figure 1-49
Sebaceous adenoma on the upper eyelid; blepharitis on the lower eyelid. A mass is present on the skin of the medial canthus. Eyelid sebaceous adenomas are the most common eyelid tumors seen in dogs.

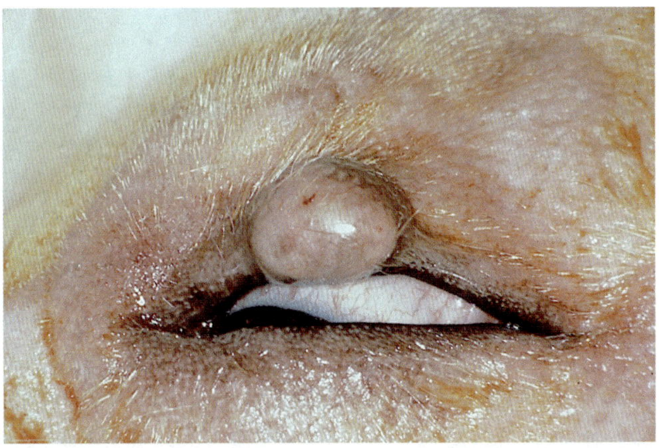

Figure 1-50
Sebaceous adenoma on the upper eyelid of a Lhasa apso.

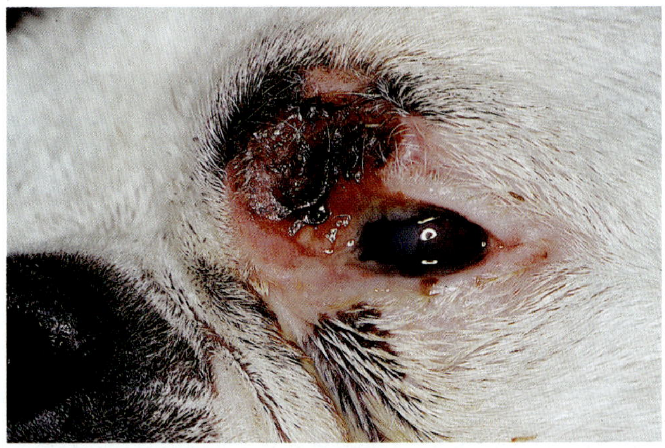

Figure 1-51
Erosive squamous cell carcinoma in the medial canthus of a 10-year-old Boston terrier.

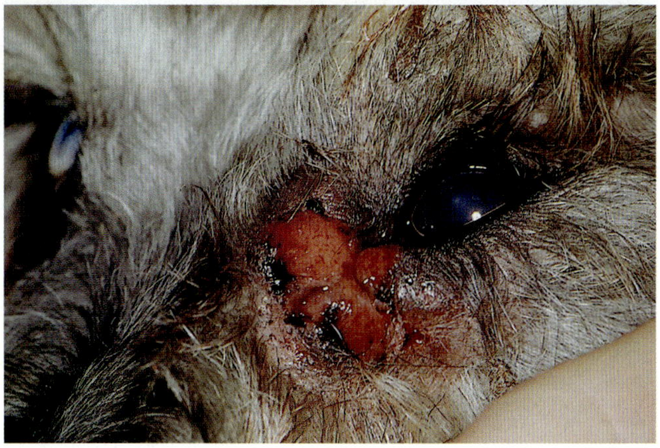

Figure 1-52
Malignant melanoma involving the medial canthus of a dog.
(Courtesy Dr. Dennis Brooks.)

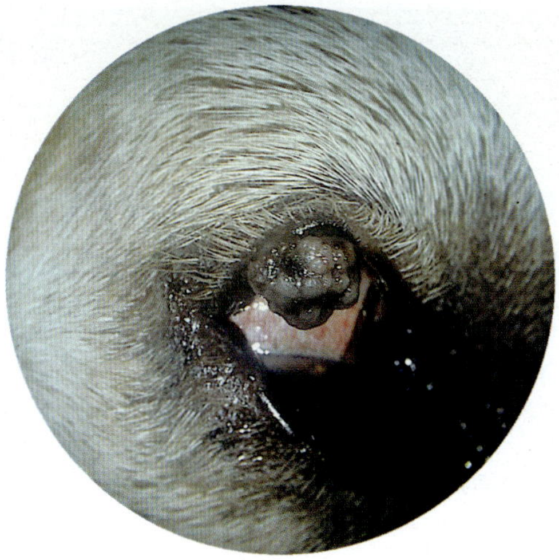

Figure 1-53
Meibomian gland adenoma of the upper eyelid of a dog.

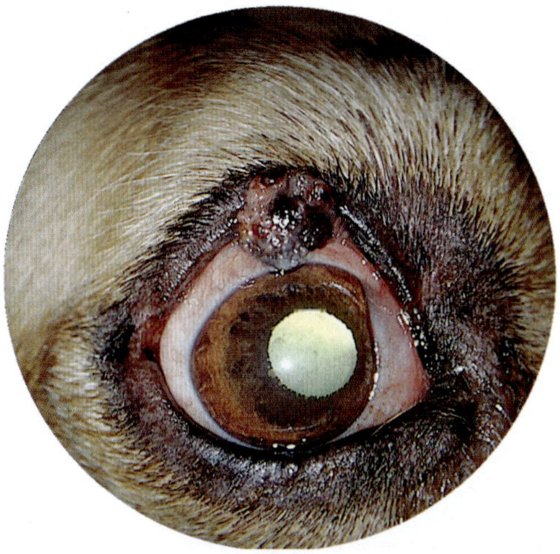

Figure 1-54
Papilloma of a dog's eyelid.

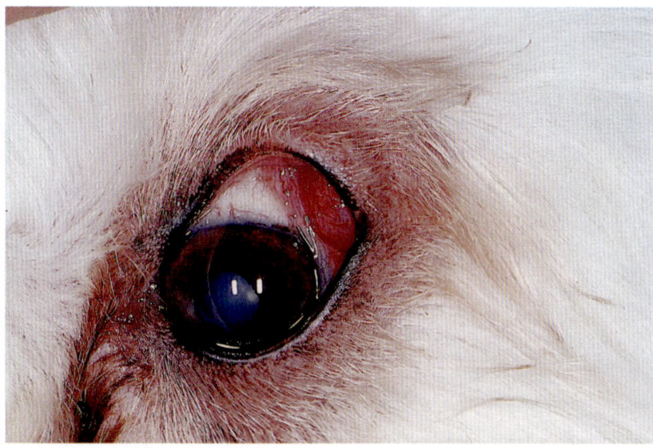

Figure 1-55
Adenocarcinoma of the upper lid of a dog.

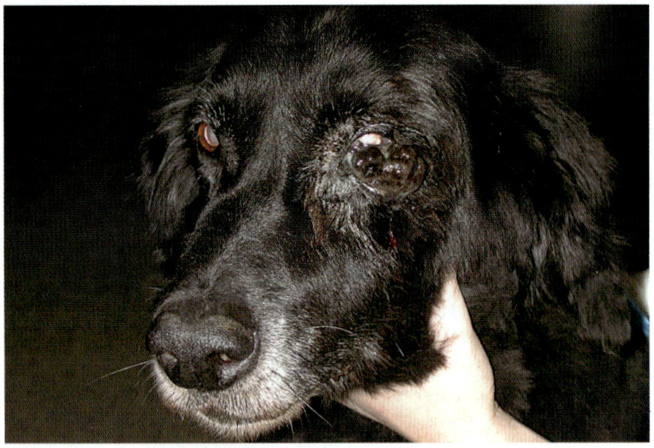

Figure 1-56
Eyelid melanoma.

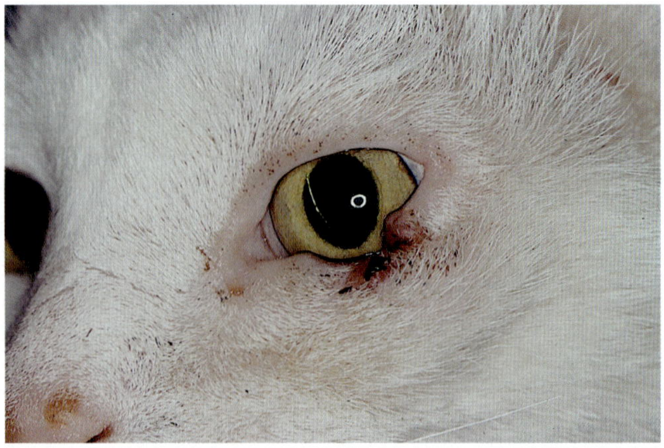

Figure 1-57
Squamous cell carcinoma eroding the lower eyelid of a white cat.

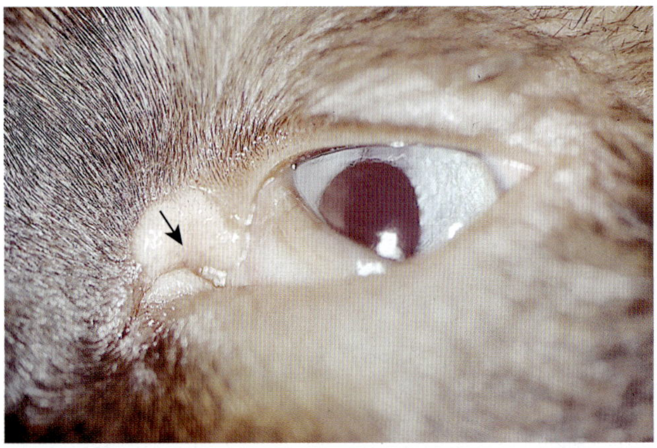

Figure 1-58
Mast cell tumor of the medial canthus of a cat.

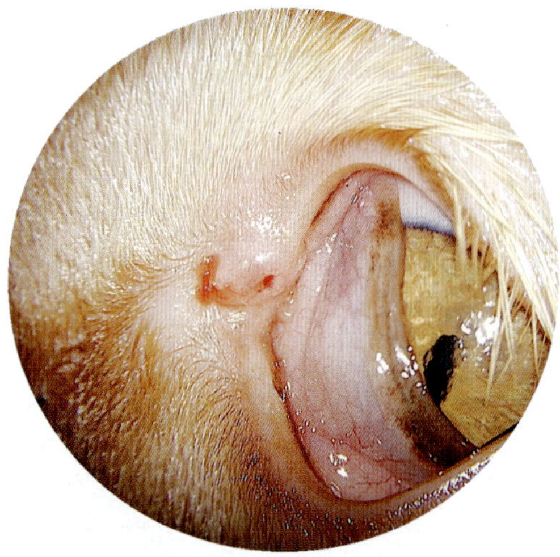

Figure 1-59
Mast cell tumor involving the medial canthus of a cat.

Chapter 2

Conjunctiva

INTRODUCTION

The conjunctiva is a highly vascular layer on the surface of the eye and eyelids. It functions in some respects as a lymph node does, reacting to antigens to which the ocular surface is exposed. The most frequently diagnosed condition is conjunctivitis, which may have various causes (e.g., infectious, allergic). Infectious conjunctivitis and its sequelae are seen commonly in cats. Conjunctival lesions in dogs and cats, including neoplasia, are illustrated in this chapter.

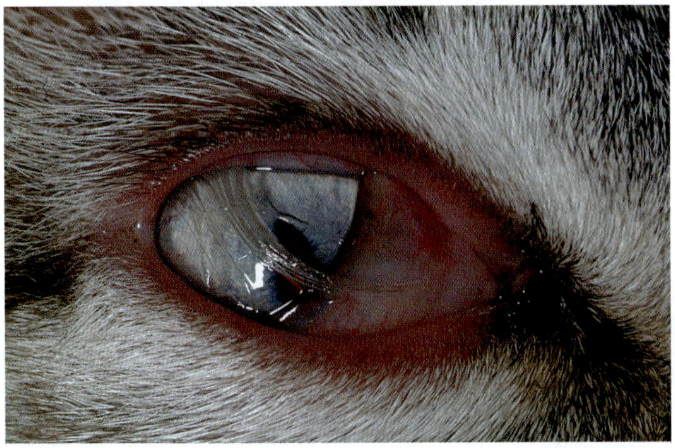

Figure 2-1
Dermoid arising from the dorsal conjunctiva in a 5-month-old Siamese cat. A dermoid is an occurrence of normal, haired skin in an abnormal location. Dermoids are found on eyelid margins, conjunctiva, and corneas.

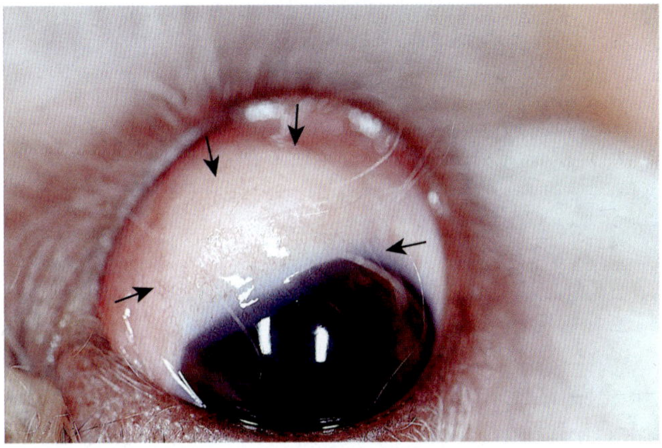

Figure 2-2
Large conjunctival dermoid in a young dog. Most of the dermoid is not haired.

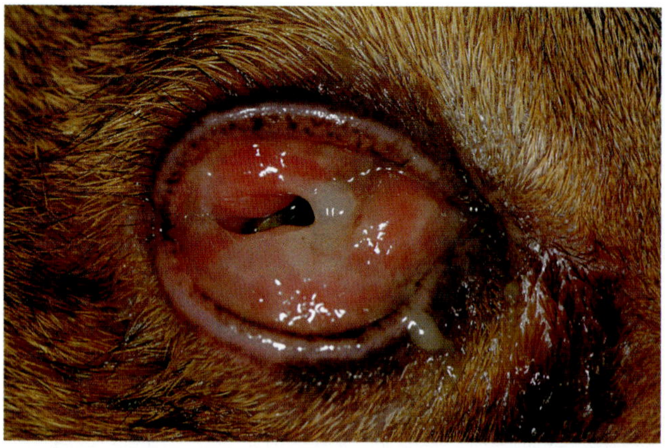

Figure 2-3
Severe herpesvirus conjunctivitis in a cat. Note the marked conjunctival swelling (chemosis) and pseudodiphtheritic membrane formation.

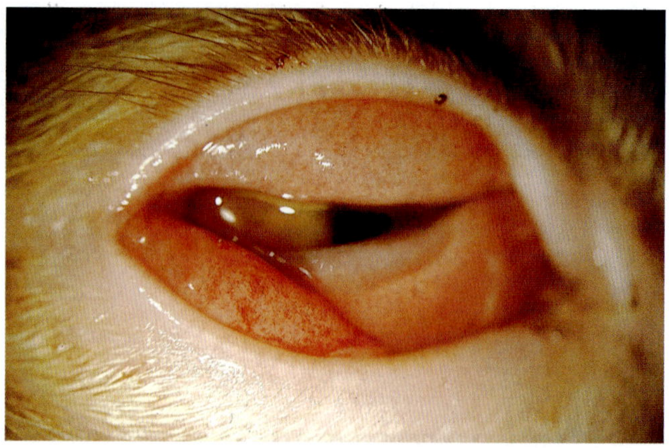

Figure 2-4
Conjunctivitis with chemosis and petechia in a cat with herpesvirus infection.

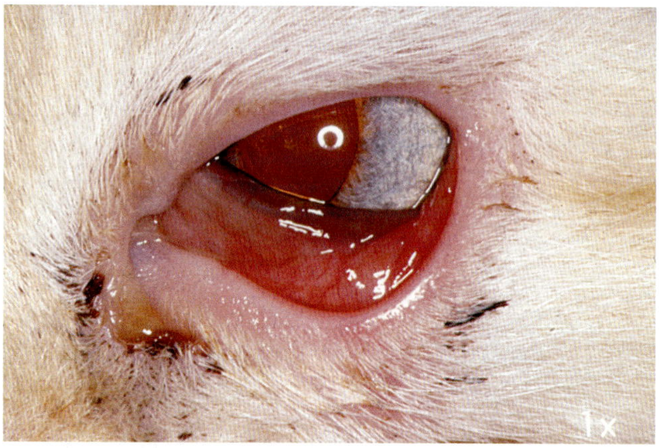

Figure 2-5
Conjunctivitis associated with feline herpesvirus infection in an adult cat. Chemosis, conjunctival injection, and mild mucopurulent ocular discharge are present.

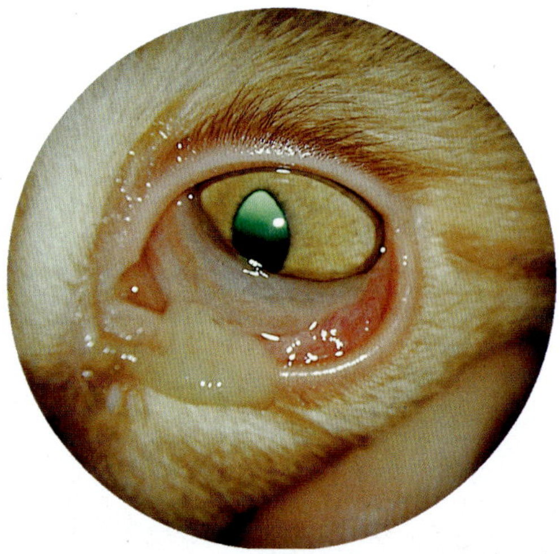

Figure 2-6
Conjunctivitis associated with feline herpesvirus infection in a cat. Upper respiratory tract infection, chemosis, conjunctival injection, and mucopurulent ocular discharge are present.

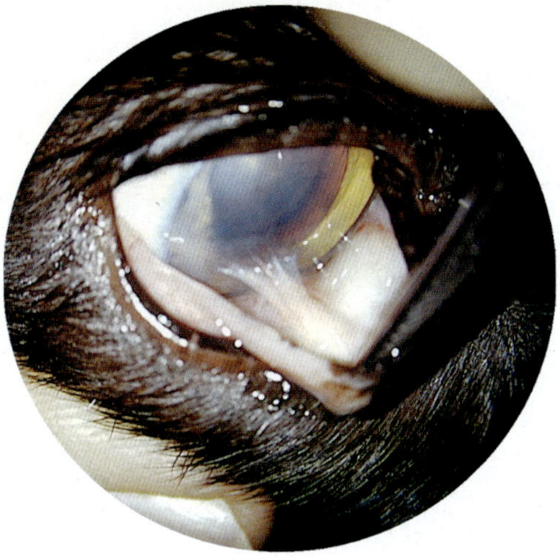

Figure 2-7
Symblepharon caused by a resolved herpesvirus infection in a cat. A symblepharon is an adhesion between structures of the eye; in this case an adhesion exists between the bulbar surface of the nictitans and the cornea.

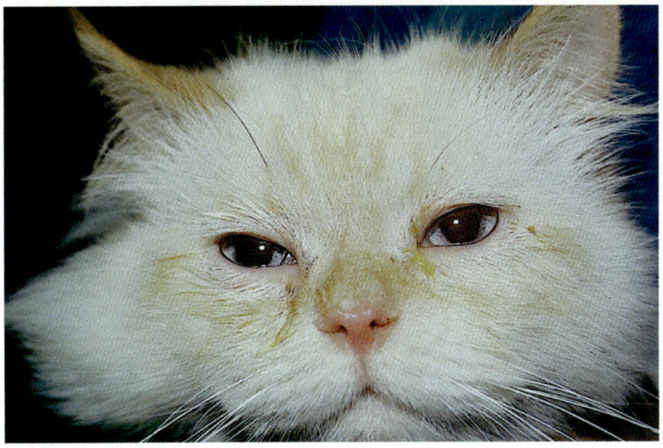

Figure 2-8
Epiphora resulting from a symblepharon and scarring of the nasolacrimal duct as a consequence of feline herpesvirus infection in a young cat. Note the tear staining on the right side of the face.

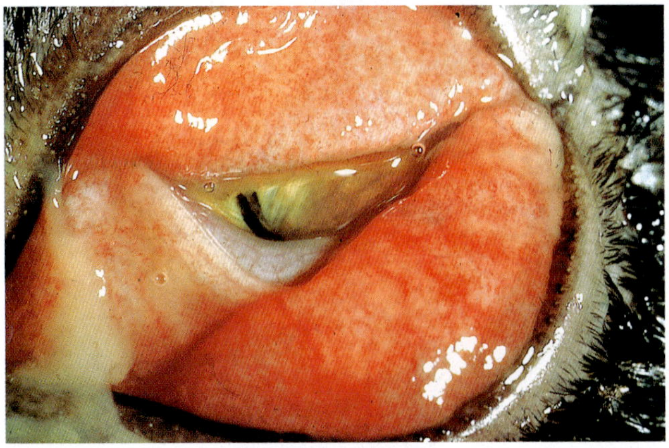

Figure 2-9
Cat with acute experimental chlamydiosis. Mucoid discharge and injected and edematous conjunctiva are present.
(Courtesy Dr. Ralph Woodland.)

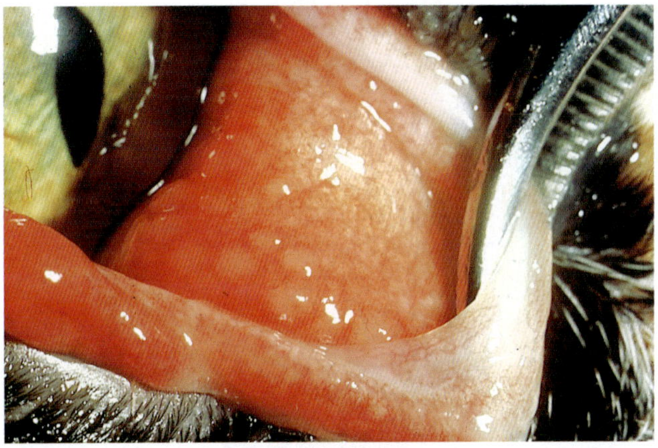

Figure 2-10
Cat with acute experimental chlamydiosis. Injected conjunctiva is present, with lymphoid follicles on bulbar surface of nictitans.
(Courtesy Dr. Ralph Woodland.)

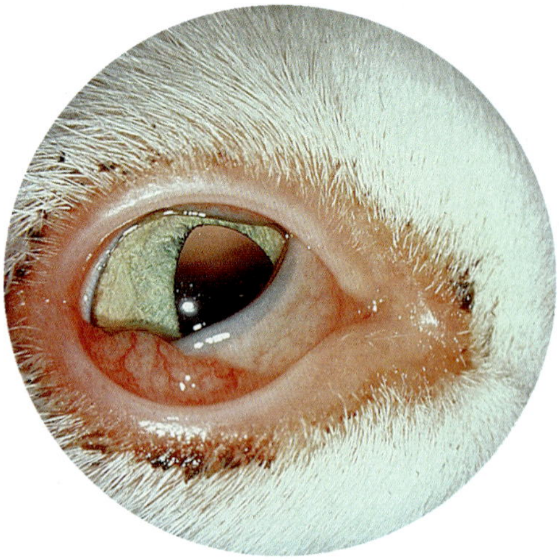

Figure 2-11
Conjunctivitis (chemosis and conjunctival injection with periocular erythema and tear staining) resulting from chlamydial infection.
(Courtesy Dr. Robert Playter.)

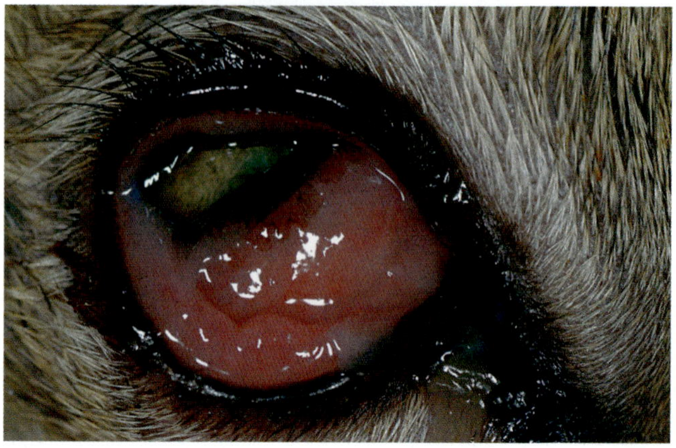

Figure 2-12
Eosinophilic conjunctivitis in a cat.

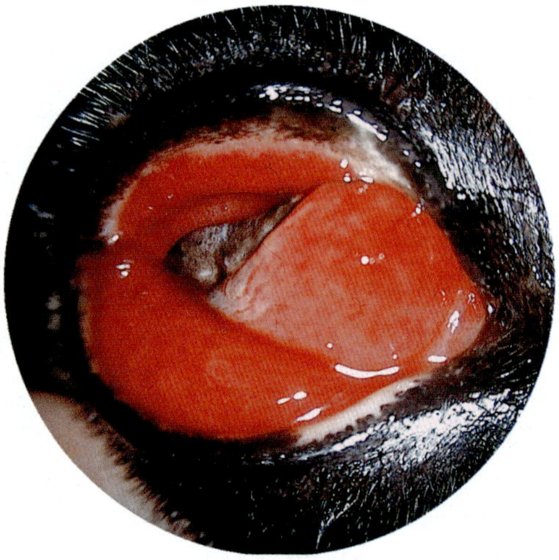

Figure 2-13
Dog that was bitten in the conjunctiva by a pygmy rattlesnake.

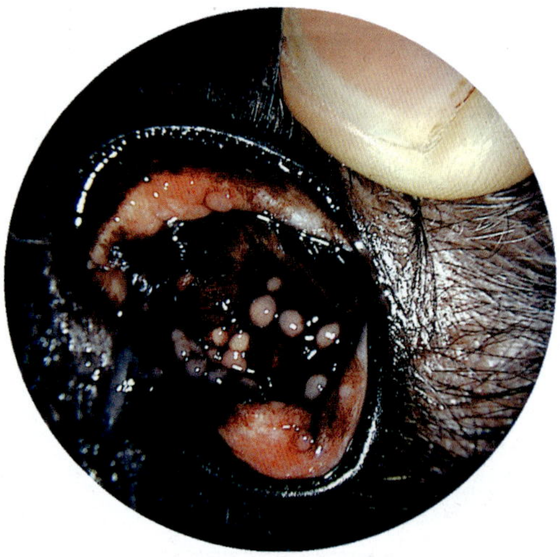

Figure 2-14
Follicular conjunctivitis of the anterior surface of the nictitans. Lymphoid follicles are seen on both sides of the nictitans and occasionally on the bulbar and eyelid conjunctiva. A mucoid conjunctivitis accompanies this disease. Allergic reactions are postulated to be the cause.
(Courtesy Dr. Robert Playter.)

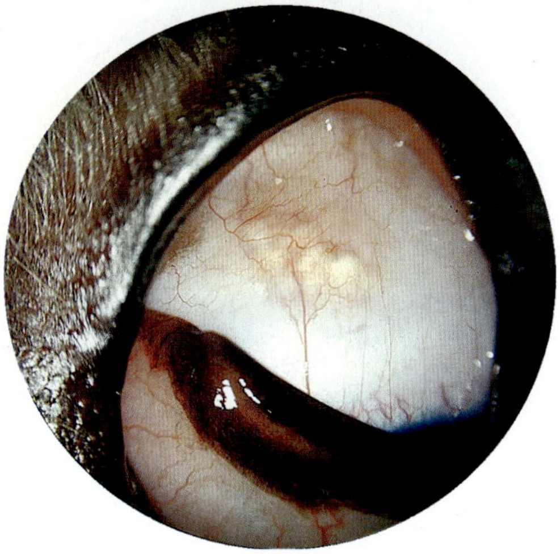

Figure 2-15
Subconjunctival plaque caused by subconjunctival injection of a long-acting corticosteroid preparation.

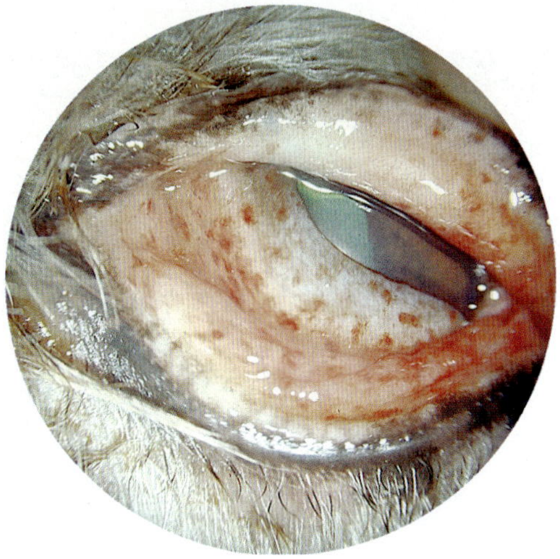

Figure 2-16
Multifocal conjunctival petechiae caused by immune-mediated thrombocytopenia.

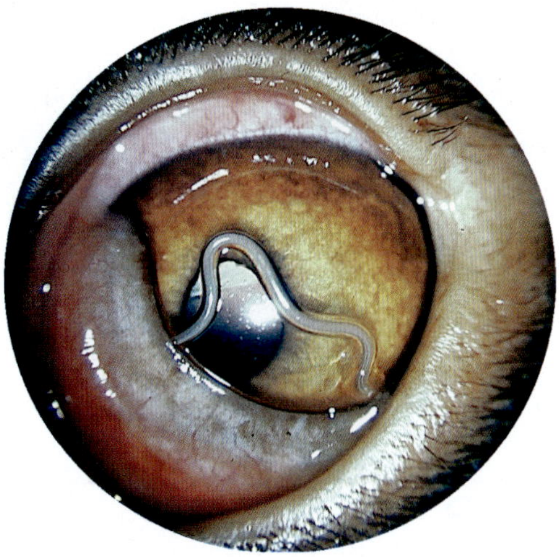

Figure 2-17
Thelazia in a dog's conjunctival sac.
(Courtesy Dr. Dennis Brooks.)

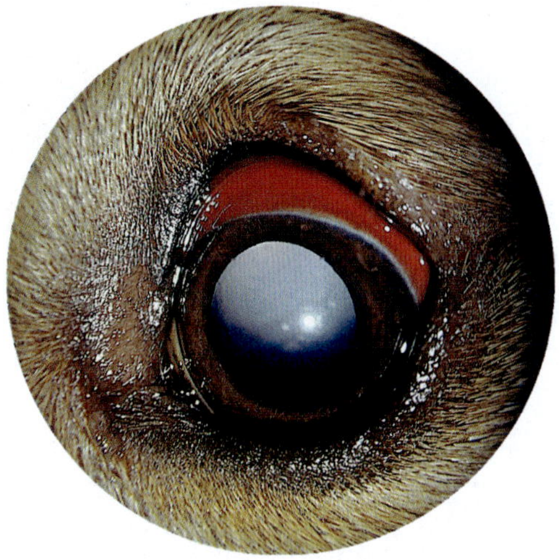

Figure 2-18
Traumatic subconjunctival hemorrhage.

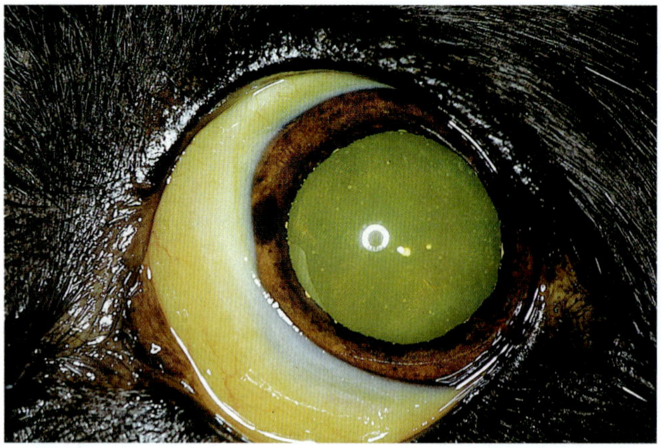

Figure 2-19
Icterus resulting from immune-mediated hemolytic anemia in an English cocker spaniel.

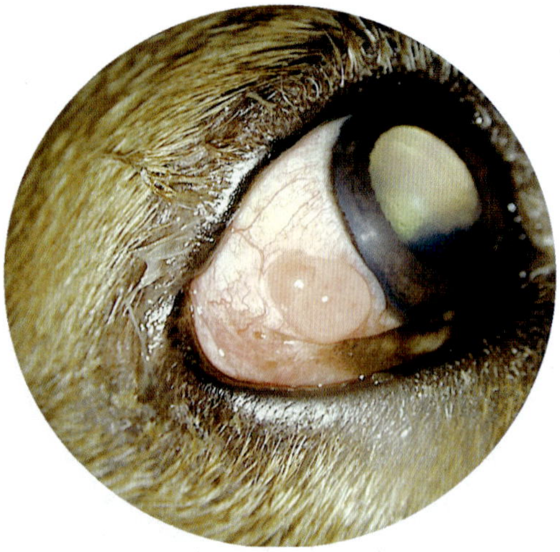

Figure 2-20
Conjunctival cyst in a dog.

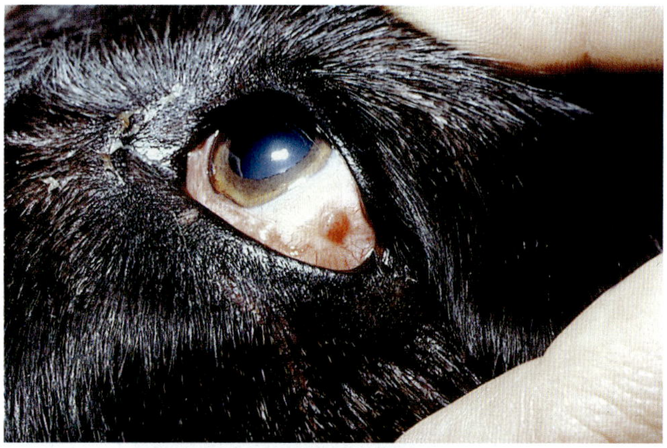

Figure 2-21
Conjunctival hemangioma in a dog.

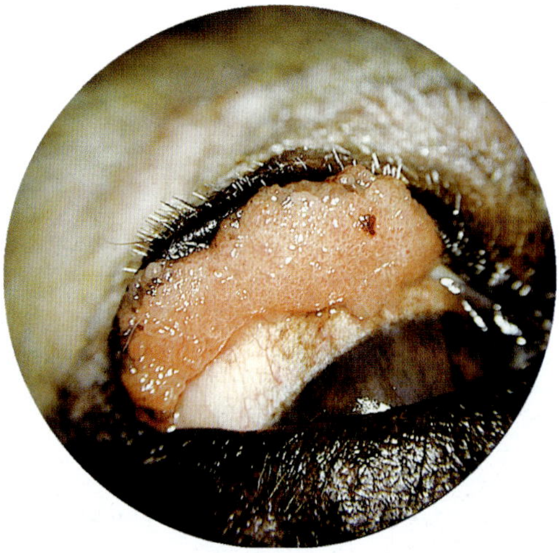

Figure 2-22
Conjunctival papilloma in a Lhasa apso.

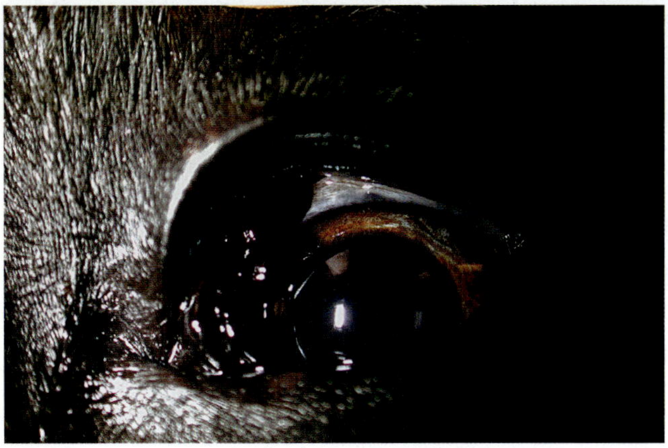

Figure 2-23
Conjunctival melanocytoma in a Labrador retriever involving the palpebral, bulbar, and third eyelid conjunctiva.

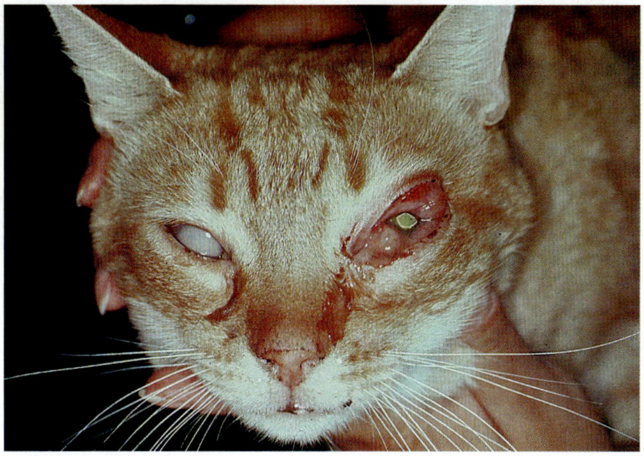

Figure 2-24
Conjunctival lymphosarcoma in the left eye of a cat.
(Courtesy Dr. Nancy Bromberg.)

Chapter 3

Third Eyelid

INTRODUCTION

The third eyelid (membrana nictitans) is composed of a T-shaped cartilage with the third eyelid lacrimal gland at its base, entirely covered with conjunctiva. The third eyelid is often affected when conjunctivitis is present. Hereditary nictitans diseases in dogs, including scrolled cartilage and prolapsed gland of the third eyelid (cherry eye), are illustrated in this chapter. Other miscellaneous conditions affecting the nictitans also are shown.

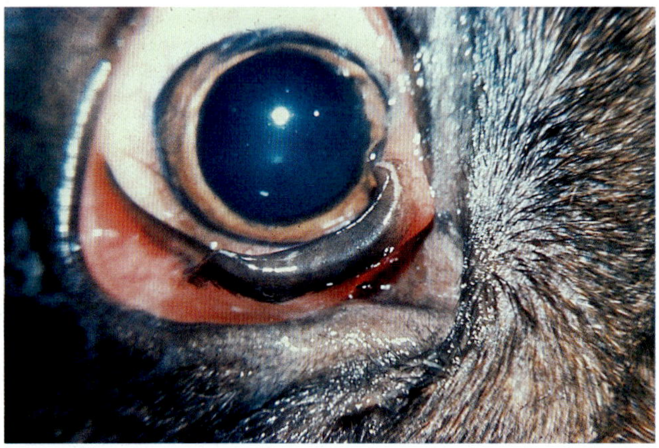

Figure 3-1
Scrolled nictitans. Abnormalities of cartilage growth cause the nictitans to scroll outward rather than lying flat on the globe. Correction involves removal of the abnormal cartilage while preserving the conjunctiva of the nictitans. A breed predisposition to this condition exists. (Courtesy Dr. Robert Playter.)

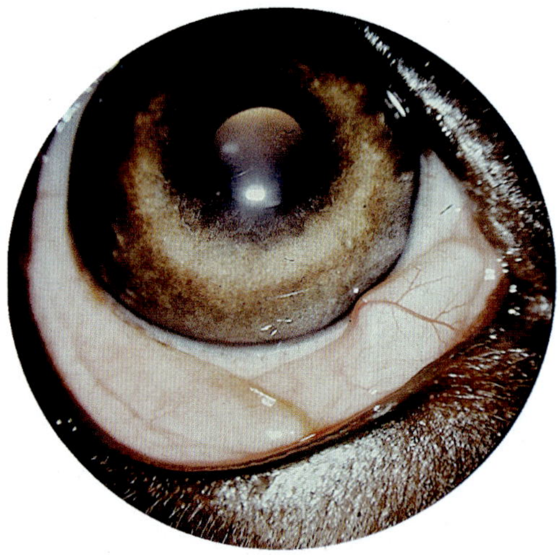

Figure 3-2
Scrolled nictitans. The middle of the T-piece of this cartilage is bent and can be seen in the medial canthus. The leading edge of the nictitans is hidden by the lower eyelid.

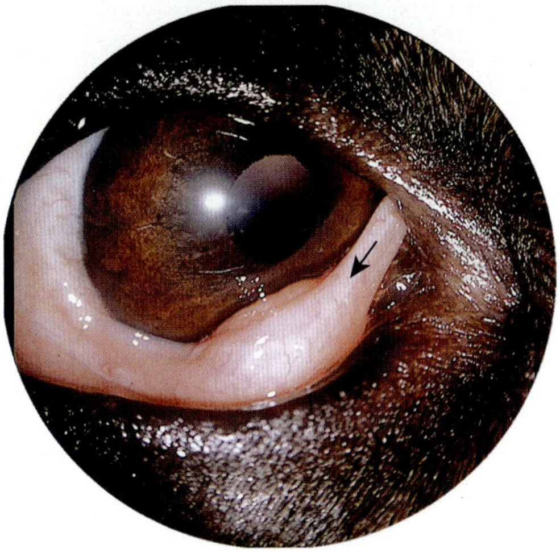

Figure 3-3
Scrolled nictitans. In dogs with a scrolled nictitans the third eyelid cannot be repositioned manually, in contrast to those with a cherry eye (prolapsed gland of the third eyelid; see Figure 3-4), which can be repositioned, at least temporarily.

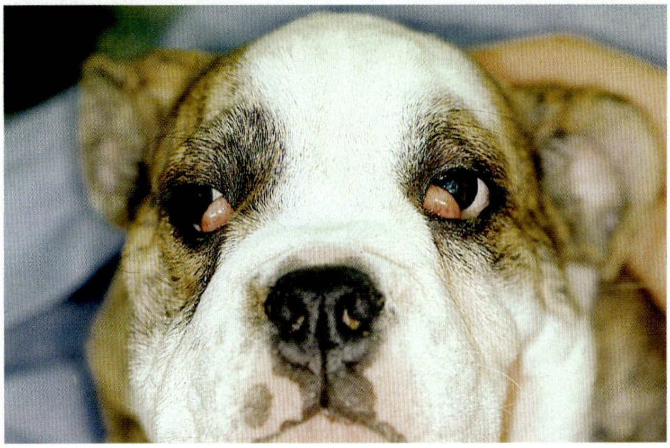

Figure 3-4
English bulldog puppy with bilateral cherry eye. A breed predisposition to this condition exists in bulldogs and other breeds. Treatment involves repositioning the gland and suturing it in place. Removal of the gland can lead to keratoconjunctivitis sicca (KCS), as can no repair.

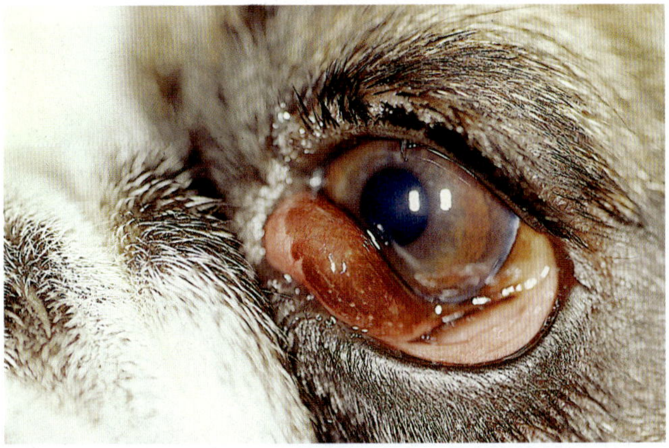

Figure 3-5
Cherry eye in an adult English bulldog.

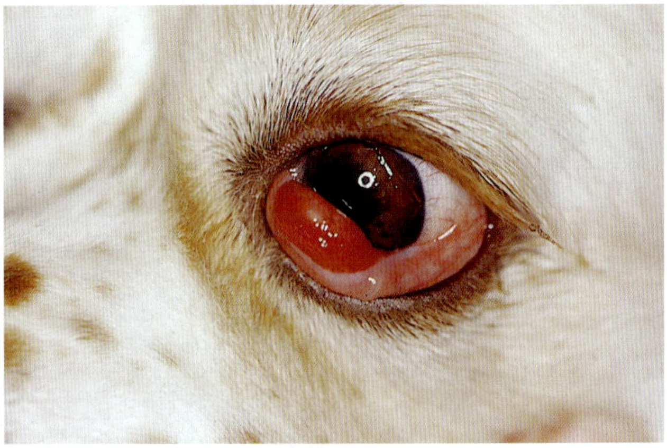

Figure 3-6
Cherry eye in a 2-year-old American cocker spaniel. Note the intumescent, hyperemic appearance of the gland, which can be seen through the bulbar surface of the third eyelid conjunctiva.

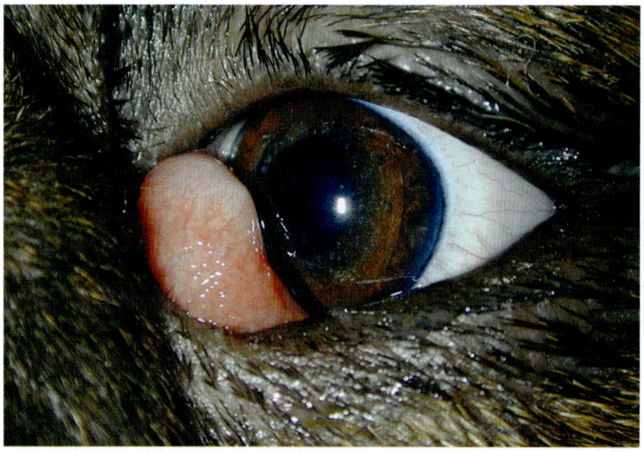

Figure 3-7
Cherry eye and facial fold or medial entropion in an English bulldog. The gland is enlarged, and lymphoid follicular enlargement is seen on the conjunctival surface.

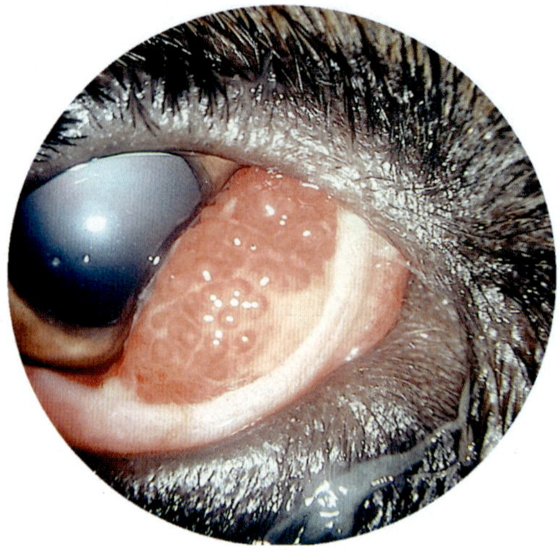

Figure 3-8
Cherry eye and follicular conjunctivitis in a dog.

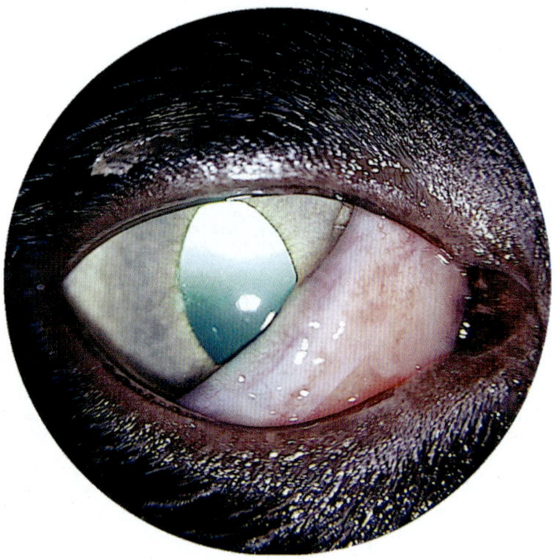

Figure 3-9
Eosinophilic and lymphocytic infiltrate of the nictitans in a 3-year-old cat. Thickened plaque on the anterior surface of the nictitans and depigmentation of the leading edge are present.

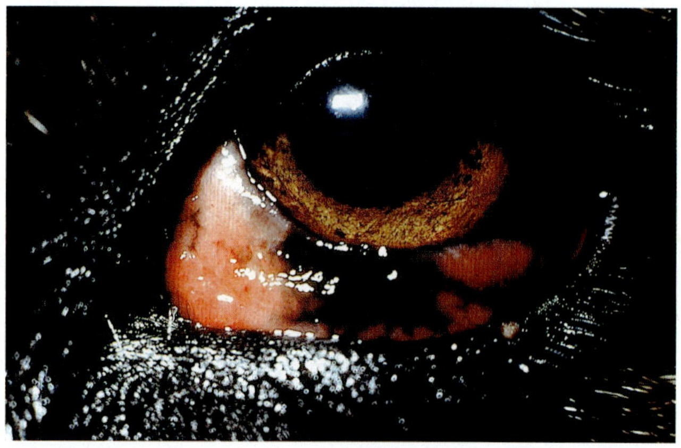

Figure 3-10
Atypical pannus in a German shepherd dog. Pannus is typically a lymphocytic or plasmacytic corneal infiltrate seen mostly in German shepherd dogs. Occasionally the cellular infiltrate is seen in the nictitans, as shown here, rather than in the cornea.

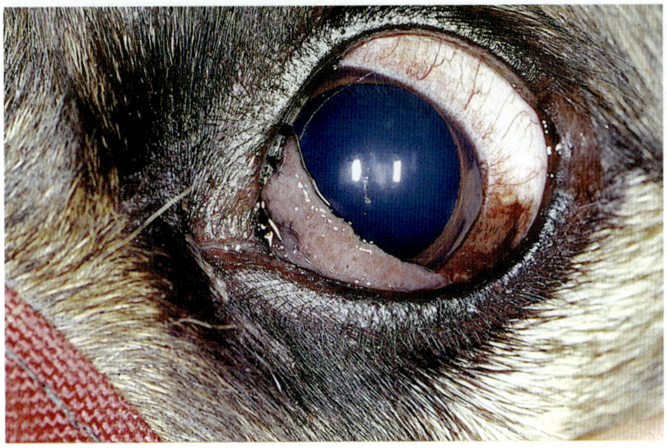

Figure 3-11
Atypical pannus involving the third eyelid of a German shepherd dog.

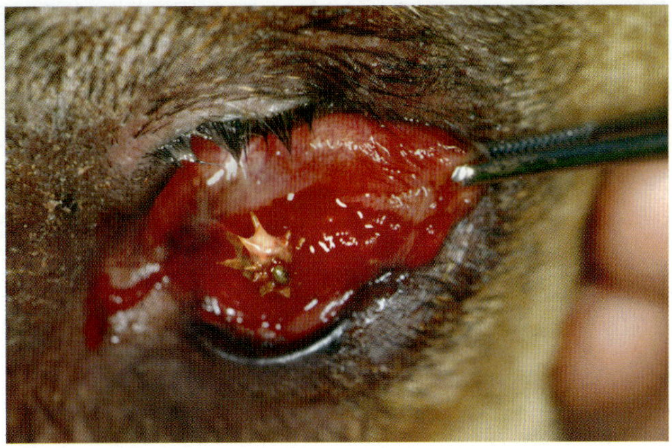

Figure 3-12
Plant seed foreign body on the palpebral surface of the nictitans. The nictitans is elevated with forceps after application of topical anesthesia.

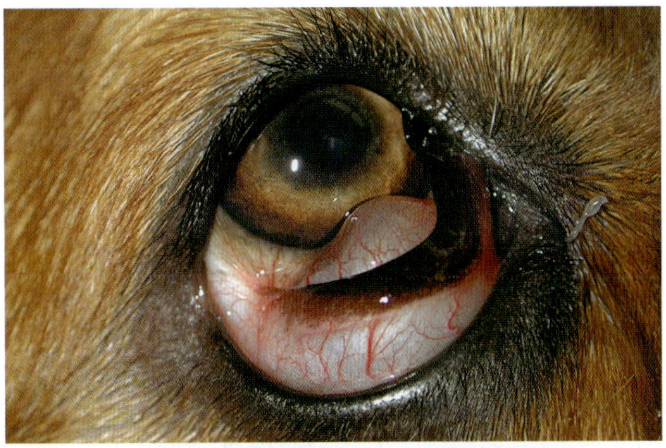

Figure 3-13
Cyst of the nictitans gland.

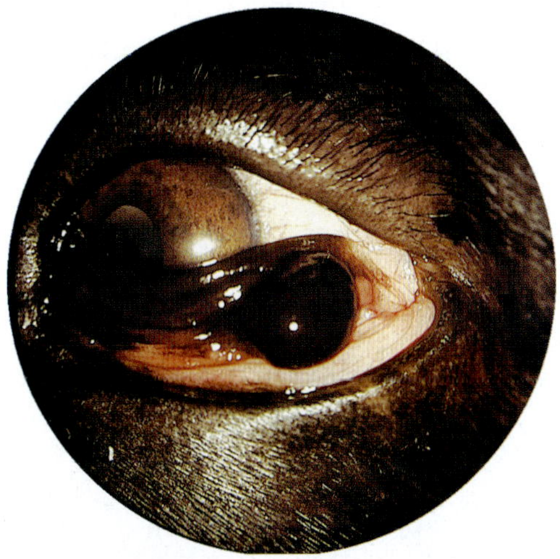

Figure 3-14
Melanoma on the anterior surface of the nictitans.

Chapter 4

Lacrimal System

INTRODUCTION

Conditions of the nasolacrimal system affect the lacrimal secretions, particularly the aqueous phase of the tear film secreted by the lacrimal and third eyelid glands and the lipid secretions of the meibomian gland. Keratoconjunctivitis sicca (KCS) is undoubtedly the most important disease of lacrimal secretion that occurs commonly in dogs of numerous breeds; the incidence in cats is much lower. For a variety of reasons, the majority of problems involving nasolacrimal drainage manifest as limited tear drainage, often resulting in epiphora.

A

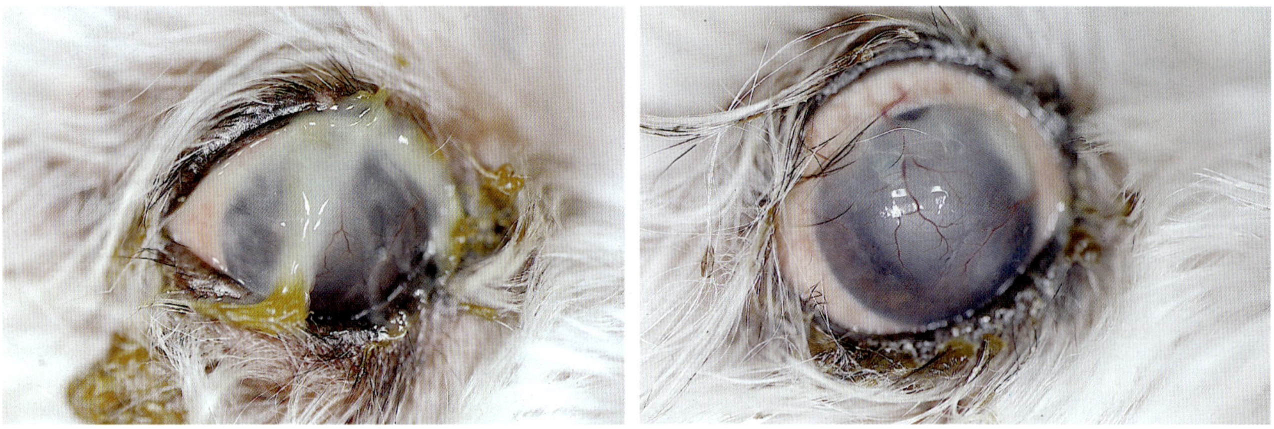

B

Figure 4-1 A-B
A, Chronic KCS has caused corneal scarring, neovascularization, and increased mucous discharge. Note the mucopurulent discharge adhering to the eyelids and cornea. **B,** the eye after it was cleaned of discharge.

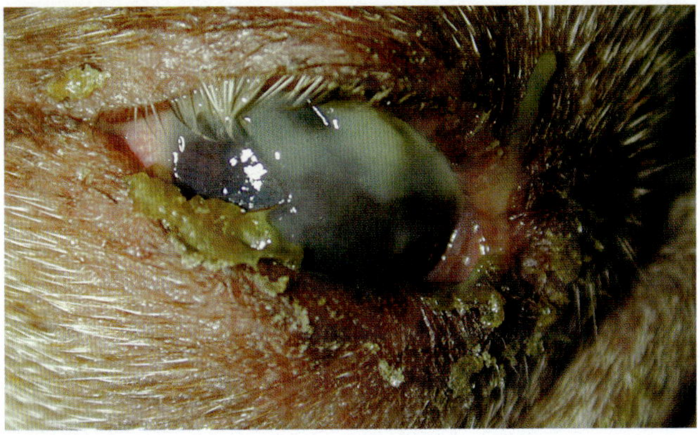

Figure 4-2
Mucopurulent discharge adherent to the eyelids and cornea and corneal neovascularization as a result of KCS.

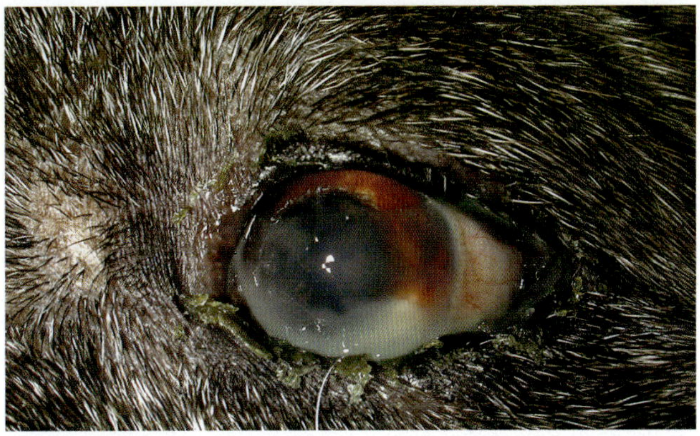

Figure 4-3
KCS in an Australian heeler. Mucopurulent discharge and corneal neovascularization are marked.

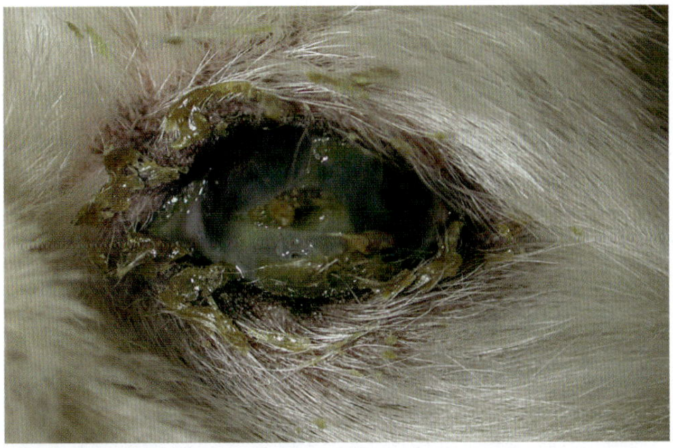

Figure 4-4
KCS in a shih tzu. Mucopurulent discharge and corneal edema and vascularization are present.

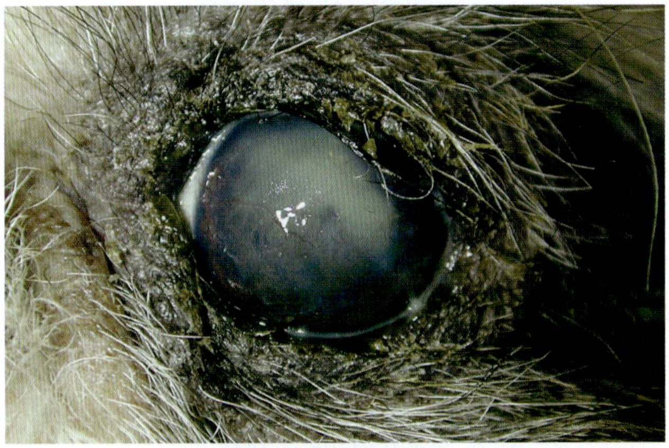

Figure 4-5
Chronic KCS in a Lhasa apso. Periocular dermatitis is present, and crusted discharge is attached to the eyelid cilia. Mucopurulent discharge adheres to the corneal surface.

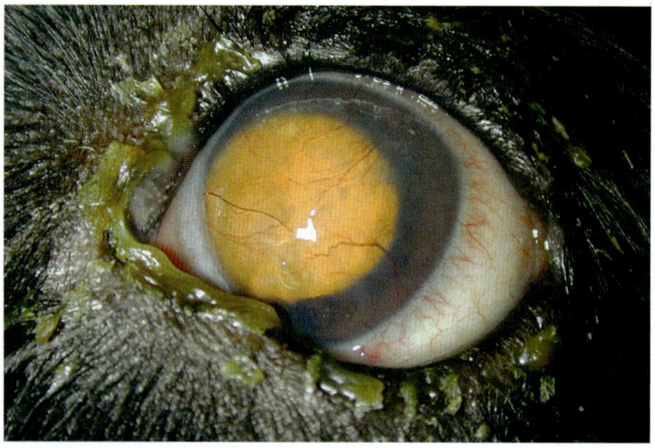

Figure 4-6
KCS in a springer spaniel. Mucopurulent discharge, conjunctival injection, corneal edema, and superficial neovascularization are present.

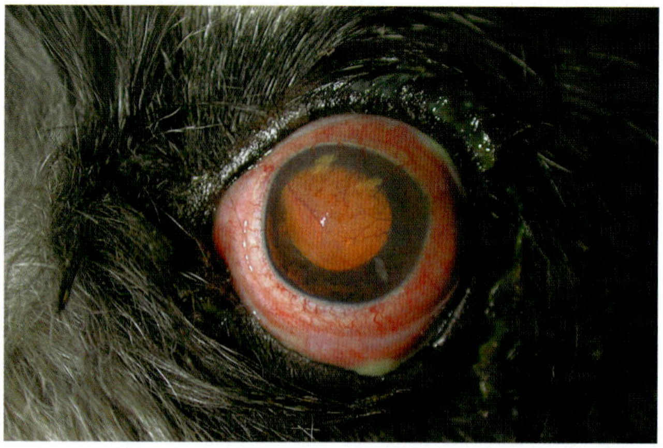

Figure 4-7
KCS in an American cocker spaniel. Note marked conjunctivitis, corneal edema and neovascularization, and mucopurulent discharge.

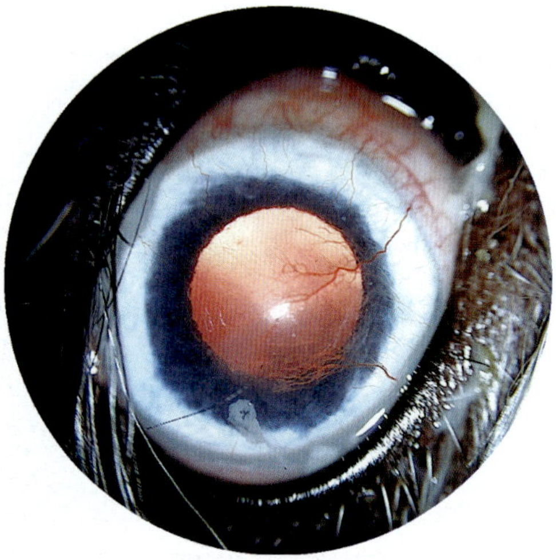

Figure 4-8
KCS in a Siberian husky. Mucoid discharge adheres to the cornea and eyelids, and corneal vascularization is present.

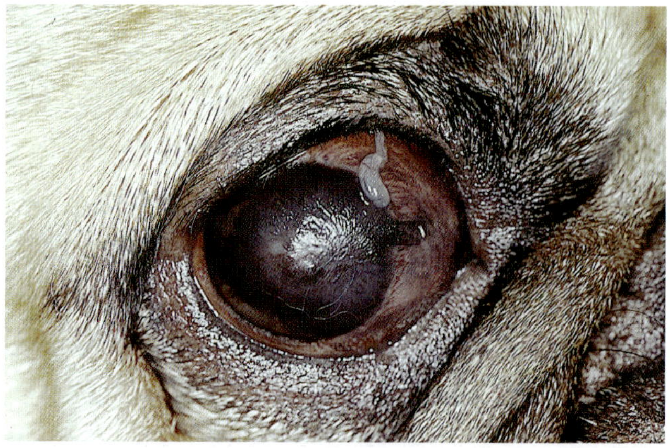

Figure 4-9
Close-up of chronic KCS that is causing corneal pigmentation and scarring in a pug.

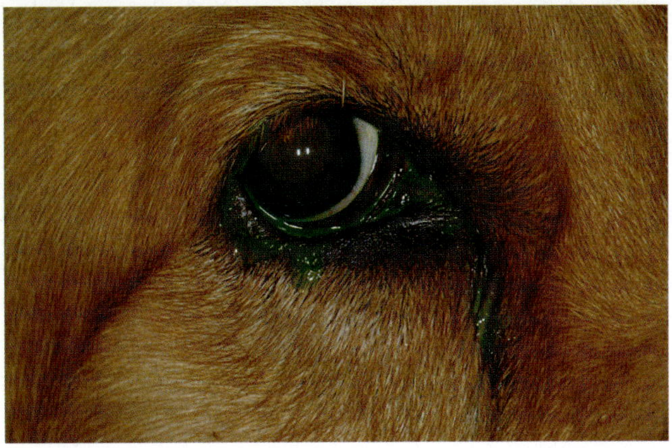

Figure 4-10
Epiphora in a golden retriever with an imperforate lower nasolacrimal punctum. Fluorescein dye that has been placed into the eye is spilling onto the eyelids and medial canthus. No dye is seen at the external nares.

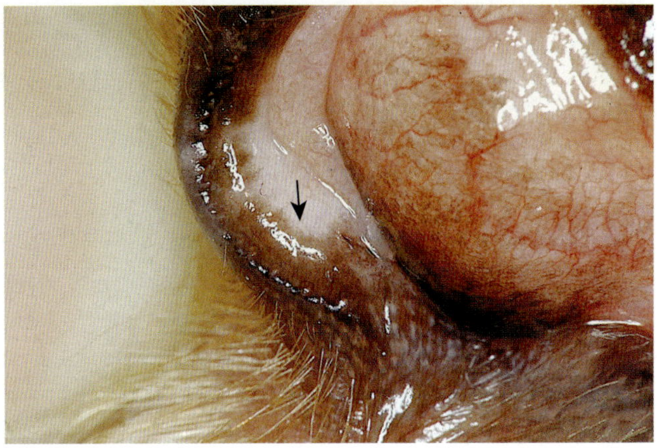

Figure 4-11
Imperforate punctum in the lower eyelid of a dog. Opening of punctum is covered by conjuctiva.

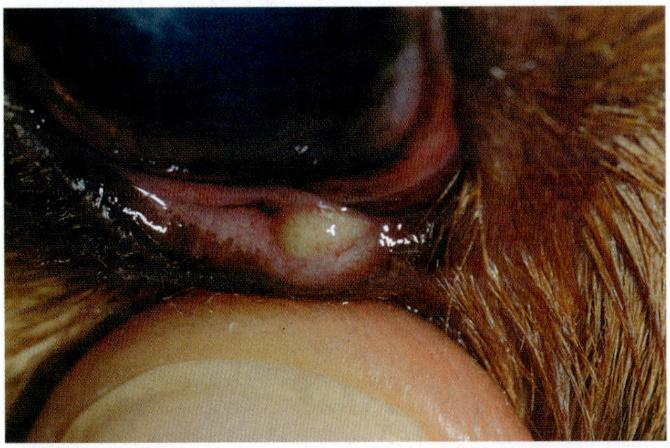

Figure 4-12
Congenitally imperforate lower nasolacrimal punctum in a 2-year-old American cocker spaniel with a history of chronic epiphora. Purulent material (seen through the conjunctiva) was released when the conjunctiva covering the punctum was incised to correct the problem.

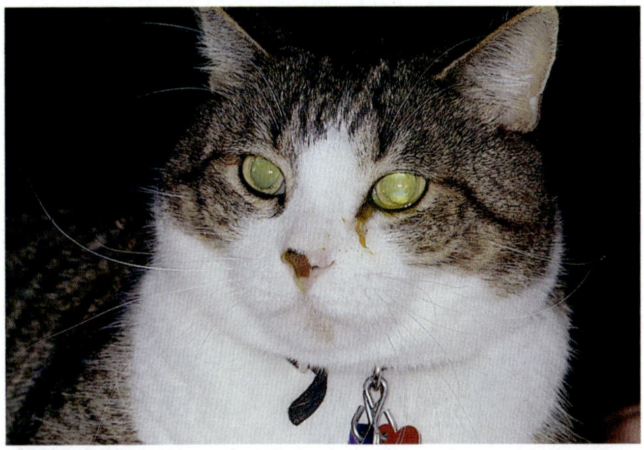

Figure 4-13
Cat with epiphora from the left eye. Fluorescein dye was placed in both eyes. Fluorescein dye stains the left side of the face but not the right and is seen at the right external nares but not the left. This indicates that the left nasolacrimal duct is not draining tears.

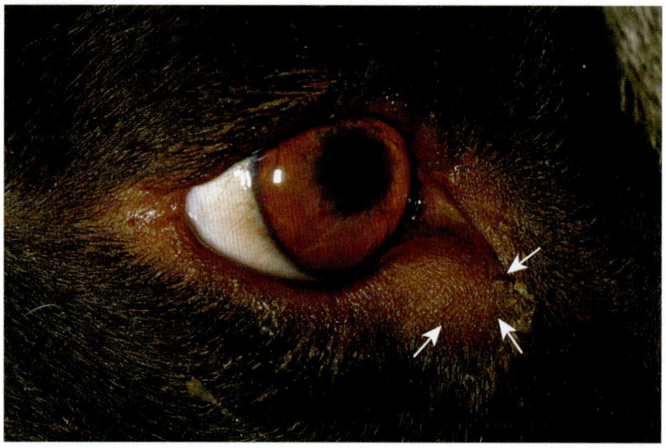

Figure 4-14
Nasolacrimal duct cyst in a 1-year-old German shorthaired pointer. This cyst communicated with the nasolacrimal duct and fluctuated in size. Careful dissection and removal of the cyst was curative.

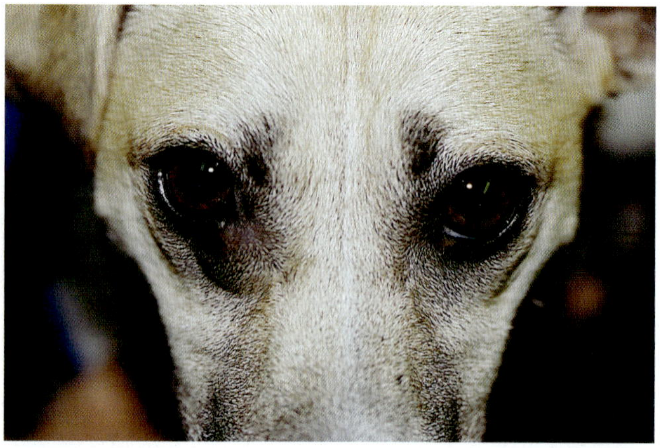

Figure 4-15
Nasolacrimal duct cyst at the right medial canthus in a terrier. The mass was firm and did not fluctuate in size or communicate with the nasolacrimal duct.

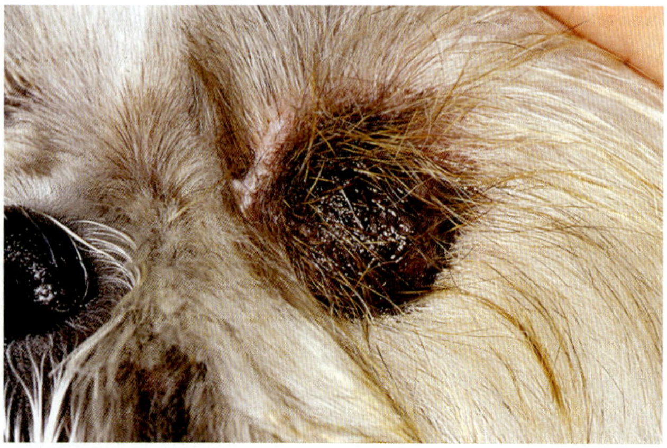

Figure 4-16
Postenucleation lacrimal cyst resulting from failure to remove lacrimal tissue at surgery. The cyst was easily dissected from the orbit.

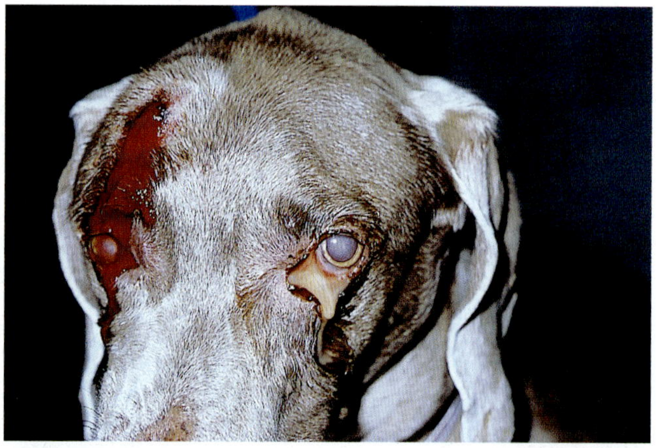

Figure 4-17
Severe dacryocystitis in a weimaraner with multifocal cutaneous draining tracts.

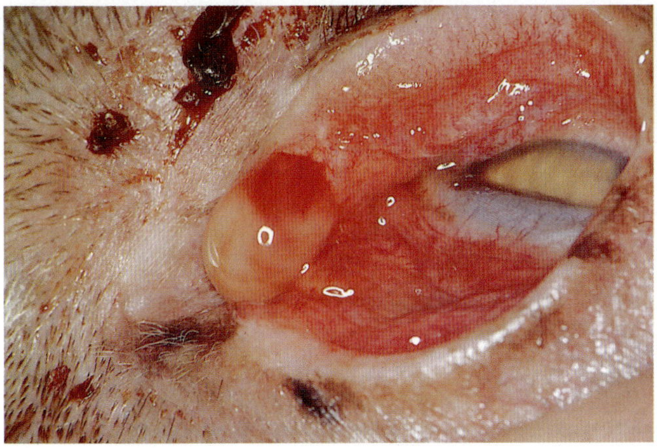

Figure 4-18
Close-up of weimaraner shown in Figure 4-17. Pus drains from the lacrimal puncta.

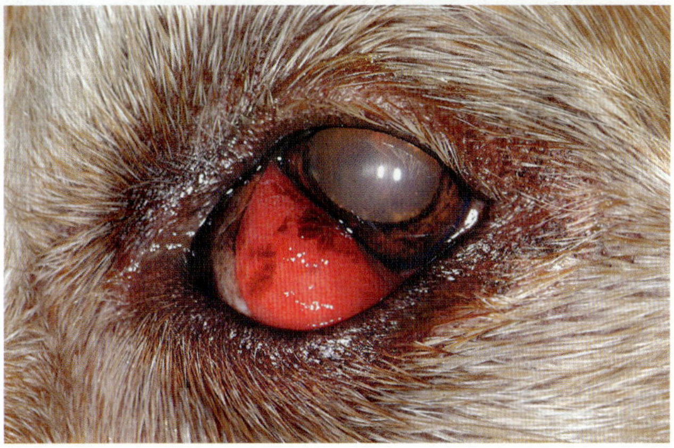

Figure 4-19
Nictitans gland adenocarcinoma in a geriatric golden retriever.

Chapter 5

Cornea

INTRODUCTION

The cornea is a vital part of the eye. Lesions of the cornea are often readily obvious to pet owners, because these lesions may be easily observed and frequently manifest as painful conditions for the animal. The transmission and refraction of light in the eye require that the cornea be transparent; any pathologic problem that affects corneal transparency can significantly reduce vision. Some corneal lesions (notably ulceration) can affect the integrity of the entire eye. For these reasons corneal diseases are a very important part of veterinary ophthalmology. Corneal ulcers, from superficial to deep, are illustrated in this chapter. Other conditions that affect the cornea, such as eosinophilic keratitis and sequestra in cats, pannus and corneal dystrophies in dogs, and mass lesions in the cornea, are also illustrated here.

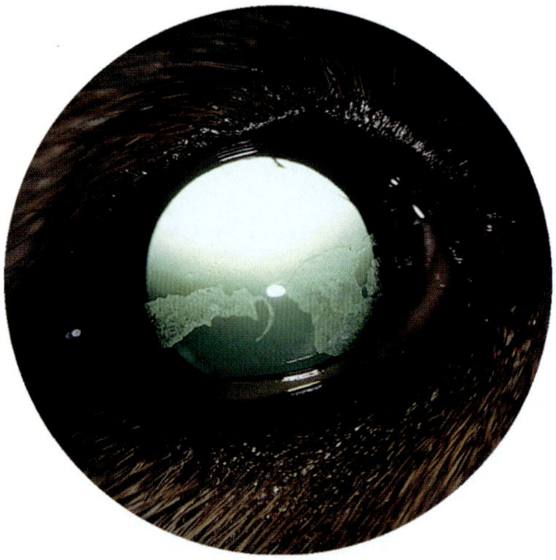

Figure 5-1
Superficial corneal opacification in the interpalpebral fissure region in a puppy. This finding is normal in young puppies after the eyelids have opened. The cornea becomes normal as the dog ages.

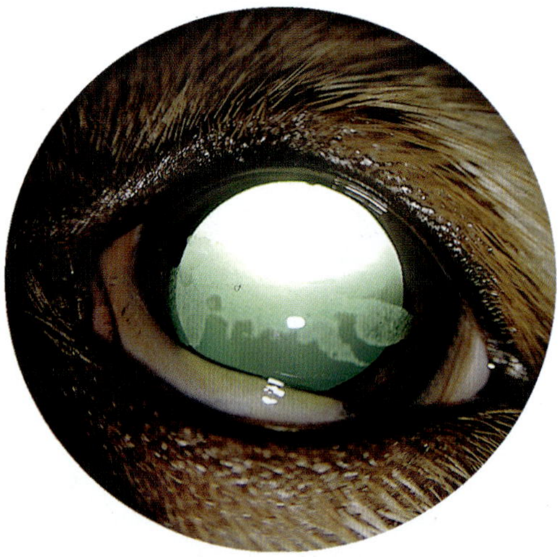

Figure 5-2
Normal superficial corneal opacification in the interpalpebral fissure region in a 5-week-old golden retriever. The opacity clears as a dog ages.

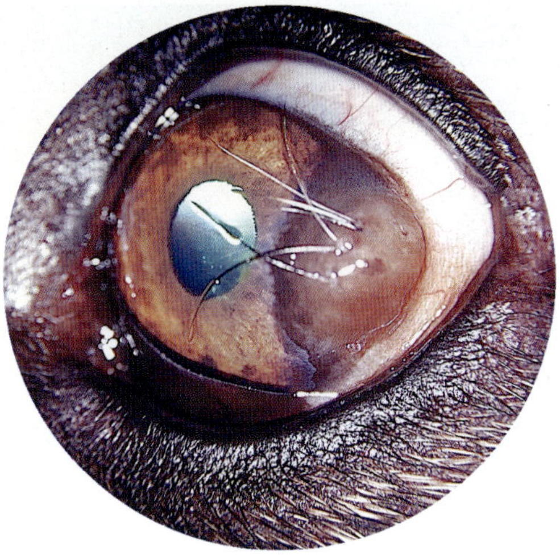

Figure 5-3
Corneal dermoid with hairs.

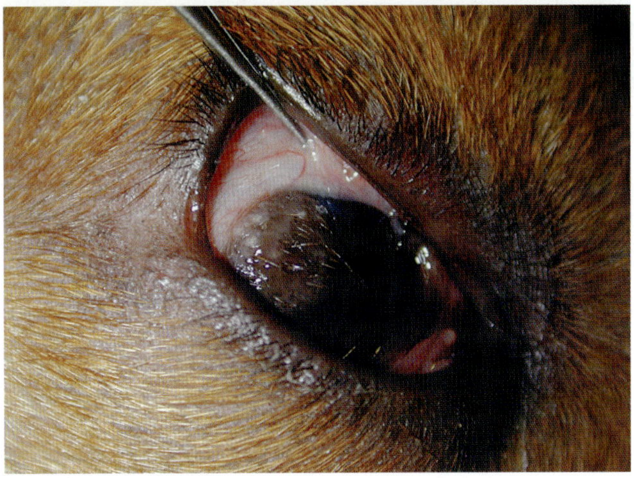

Figure 5-4
Corneal dermoid in a dachshund puppy.

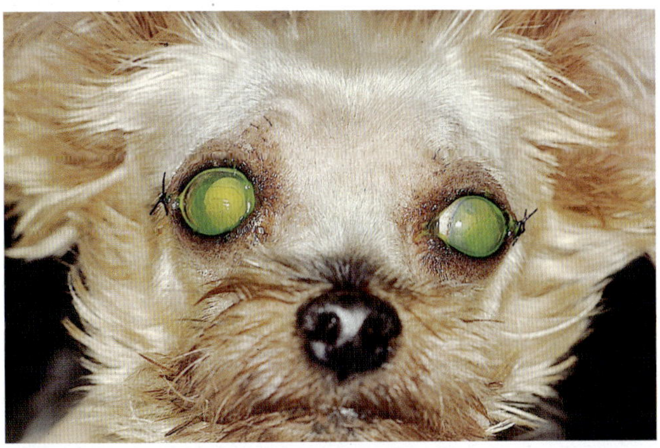

Figure 5-5
Yorkshire terrier with bilateral superficial ulcers stained with fluorescein dye 24 hours after cataract surgery. The eyes dried after surgery, which resulted in the ulceration.

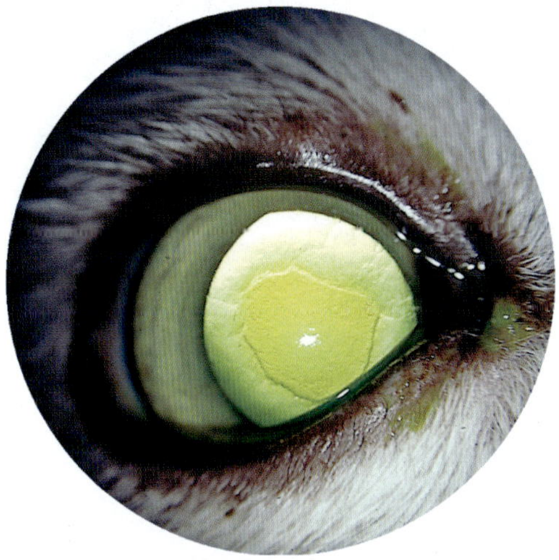

Figure 5-6
Superficial corneal ulcer in a cat. The ulcer resulted from corneal drying while the cat was under general anesthesia without corneal lubrication or moistening.

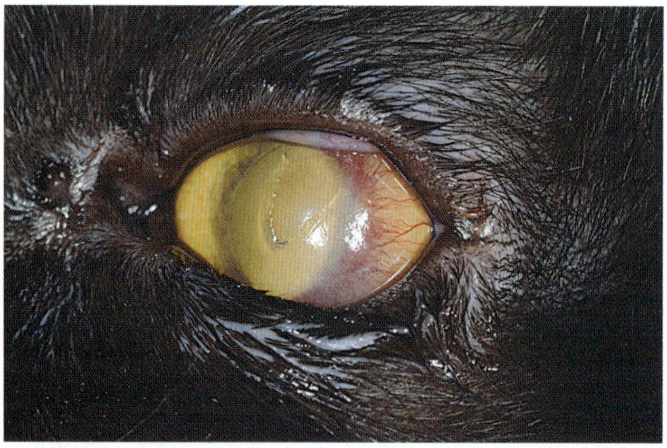

Figure 5-7
Lower eyelid entropion in a domestic shorthair cat, which resulted in a chronic corneal ulcer and neovascularization.

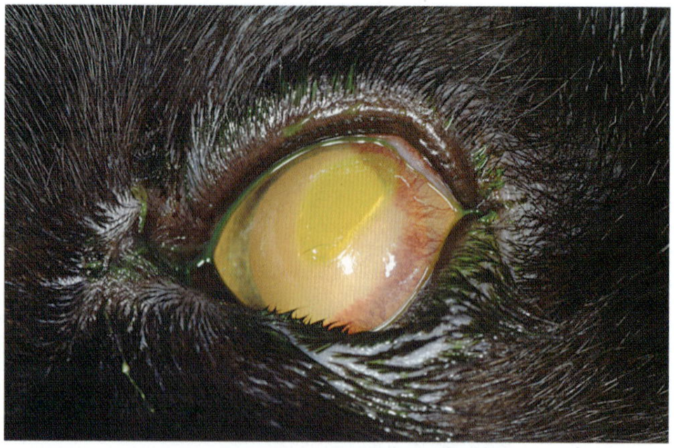

Figure 5-8
Same cat as in Figure 5-7. Corneal ulcer stained with fluorescein dye.

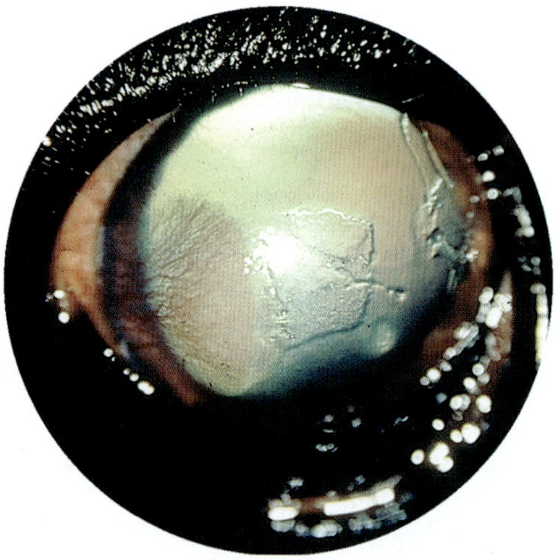

Figure 5-9
Nonhealing (refractory, indolent) corneal ulcer with neovascularization. Note tag of epithelium in ulcerated area. Nonhealing corneal ulcers are seen in eyes with basement membrane defects. Superficial corneal ulcers do not heal because migrating epithelium does not adhere to the basement membrane.
(Courtesy Dr. Robert Playter.)

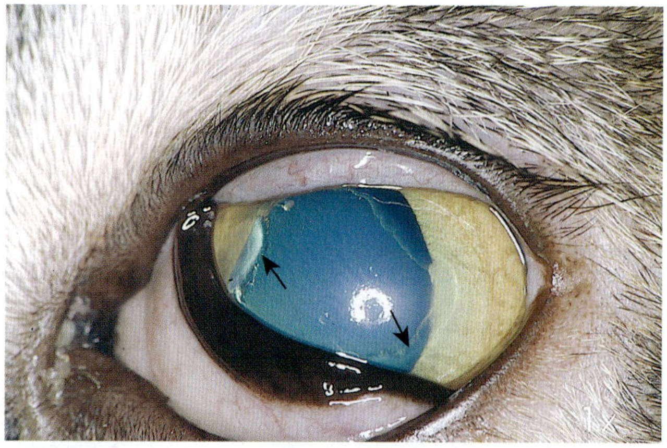

Figure 5-10
Superficial nonhealing corneal ulcer in a cat. Note the loose edges of epithelium *(arrows)*.

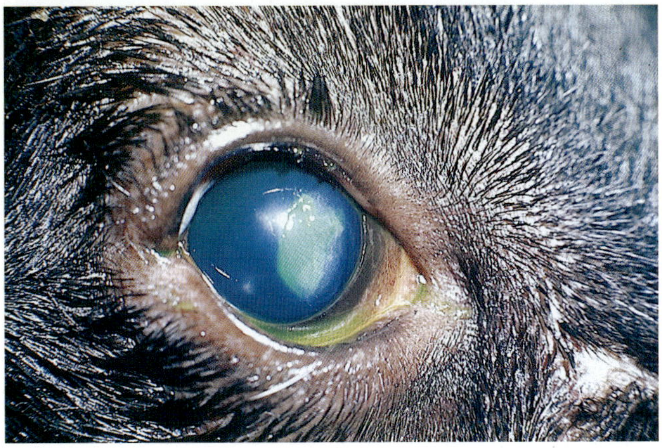

Figure 5-11
Nonhealing superficial ulcer stained with flourescein dye. Note the tags of epithelium across the ulcer and the stain beyond the edges of the ulcer.
(Courtesy Dr. Robert Playter.)

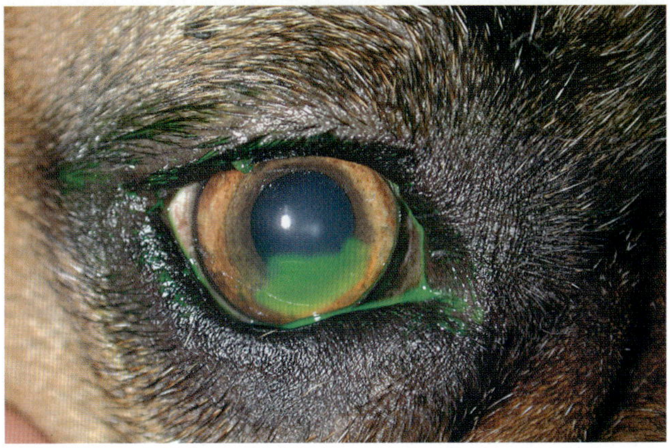

Figure 5-12
Nonhealing superficial corneal ulcer that had been present for several weeks in this boxer. The ulcer is stained with fluorescein dye. Note the lack of corneal vascularization and the lip of epithelium at the edge of the ulcer, which is underrun by fluorescein.

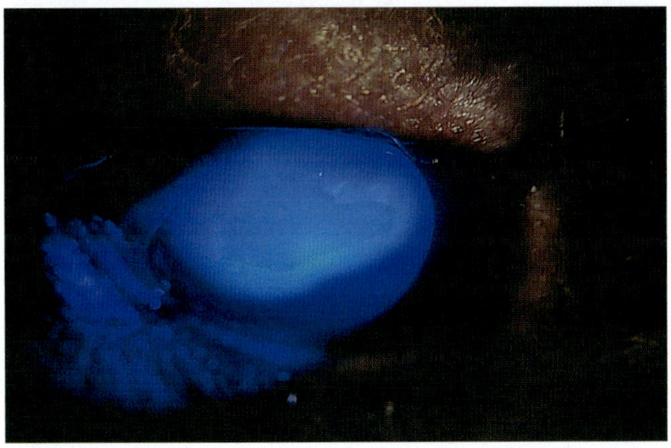

Figure 5-13
Nonhealing corneal ulcer stained with fluorescein and photographed under a blue light. Note the stain that is migrating beyond the edges of the ulcer.

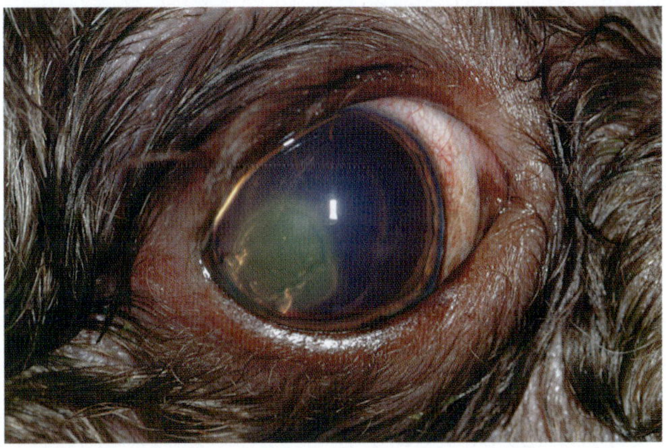

Figure 5-14
Nonhealing superficial ulcer. Note the loose tags of epithelium at the edge of the ulcer.

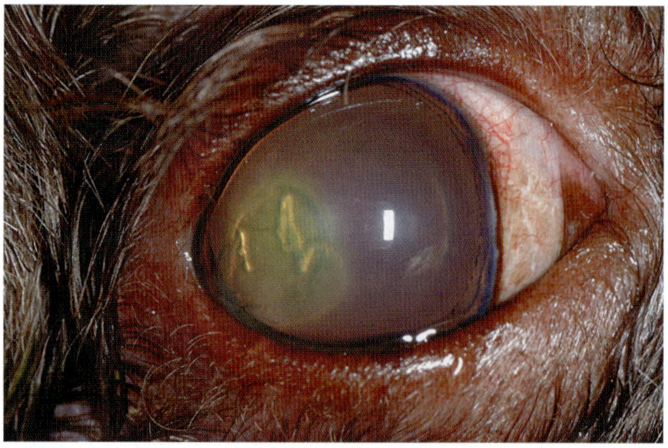

Figure 5-15
Nonhealing ulcer. Note the loose tags of epithelium.

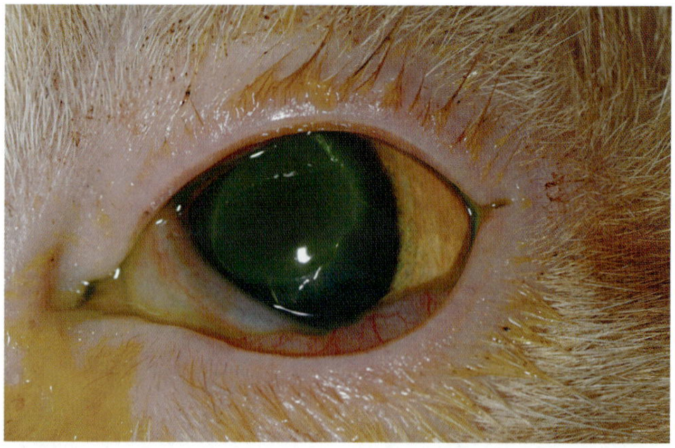

Figure 5-16
Indolent ulcer with loose lip of epithelium in a cat.

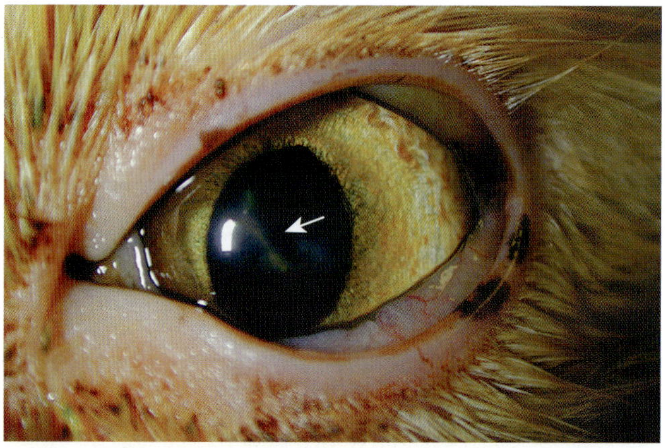

Figure 5-17
Dendritic ulcer (a thin, meandering, often arborizing epithelial defect) in the cornea of a cat with herpesvirus infection.

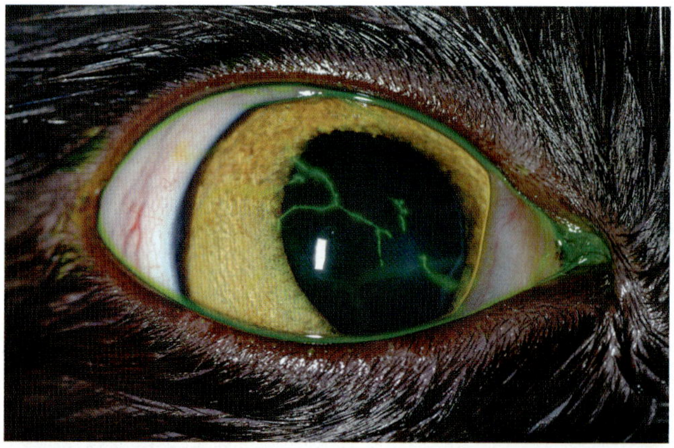

Figure 5-18
Dendritic ulcer caused by herpes in a cat. The ulcer is stained with fluorescein.

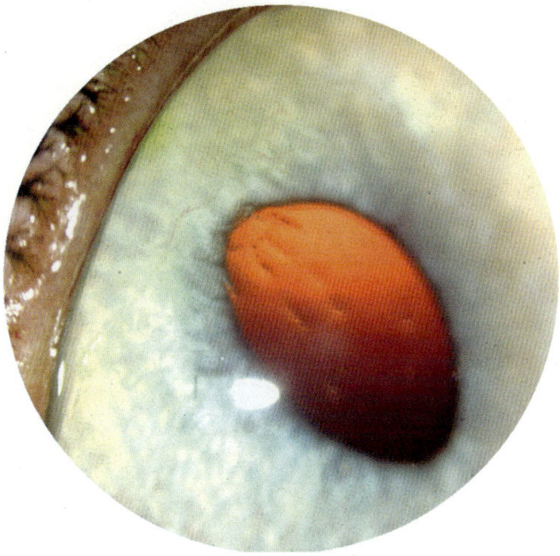

Figure 5-19
Herpesvirus keratitis (unstained) in a cat.

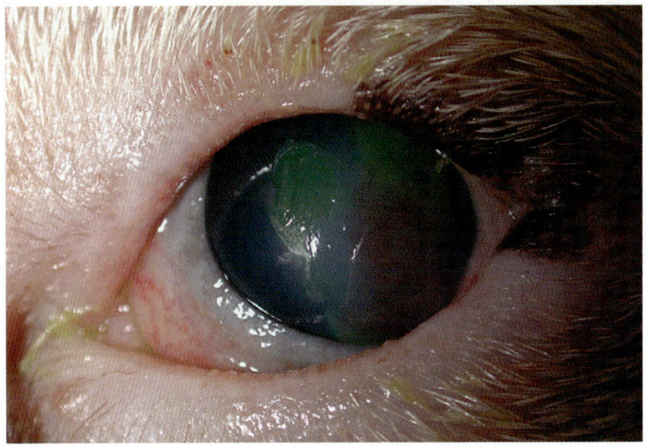

Figure 5-20
Feline herpesvirus keratitis. Corneal ulceration, edema, and vascularization are present.

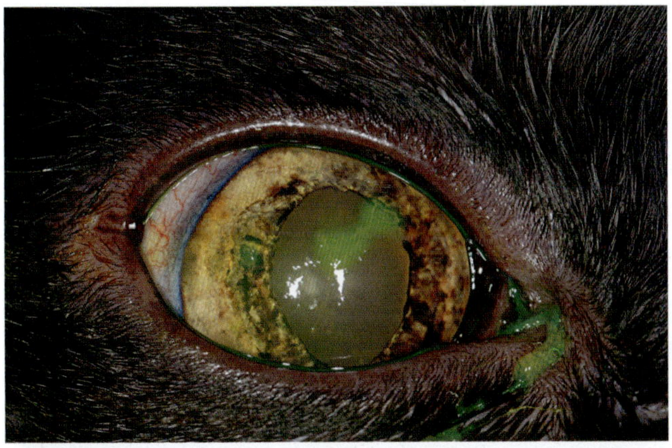

Figure 5-21
Nonhealing corneal ulcer in a cat that tested positive for herpesvirus. Iris atrophy and increased pigmentation are present.

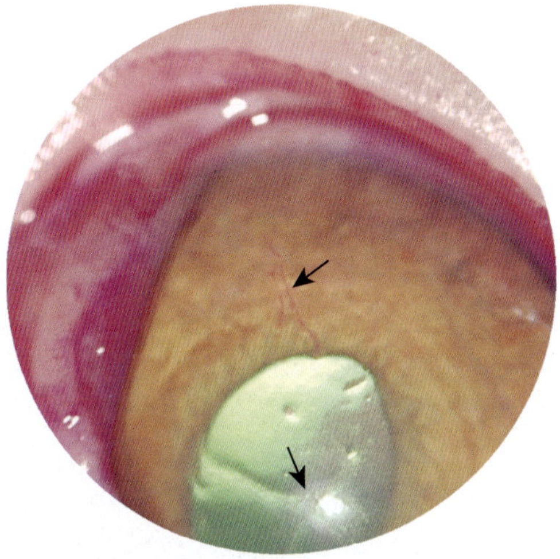

Figure 5-22
Herpesvirus keratitis stained with rose bengal in a cat. Faint, linear, red-stained lesions can be seen.

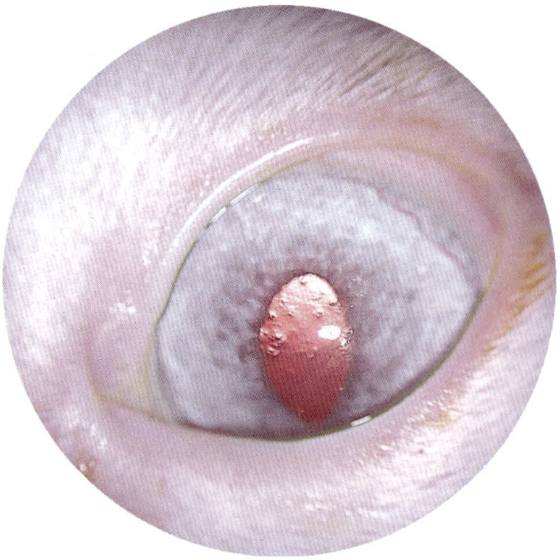

Figure 5-23
Multifocal areas of keratitis associated with herpesvirus infection in a cat.

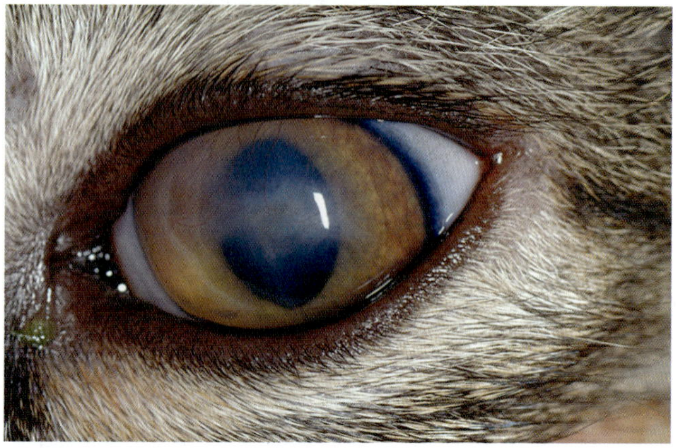

Figure 5-24
Corneal scarring in a cat undergoing treatment with trifluridine and oral lysine for herpesvirus infection.

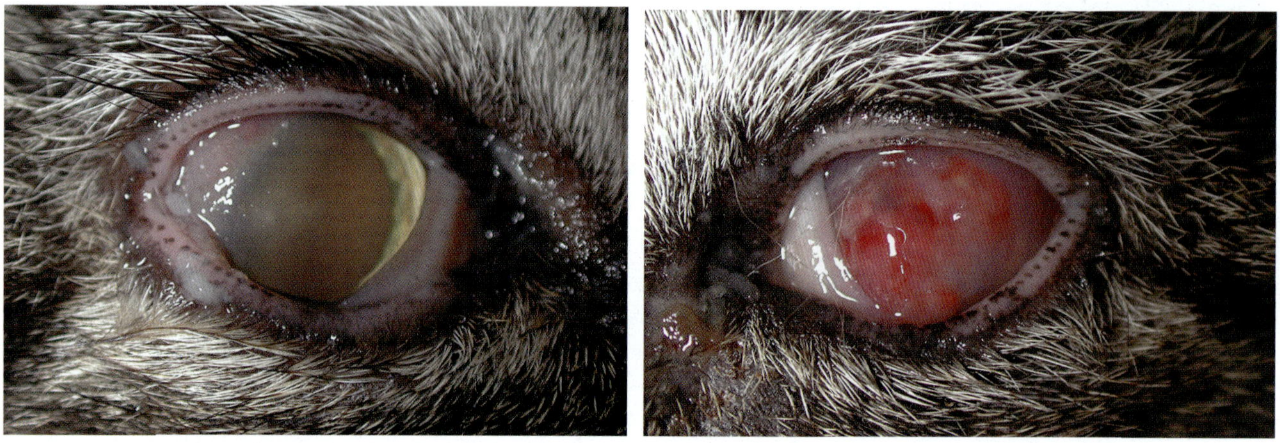

Figure 5-25
Bilateral eosinophilic and herpesvirus keratoconjunctivitis in a cat. Cellular infiltration is present in the cornea with mixed inflammatory cell populations with high eosinophil numbers.

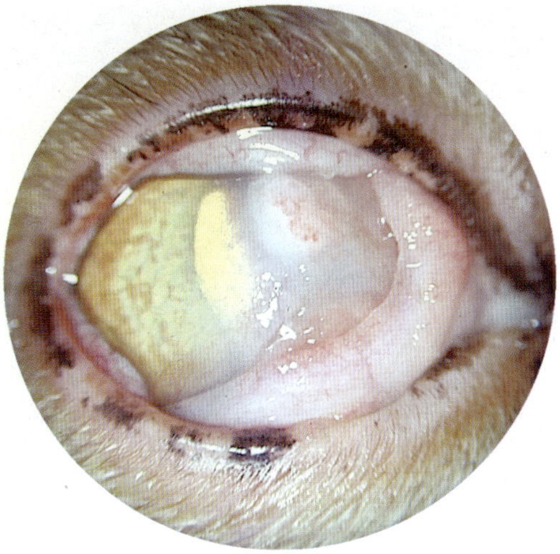

Figure 5-26
Neovascularization and cellular infiltrate in the cornea and nictitans of a cat with eosinophilic keratitis.

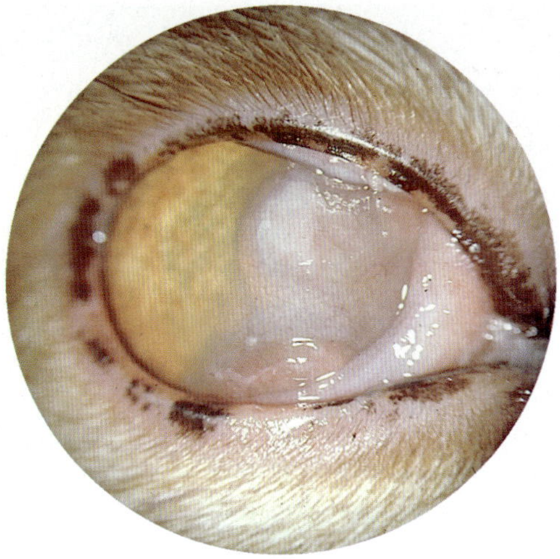

Figure 5-27
Eosinophilic keratitis in a cat.

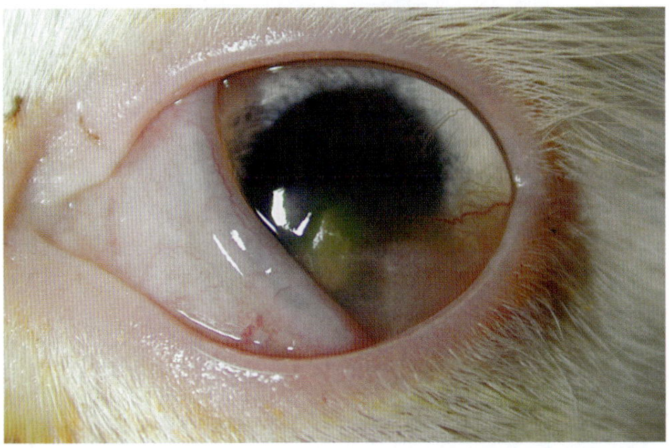

Figure 5-28
Herpesvirus keratitis and eosinophilic keratitis. This cat was being treated with topical trifluridine and corticosteroids.

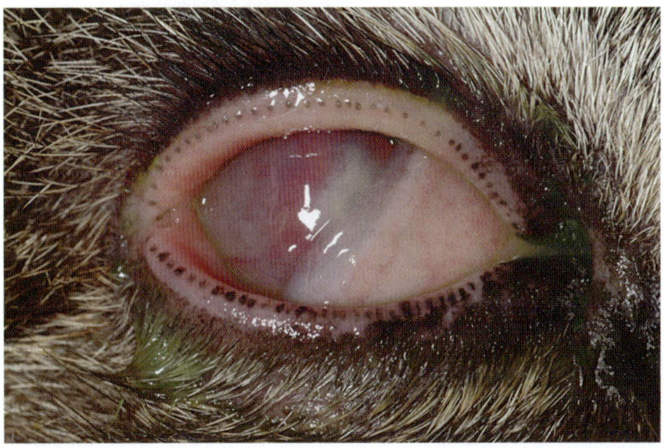

Figure 5-29
Eosinophilic keratitis and blepharitis in a cat with a positive result on polymerase chain reaction testing for herpesvirus infection. Lesions responded to topical trifluridine and dexamethasone.

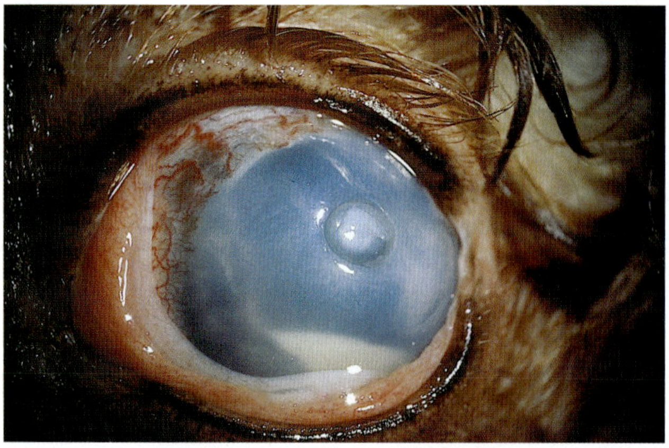

Figure 5-30
Deep corneal ulcer resulting from *Candida* species infection. "Red eye," corneal edema, hypopyon, and anterior synechiae at the 6- to 8-o'clock position are present.

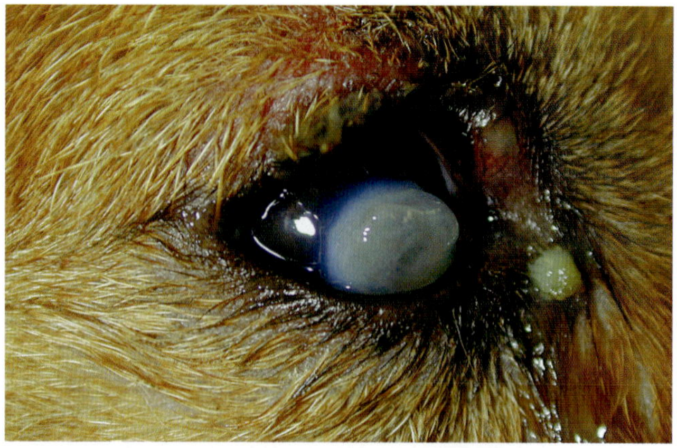

Figure 5-31
Melting corneal ulcer secondary to a bite from a copperhead snake to the upper eyelid, which penetrated, but did not perforate, the cornea.

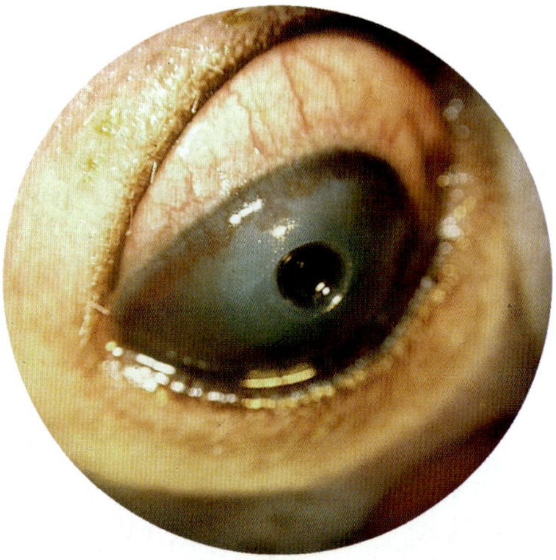

Figure 5-32
Descemetocele in a dog. The base of the ulcer looks black because the image appears against the dark iris. If the photograph had been taken against the tapetal reflex, the image would have resembled Figure 5-33. Corneal neovascularization is present.

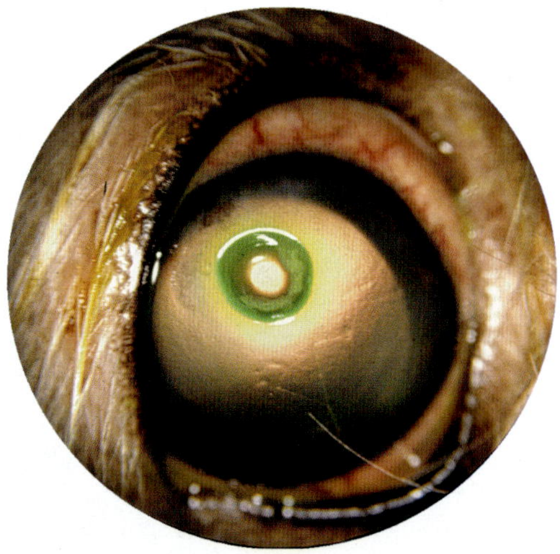

Figure 5-33
Descemetocele stained with fluorescein. Edges of the ulcer stain positively, because exposed stroma is present. The base of the ulcer does not stain, because Descemet's membrane is lypophilic. Because this photograph was taken against the tapetal reflex, the base of the ulcer looks clear (compare with Figure 5-32).

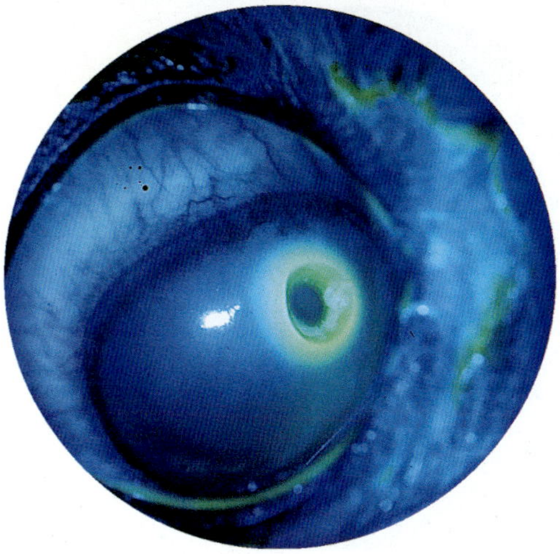

Figure 5-34
Same dog as in Figure 5-33. The descemetocele is stained with fluorescein and photographed with blue light. The edges of the ulcer stain positively, because exposed stroma is present. The base of the ulcer does not stain, because Descemet's membrane is lypophilic.

A

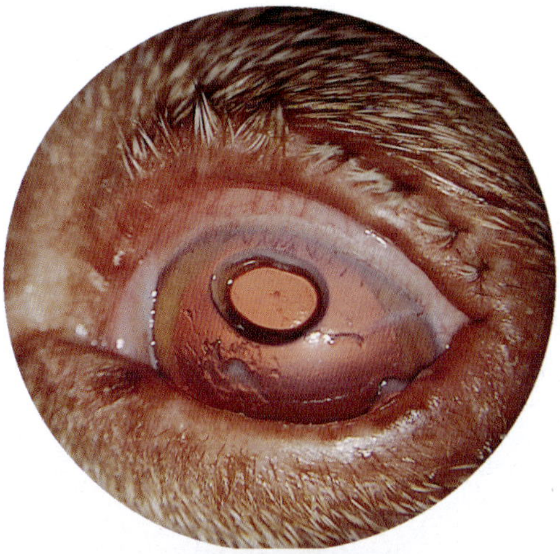

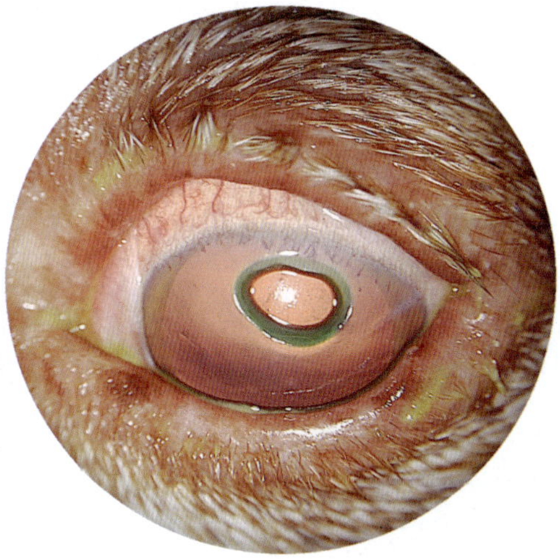

B

C

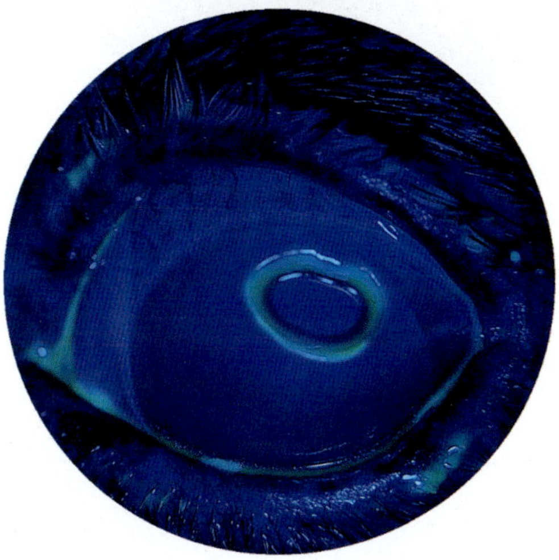

Figure 5-35 A-C
Pointer with corneal descemetocele. **A,** Unstained. **B,** Fluorescein stained. **C,** Fluorescein stained under cobalt blue light to highlight the stain. The fluorescein is taken up by the corneal stroma encircling the descemetocele. Descemet's membrane itself does not take up the fluorescein dye.

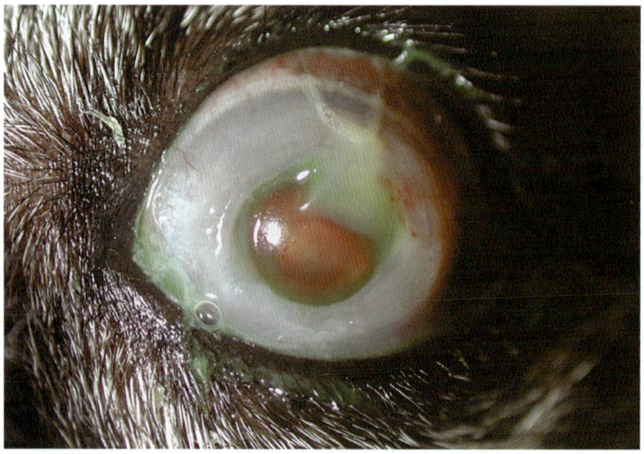

Figure 5-36
Corneal descemetocele in an Australian heeler. Corneal edema is present, along with vascularization peripherally with a deep central corneal defect.

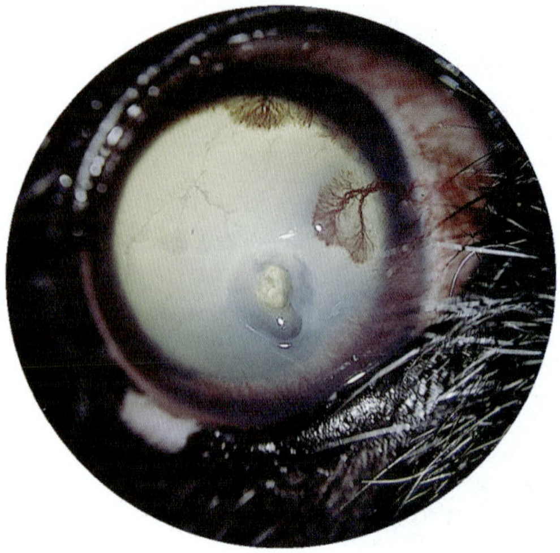

Figure 5-37
Chronic keratoconjunctivitis sicca (KCS) with healing deep corneal ulcer (see staining pattern in Figure 5-38).

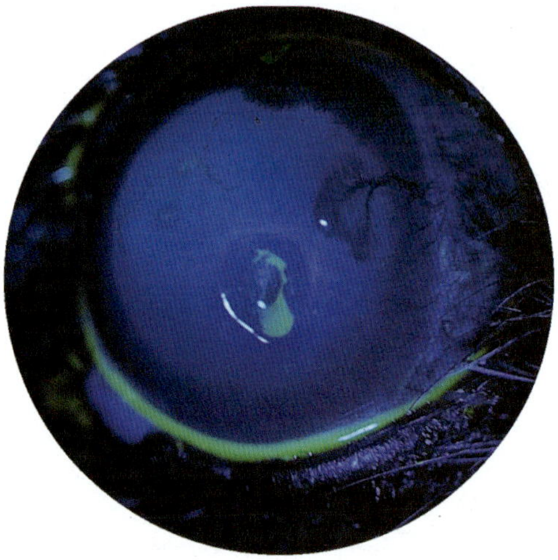

Figure 5-38
Same dog as in Figure 5-37. Eye is stained with fluorescein.

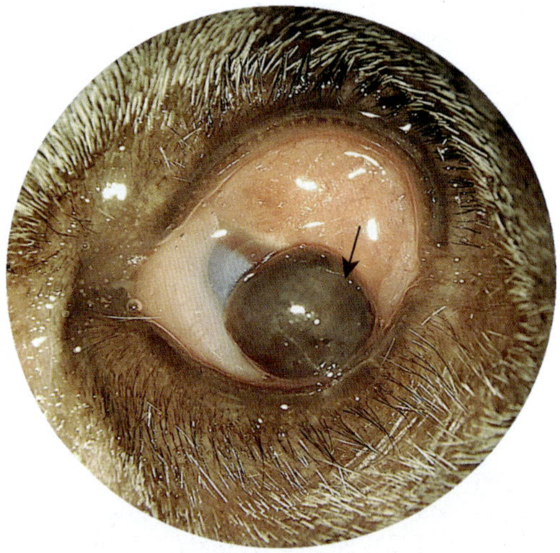

Figure 5-39
Perforated corneal ulcer with large area of protruding uvea *(arrow)*. The cornea is edematous and neovascularized, and the conjunctiva is red and swollen.

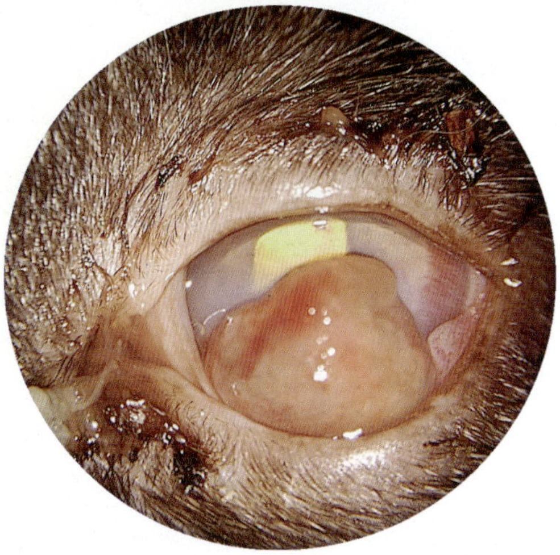

Figure 5-40
Perforated cornea in a cat. A large fibrin clot protrudes from the wound. The cornea is edematous and neovascularized.

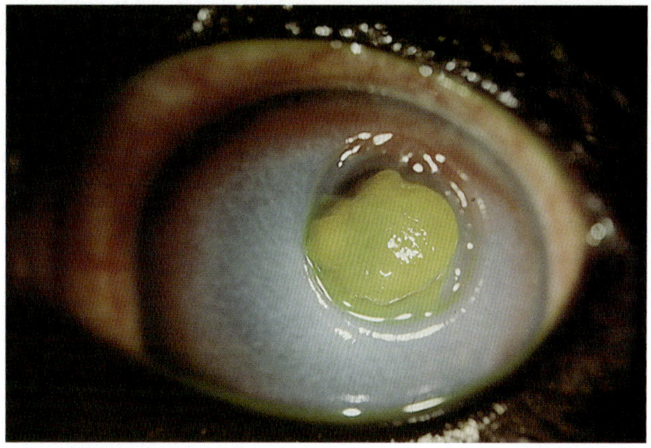

Figure 5-41
Perforated corneal ulcer stained with fluorescein in a Boston terrier. A fibrin plug is visible in the ulcer, and diffuse corneal edema and 360-degree neovascularization are present.

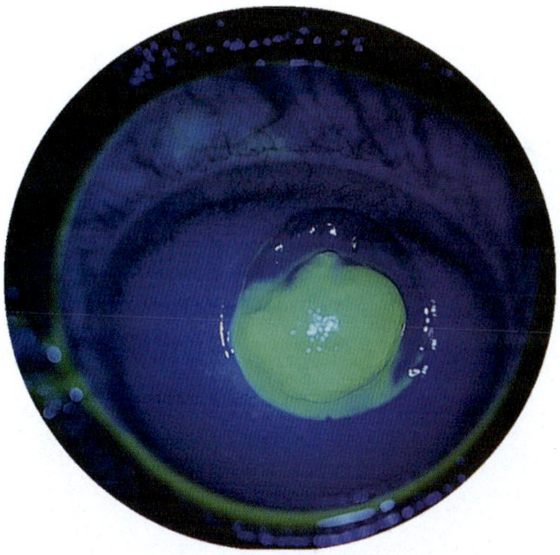

Figure 5-42
Same dog as in Figure 5-41. Perforated corneal ulcer stained with fluorescein in a Boston terrier. The ulcer was photographed under blue light. The fibrin clot has picked up the stain, but parts of the edge of the ulcer have not, indicating epithelialization of the edges.

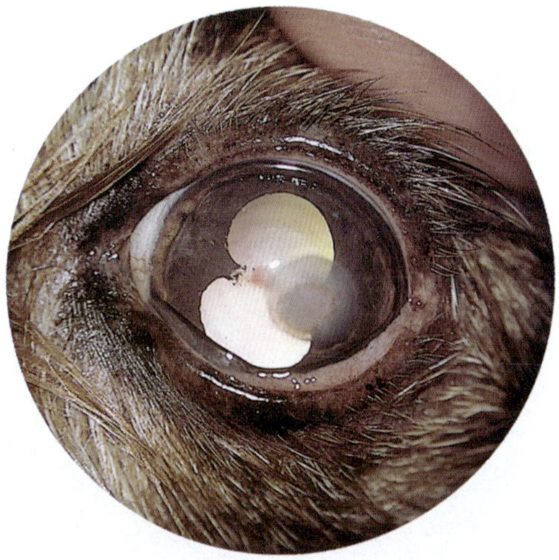

Figure 5-43
Corneal perforation in the right eye of a dog, causing posterior synechiae nasally and anterior synechiae temporally.

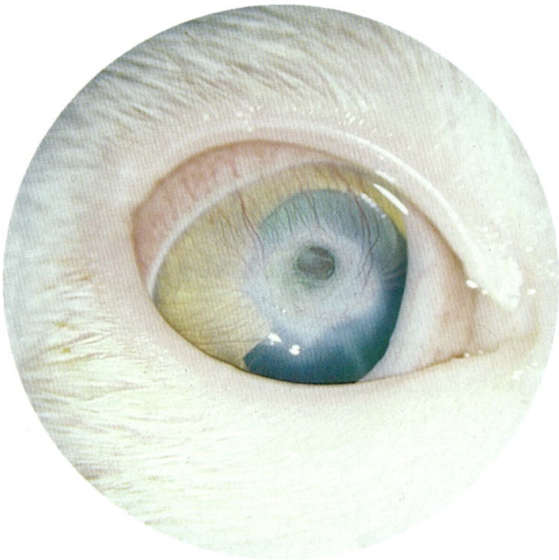

Figure 5-44
Chronic perforated descemetocele in a cat. The descemetocele is still leaking (based on a Seidel test, which is not shown). Corneal neovascularization surrounds the center of the ulcer, and anterior synechiae are present laterally.

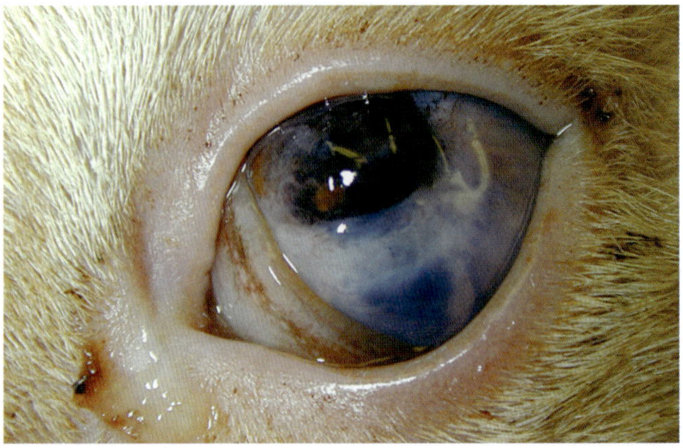

Figure 5-45
Cat with corneal perforation resulting from herpesvirus keratitis and corneal ulceration. Iris prolapse seals the cornea and maintains the anterior chamber.

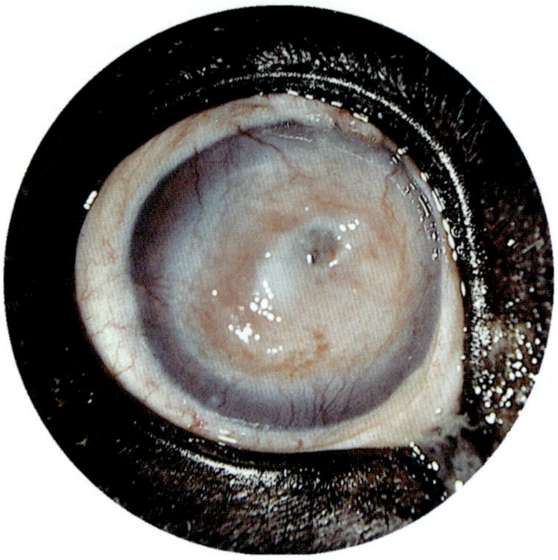

Figure 5-46
A healing perforated corneal ulcer. Approaching the center of the ulcer, 360-degree neovascularization is present.

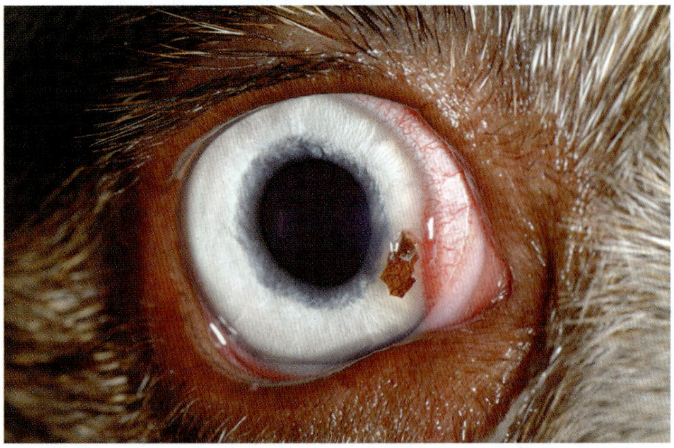

Figure 5-47
Plant material foreign body on the surface of the cornea of a Siberian husky. The foreign body had been present for 7 days.

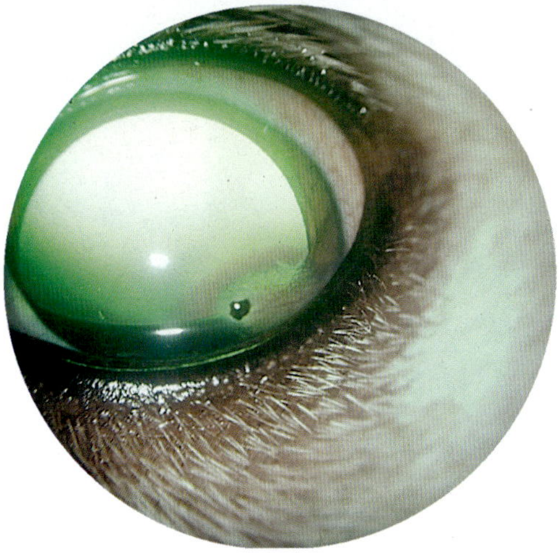

Figure 5-48
Superficial foreign body on the cornea. The foreign body had been present long enough to have caused corneal neovascularization.

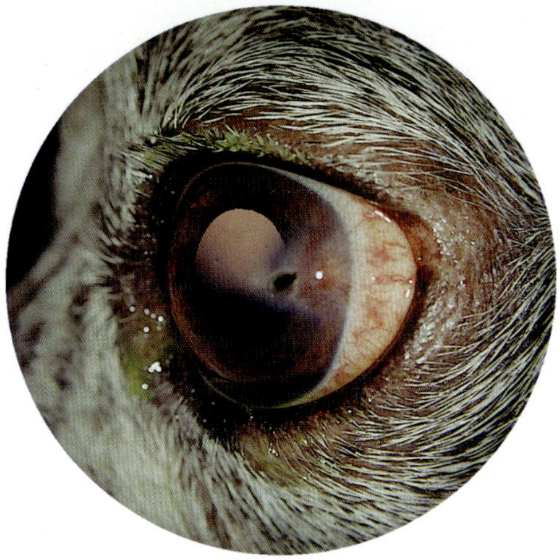

Figure 5-49
Superficial corneal foreign body that has elicited neovascularization.

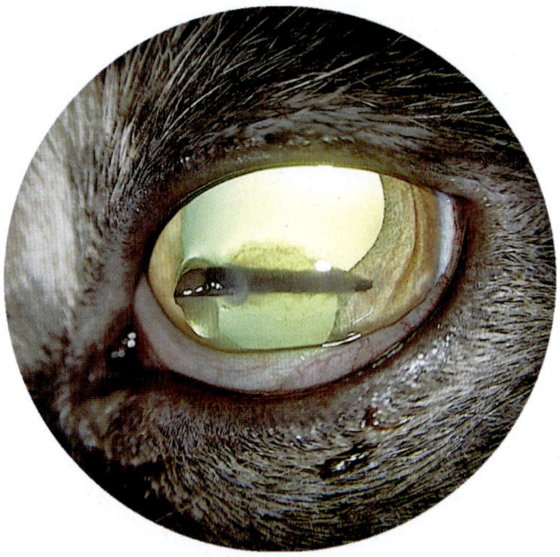

Figure 5-50
Corneal foreign body in a cat. A mesquite thorn perforated the cornea and impaled the temporal iris but not the lens. The thorn was removed and the cornea sutured. Excellent healing and minimal uveitis ensued.

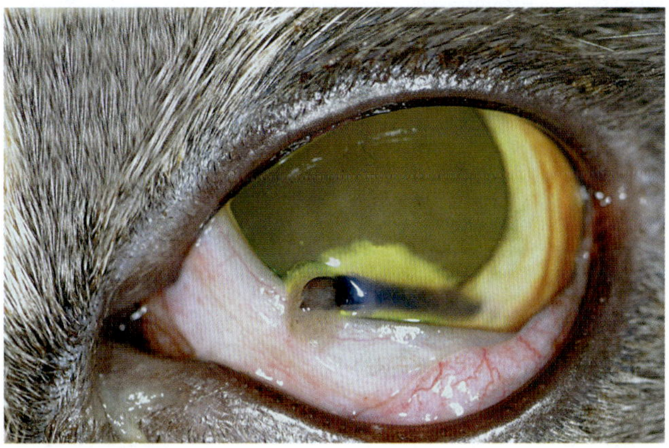

Figure 5-51
Same eye as in Figure 5-50. Close-up of a perforating foreign body in a cat cornea.

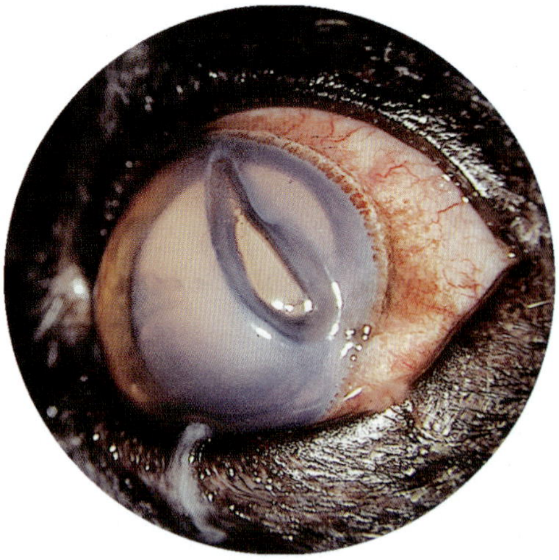

Figure 5-52
Penetrating deep laceration of the cornea.

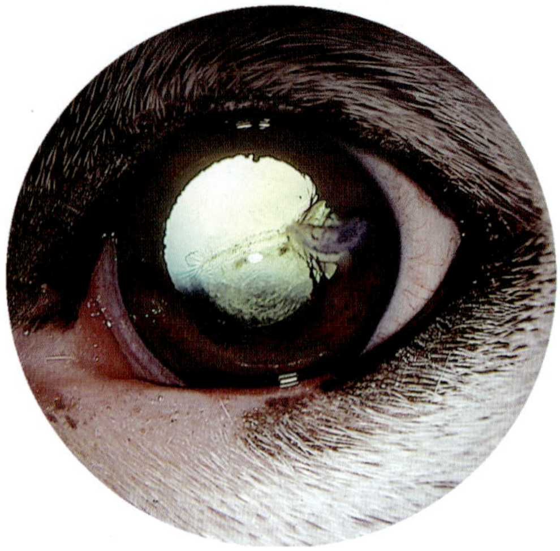

Figure 5-53
Corneal scar with anterior synechiae and cataract, presumably resulting from healed corneal perforation.

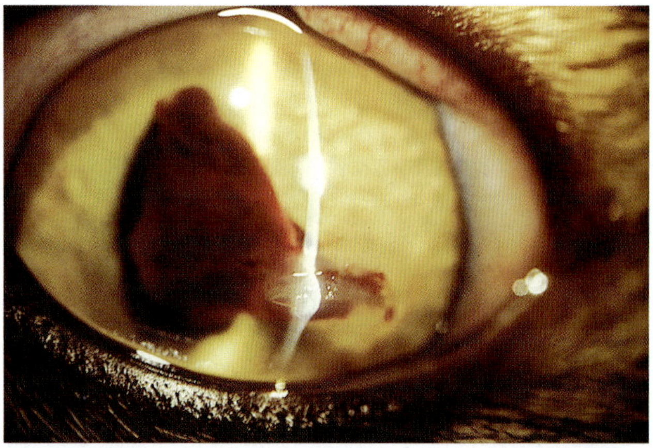

Figure 5-54
Slit lamp photograph of a perforating corneal laceration caused by a cat scratch. Hyphema is present in the pupil.

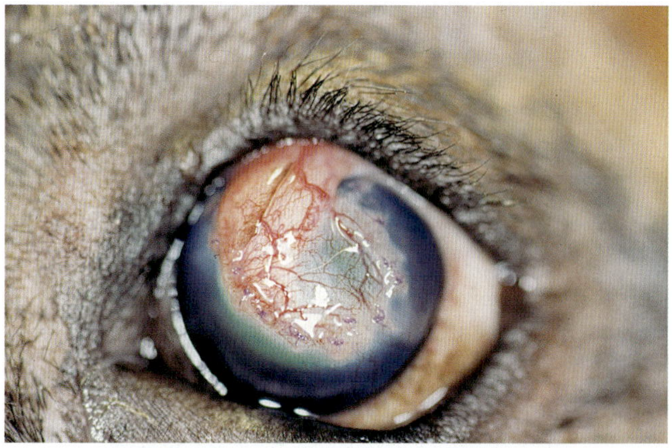

Figure 5-55
Healing corneoconjunctival transposition. Corneoconjunctival transpositions are half-thickness sliding corneoconjunctival grafts that work very well for the treatment of deep or perforated ulcers.

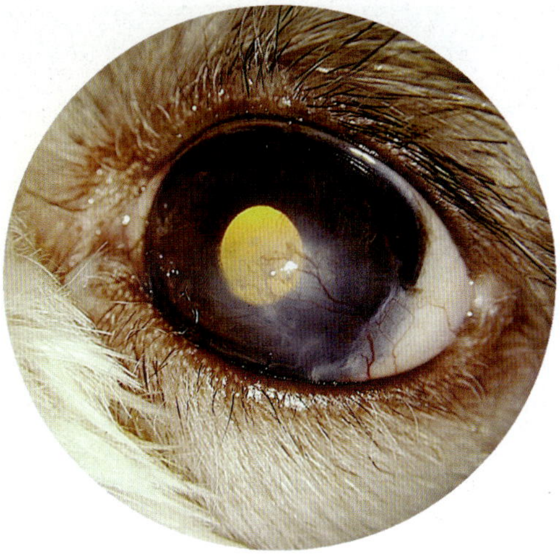

Figure 5-56
Healed corneoconjunctival transposition.

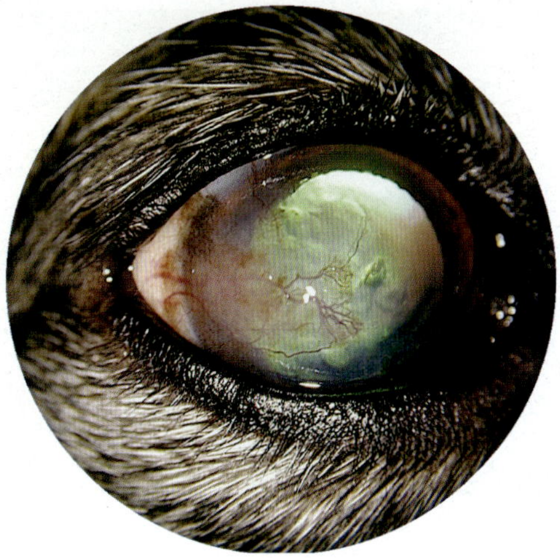

Figure 5-57
Pannus (chronic superficial keratitis) in a German shepherd dog. Corneal granulation tissue and neovascularization are seen in the temporal and central quadrants of this eye. Pannus is a lymphocytic-plasmacytic corneal infiltrate seen mostly in German shepherd dogs, usually arising from the temporal quadrant of the cornea. Pannus is a bilateral disease that is assumed to be immune mediated. Left untreated, it can lead to blindness, especially in geographic areas in which the ultraviolet index is high.

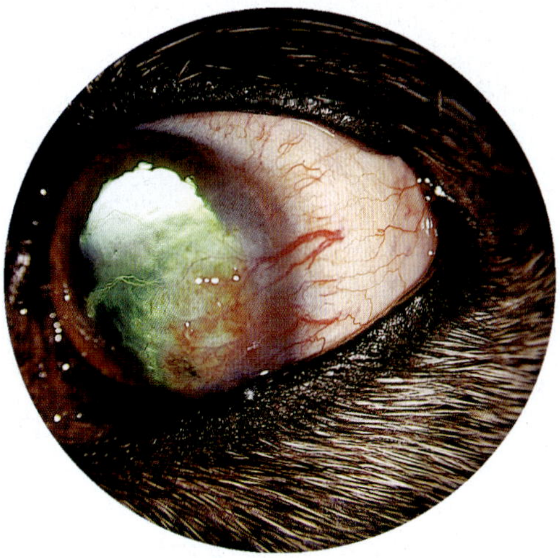

Figure 5-58
Pannus in a German shepherd dog. Neovascularization and granulation tissue are present.

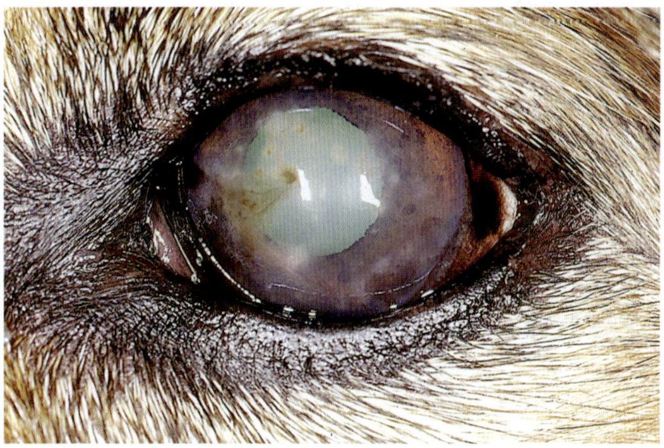

Figure 5-59
Pannus in a German shepherd dog, with corneal infiltrates and pigmentation.

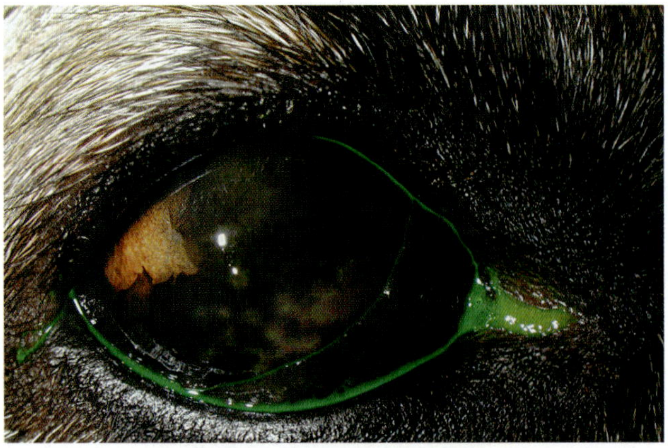

Figure 5-60
Pannus with pigmentation and inflammatory cell infiltrate in the cornea of a German shepherd dog.

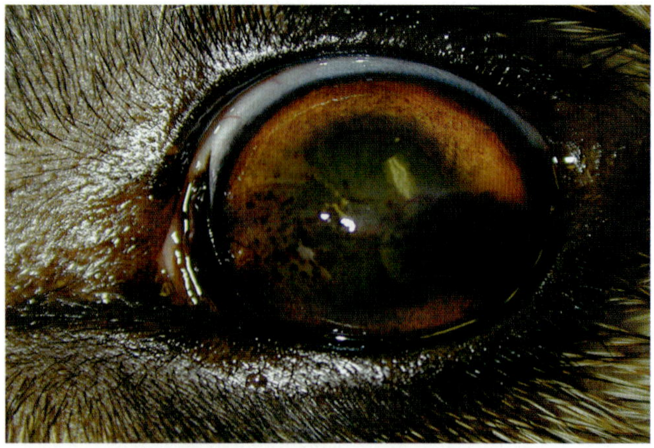

Figure 5-61
Pannus with a dense central band of corneal pigmentation in a German shepherd dog.

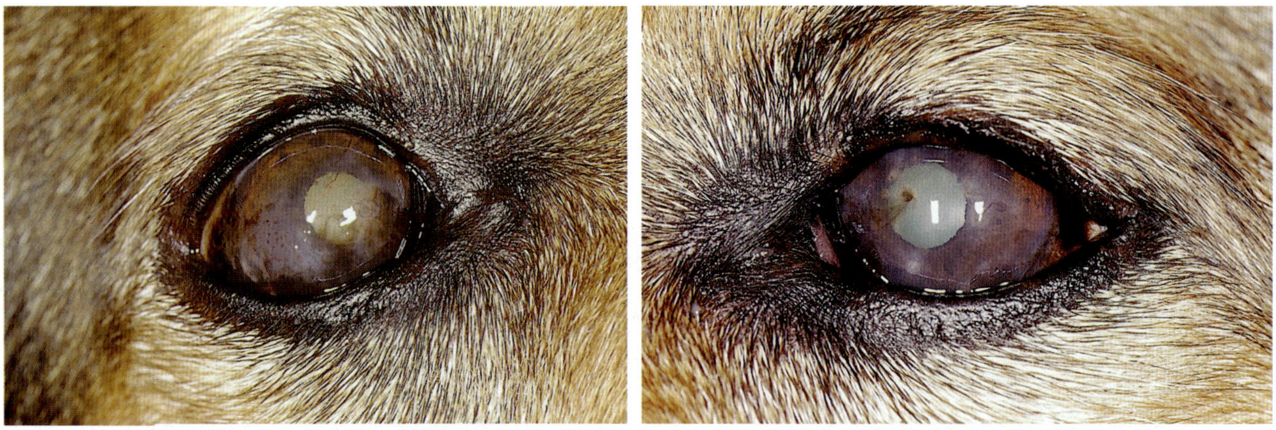

Figure 5-62
Pannus in a German shepherd dog. Note the asymmetry of the lesions.

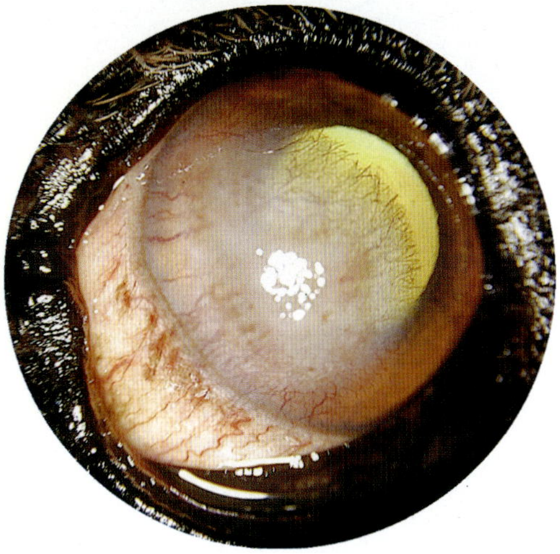

Figure 5-63
Pannus in a German shepherd dog. Neovascularization and granulation tissue are present.

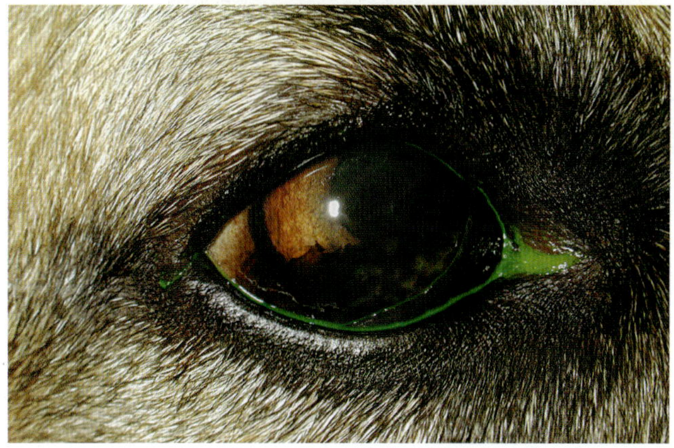

Figure 5-64
Pannus in a German shepherd dog. Pigmentation in the cornea with no fluorescein uptake after fluorescein staining.

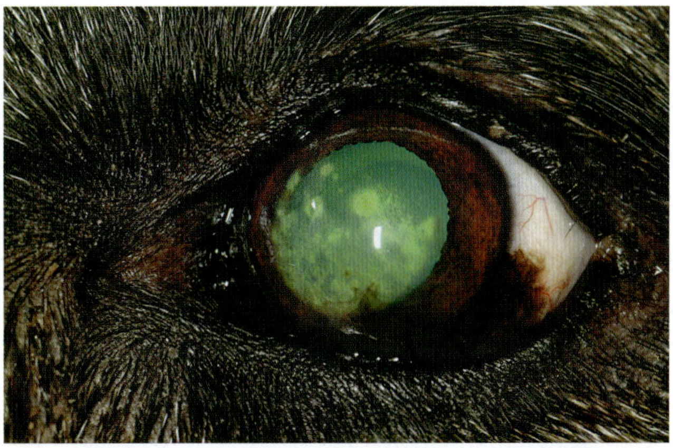

Figure 5-65
Pannus in a 5-year-old German shepherd dog being treated with topical dexamethasone.

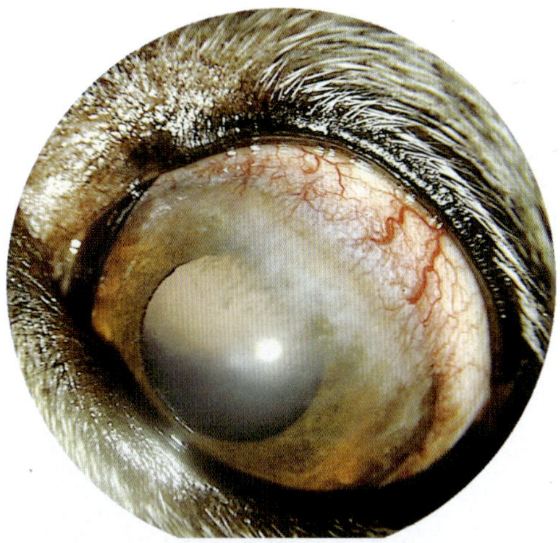

Figure 5-66
Occasionally pannus is seen in breeds other than the German shepherd. Pannus in a greyhound is shown here. Corneal scarring, neovascularization, and corneal deposit of lipid are present.

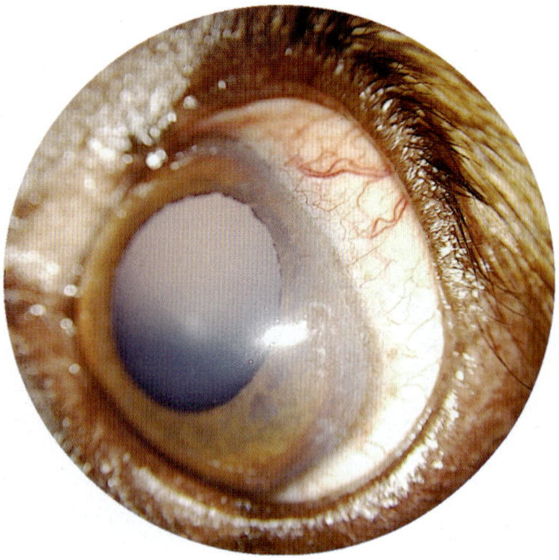

Figure 5-67
Pannus in a Pembroke Welsh corgi. Cellular infiltrates are present, as well as neovascularization in the temporal quadrant.

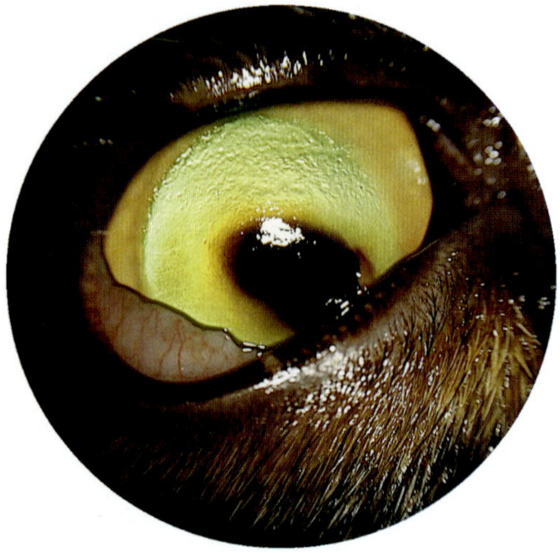

Figure 5-68
Corneal sequestrum in a cat. A corneal sequestrum is an area of necrotic stroma that takes on a brown color from the tear porphyrins. Sequestra can be associated with chronic ulceration, entropion, and herpesvirus keratitis, especially in animals undergoing treatment with corticosteroids.

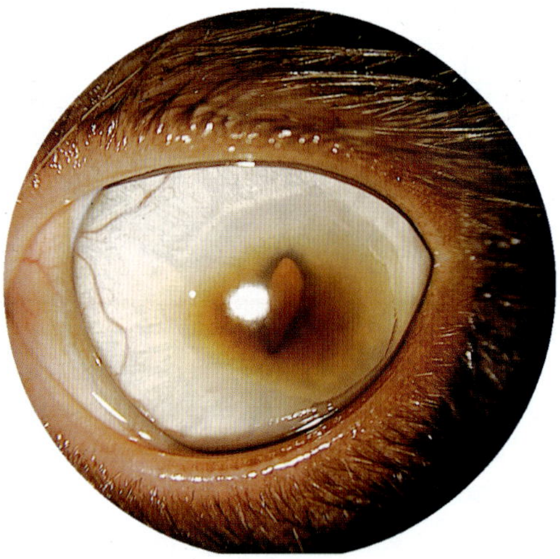

Figure 5-69
Corneal sequestrum in a cat (the faint brown opacity in the central cornea).

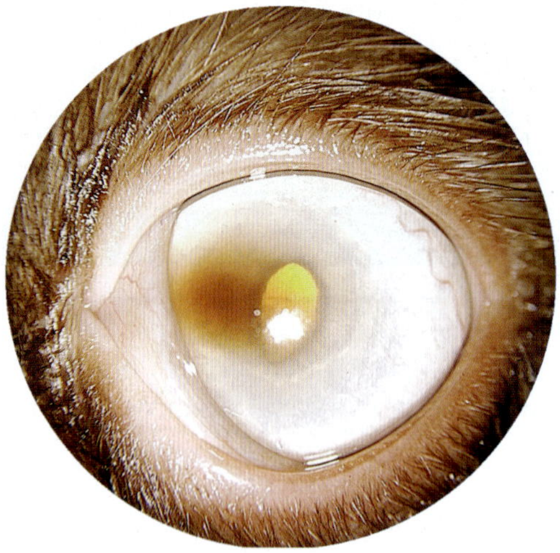

Figure 5-70
Sequestrum in a cat.

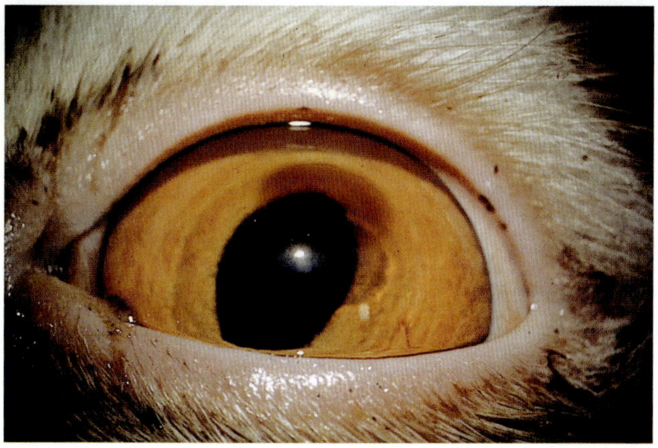

Figure 5-71
Corneal sequestrum in a cat.

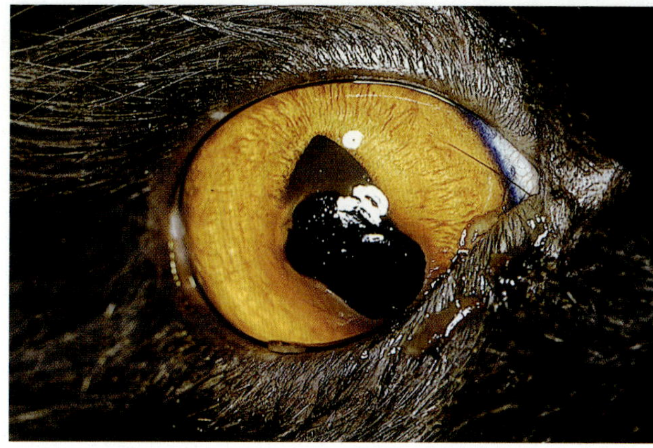

Figure 5-72
Sequestrum in a cat with lower eyelid entropion.

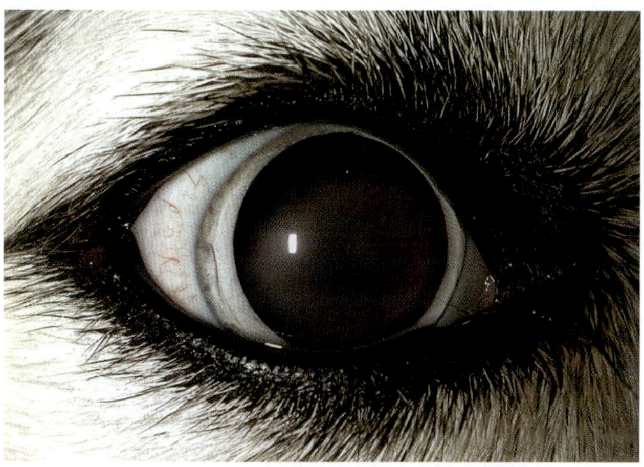

Figure 5-73
Typical doughnut-shaped inherited corneal stromal (lipid) dystrophy in a 4-year-old Siberian husky. Corneal dystrophies are a nebulous group of inherited, bilateral diseases that can affect epithelium, stroma, or endothelium. Stromal dystrophies are associated with deposition of lipids in the stroma.

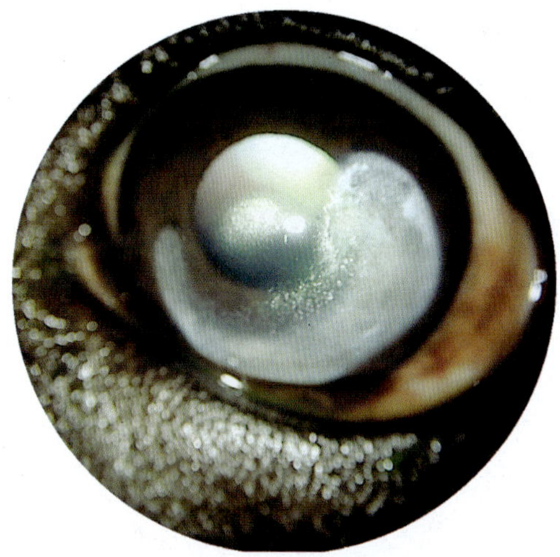

Figure 5-74
Corneal dystrophy in a Boston terrier. Lipid deposition has occurred in the central and temporal cornea.

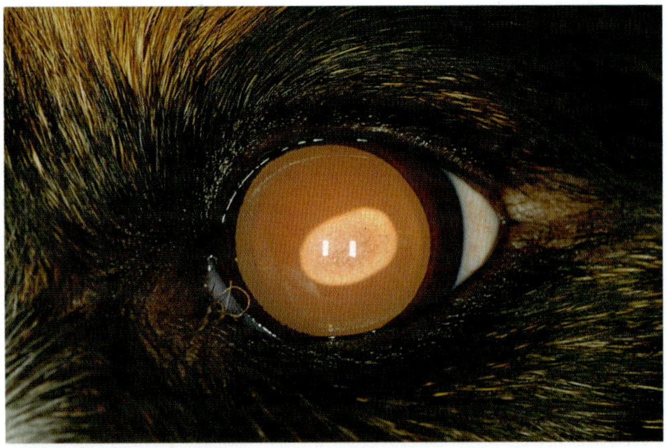

Figure 5-75
Stromal lipid dystrophy in a Shetland sheepdog.

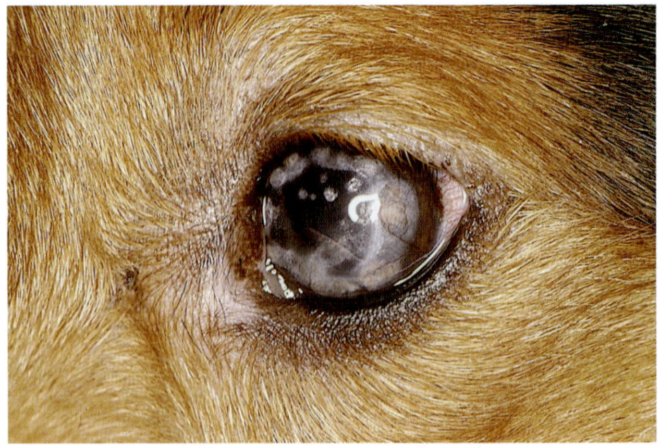

Figure 5-76
Inherited corneal dystrophy in a Shetland sheepdog. Lipid infiltrates and corneal neovascularization are present.

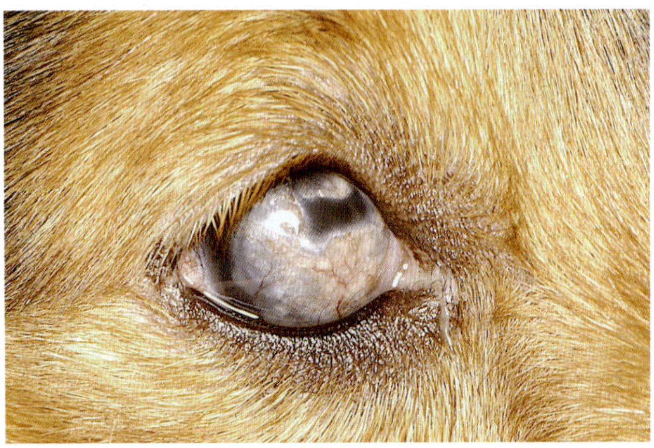

Figure 5-77
Inherited corneal dystrophy in a Shetland sheepdog. The opposite eye of the dog in Figure 5-76 is shown.

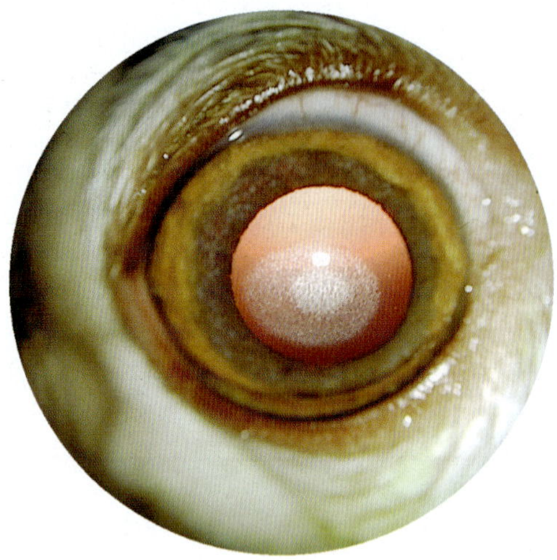

Figure 5-78
Corneal dystrophy with central anterior stromal lipid deposits in an Australian shepherd.

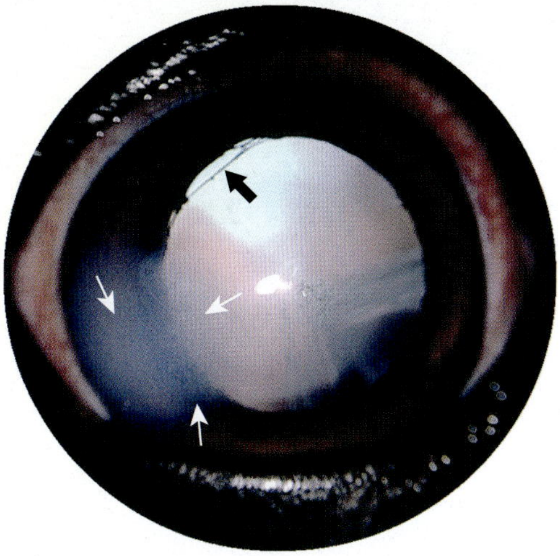

Figure 5-79
Endothelial dystrophy temporally (corneal edema *[small arrows]*), iris sphincter atrophy *(large arrow)*, and incipient anterior cortical cataract in a Boston terrier.

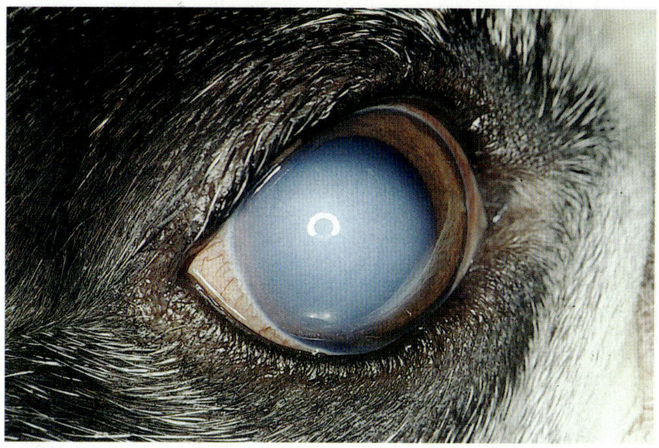

Figure 5-80
Endothelial dystrophy that is causing corneal edema in a Boston terrier.

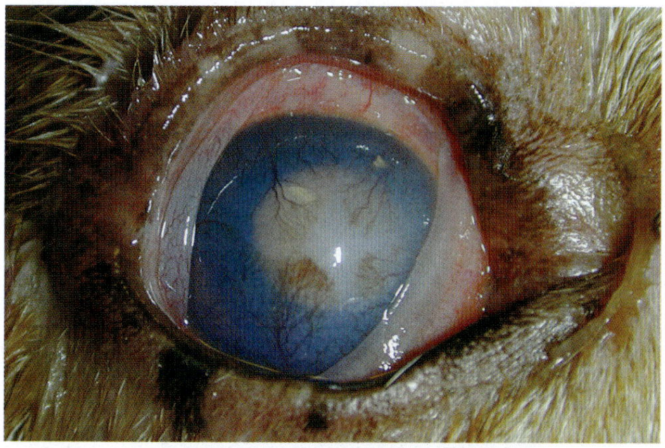

Figure 5-81
Corneal endothelial dystrophy in a basset hound. Corneal edema, vascularization, and scarring secondary to corneal erosions are present.

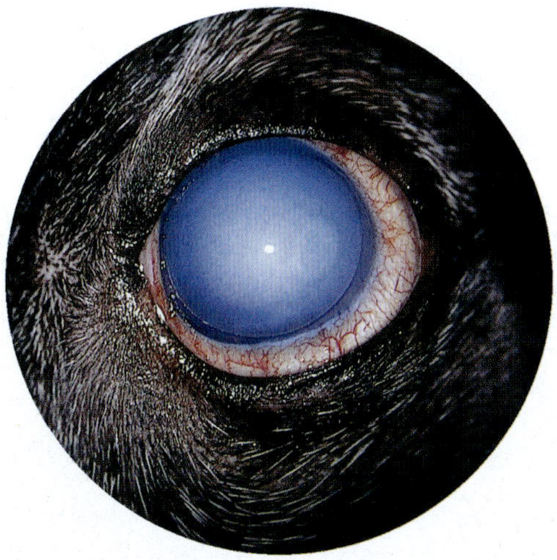

Figure 5-82
Diffuse corneal edema in a Boston terrier with endothelial dystrophy.

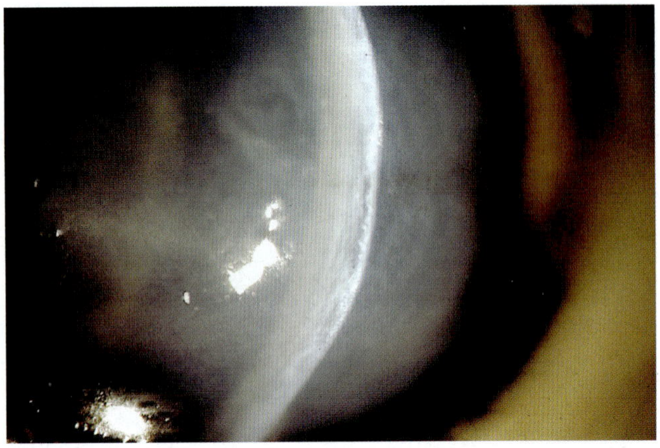

Figure 5-83
Slit lamp photograph of corneal endothelial dystrophy in a Chihuahua. Note the fluid-filled lacunae under the corneal epithelium.

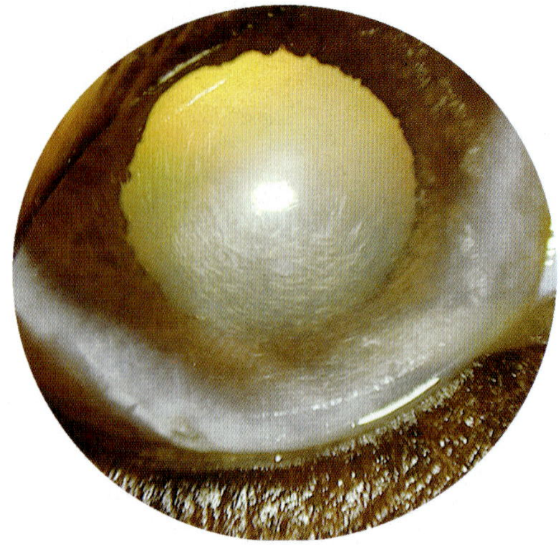

Figure 5-84
Lipid degeneration in a Shetland sheepdog crossbreed with hypothyroidism. Also present is iris sphincter atrophy. Lipid degenerations in the cornea usually appear in older dogs in which lipid or minerals are deposited in the corneal stroma.

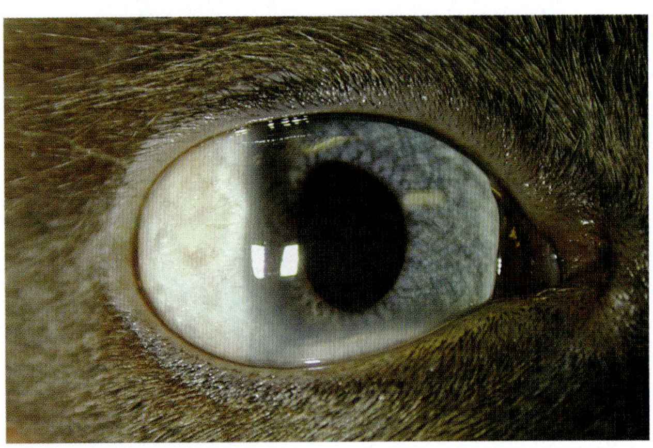

Figure 5-85
Lipid keratopathy in a Siamese cat with severe hypertriglyceridemia.

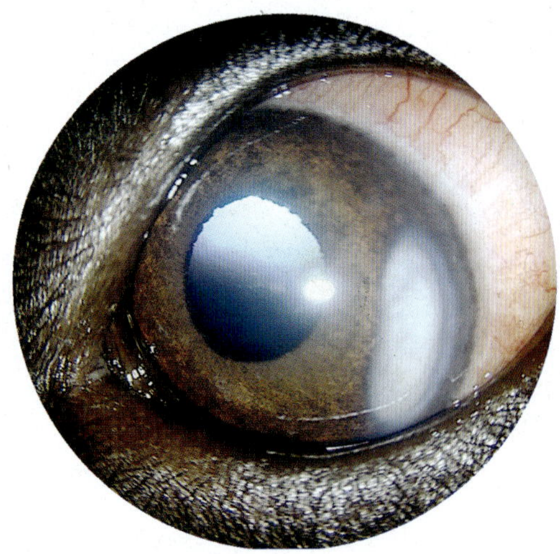

Figure 5-86
Perilimbal arcus lipoides in a German shepherd dog with hypothyroidism. Arcus lipoides is a bow-shaped area (arc) of lipid that parallels the limbus, usually with a clear area of cornea between the limbus and lipid.

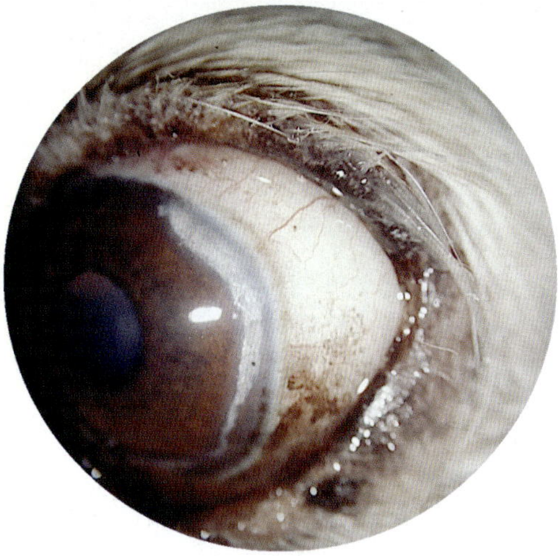

Figure 5-87
Cocker spaniel with arcus lipoides resulting from hypothyroidism.

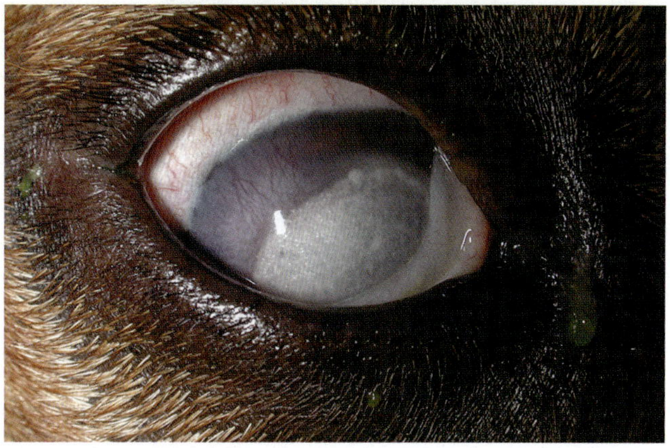

Figure 5-88
Dense infiltration of lipid in the corneal stroma with accompanying neovascularization. The cause of the condition was unknown.

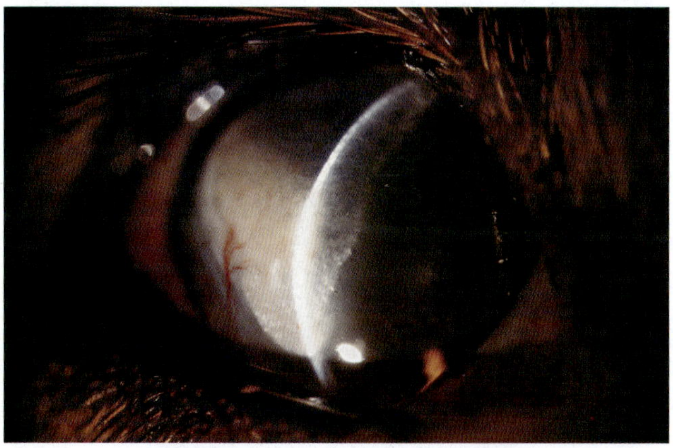

Figure 5-89
Corneal degeneration with lipid infiltrates and neovascularization, in a slit lamp photograph.

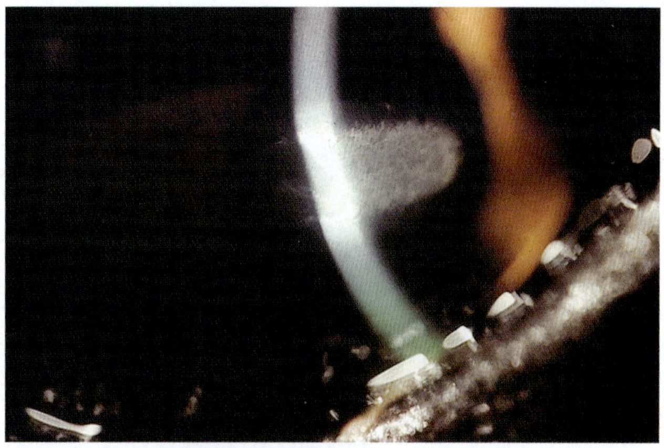

Figure 5-90
Slit lamp photograph of corneal degeneration in a dachshund. The white infiltrate is probably lipid. Flattening of the cornea has occurred centrally.

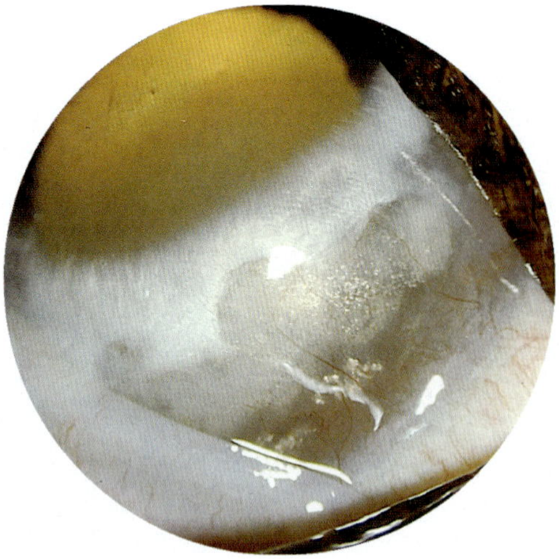

Figure 5-91
Perilimbal corneal degeneration in a Shetland sheepdog crossbreed with hypothyroidism. Lipid deposits in the stroma are present, as is neovascularization.

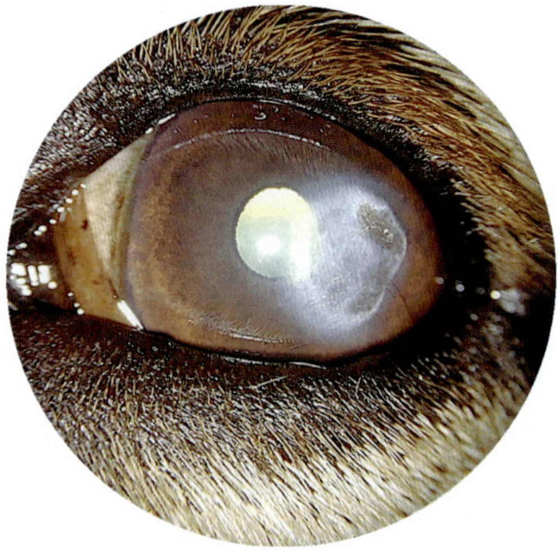

Figure 5-92
Corneal degeneration in a dog. Lipid deposition is present in the anterior corneal stroma.

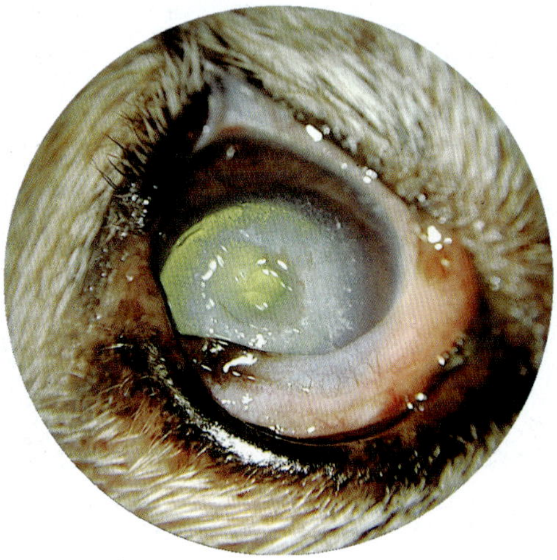

Figure 5-93
Corneal degeneration in an elderly mixed-breed dog. Thinning of the central corneal stroma with surrounding lipid and mineralization has occurred.

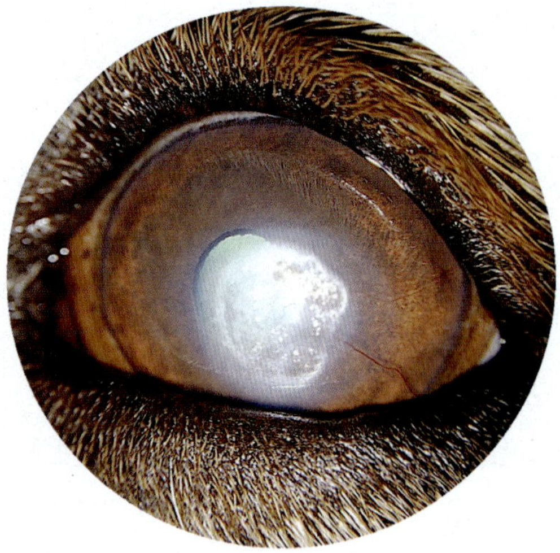

Figure 5-94
Corneal degeneration in a dog. Note the neovascularization and lipid deposition in the corneal stroma centrally.

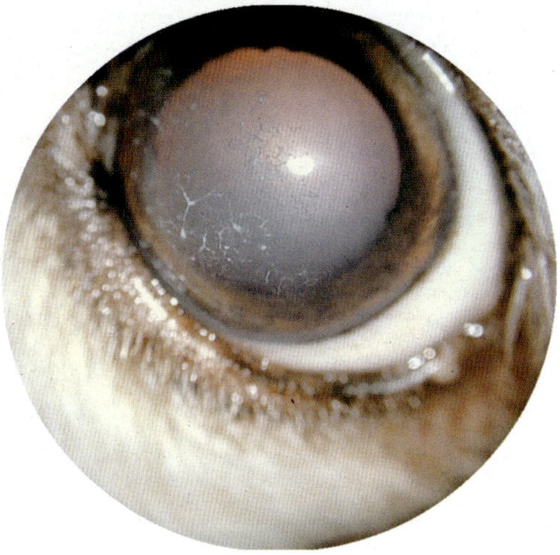

Figure 5-95
Corneal degeneration in an elderly dog. Anterior corneal stromal spicules are present. Negative fluorescein stain.

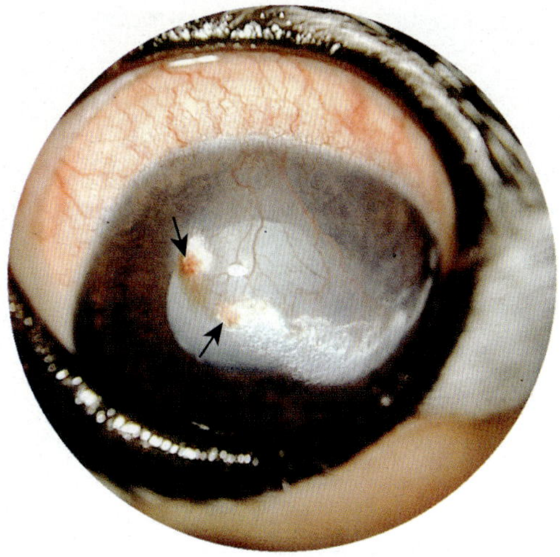

Figure 5-96
Intrastromal corneal hemorrhage *(arrows),* corneal neovascularization, and corneal lipid degeneration in a dog.

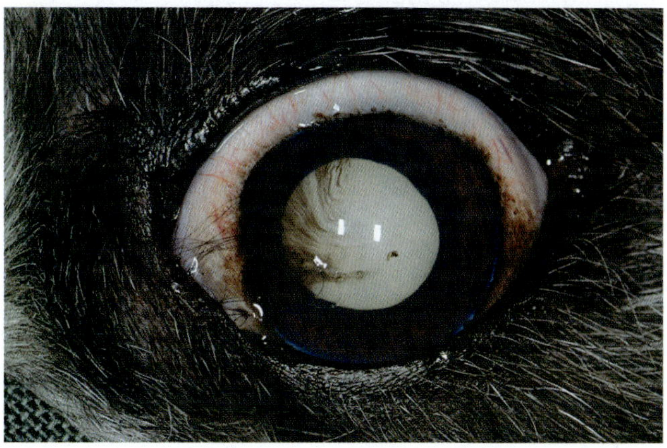

Figure 5-97
Medial trichiasis and pigmentary (superficial) keratitis. A hypermature cataract and mild lens-induced uveitis (diffuse corneal edema and dark iris pigmentation) are also present.

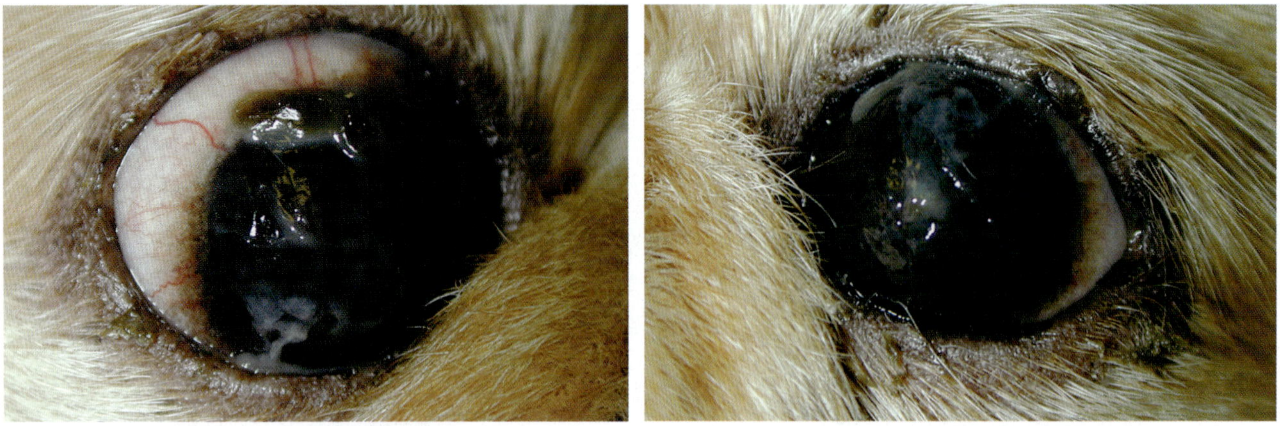

Figure 5-98
Pekingese with nasal fold trichiasis and KCS. Mucopurulent discharge adheres to the cornea, and superficial pigment has infiltrated the corneal epithelium.

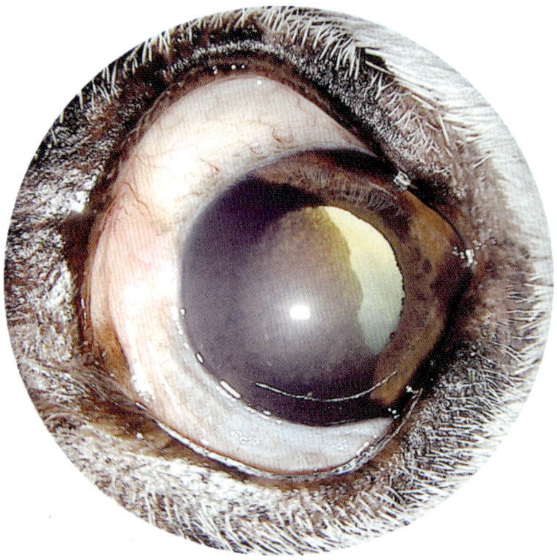

Figure 5-99
Endothelial pigmentation in an otherwise normal-appearing eye of an English pointer.

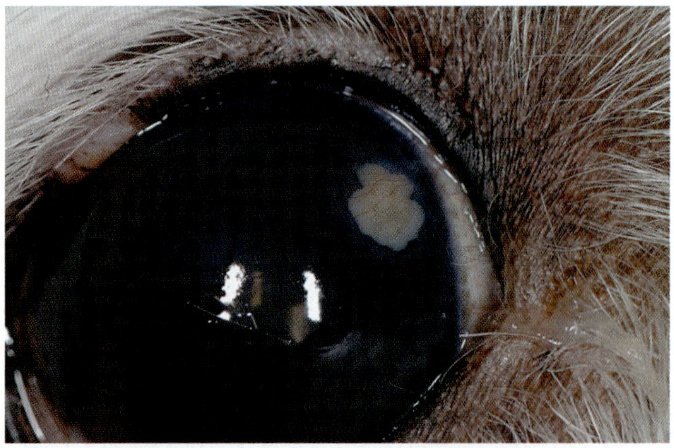

Figure 5-100
Presumed inclusion cyst at the level of Descemet's membrane in a bichon frise 1 year after cataract surgery. The lesion occurred at the site of the corneal incision.

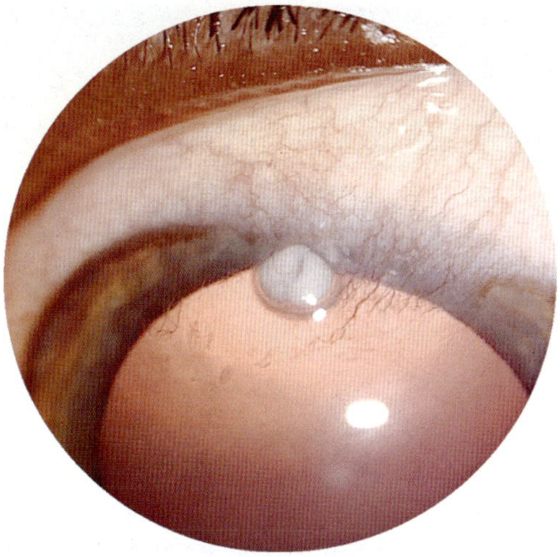

Figure 5-101
Epithelial inclusion cyst at the site of a previous corneal injury and ulceration.

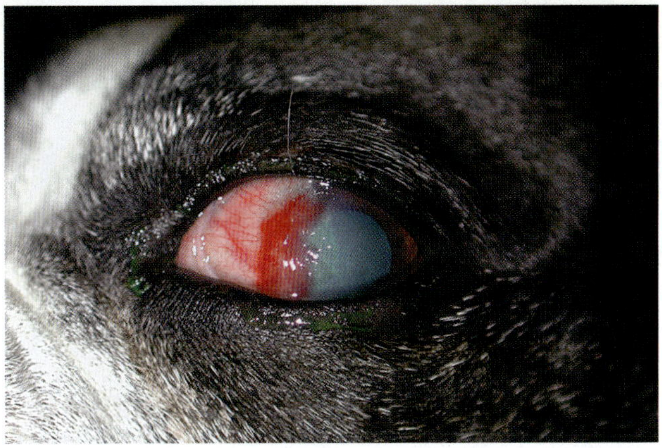

Figure 5-102
Nasal limbal hemangiosarcoma in a Boston terrier.

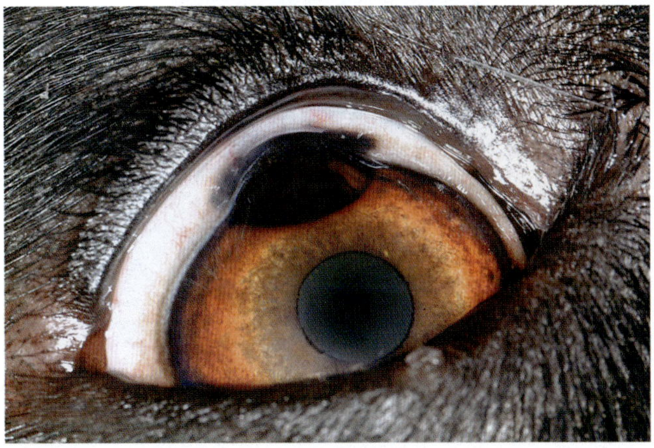

Figure 5-103
Limbal melanoma in a Labrador retriever.

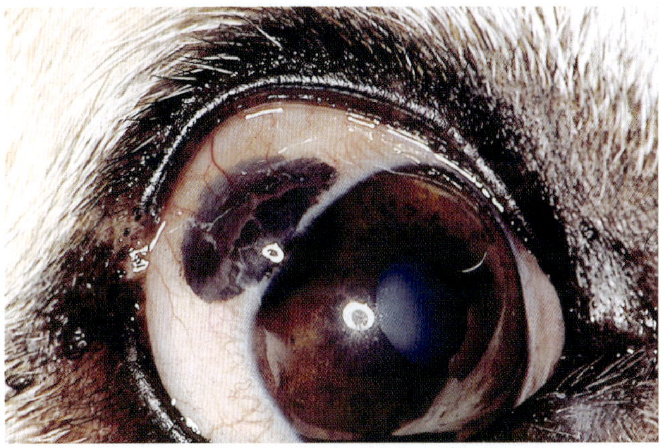

Figure 5-104
Limbal melanoma in a dog.

Chapter 6

Sclera

INTRODUCTION

The sclera is the fibrous outer coat of the eye—a continuation of the cornea, but, unlike the latter, nontransparent. Few conditions affect the sclera, and these are poorly understood. Episcleritis and nodular granulomatous episclerokeratitis are illustrated in this chapter.

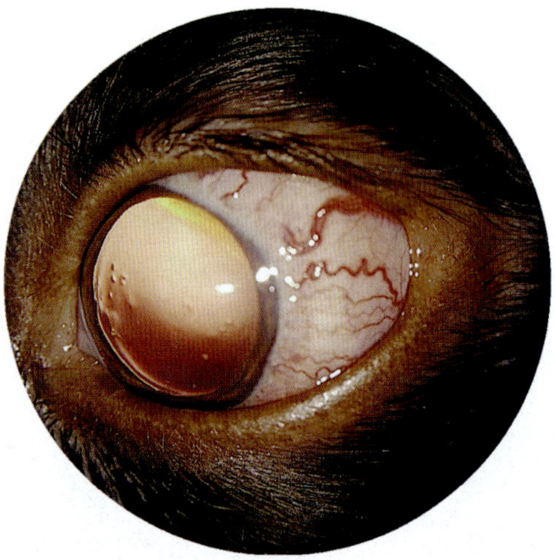

Figure 6-1
"Red eye" resulting from episcleritis. Episcleritis is an inflammation of the superficial layers of the sclera, often presumed to be immune mediated.

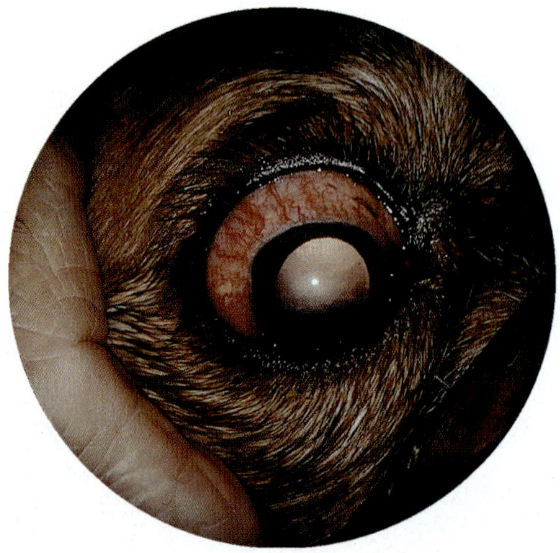

Figure 6-2
Episcleritis in an American cocker spaniel.

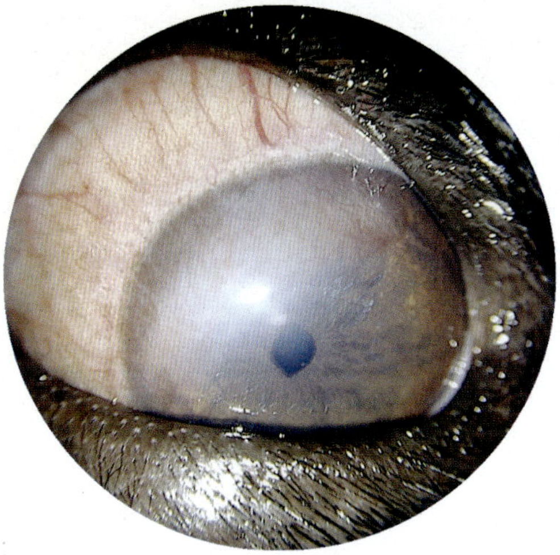

Figure 6-3
Episcleritis and associated corneal edema and neovascularization.
(Courtesy Dr. Robert Playter.)

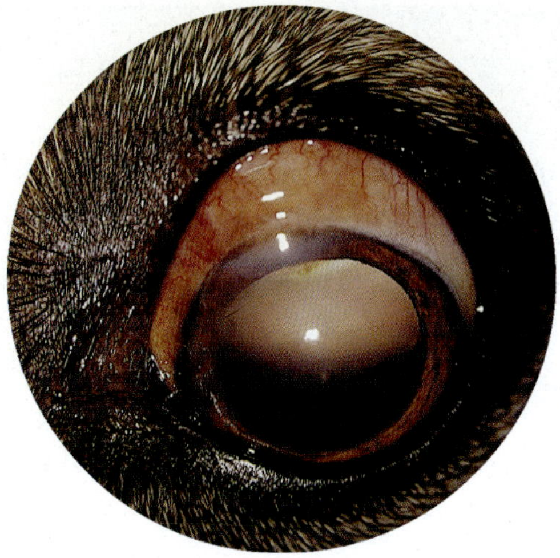

Figure 6-4
Episcleritis in a dog with associated corneal edema.

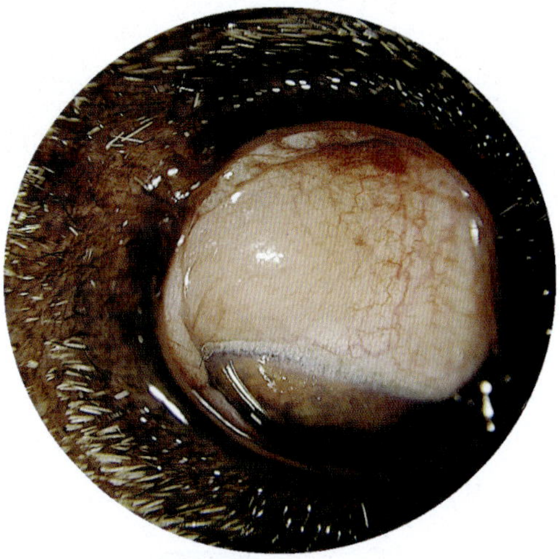

Figure 6-5
Episcleritis. Nodular swelling of the sclera is present.

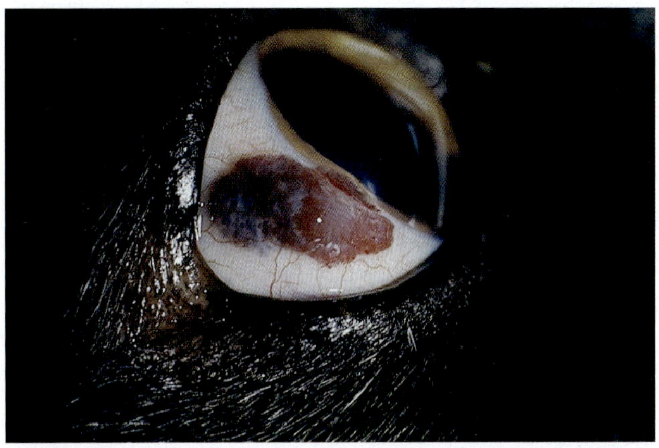

Figure 6-6
Vascular tumor in the sclera of a dog.

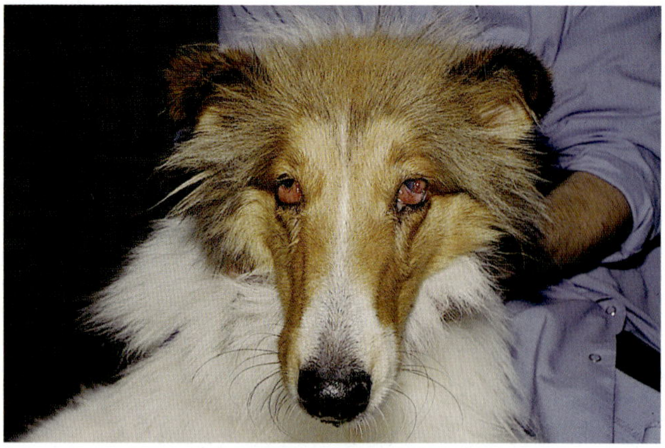

Figure 6-7
Nodular granulomatous episclerokeratitis (NGE) in a collie. NGE is a bilateral proliferative disease seen most commonly in collies and Shetland sheepdogs and is characterized by chronic granulomatous infiltrates of the sclera, eyelids, and cornea and occasionally the anterior chamber.

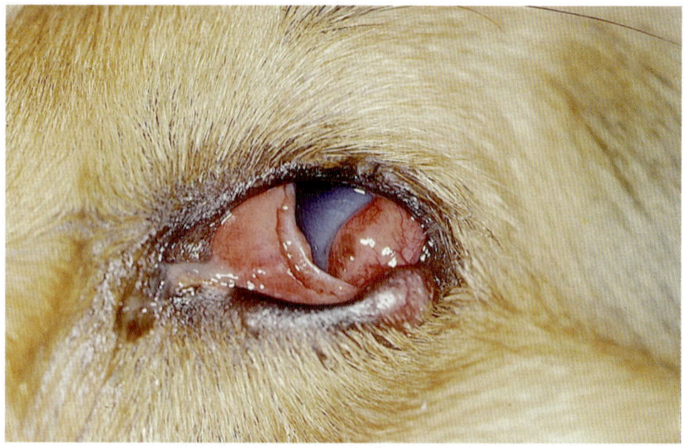

Figure 6-8
Close-up of the left eye of the collie in Figure 6-7.

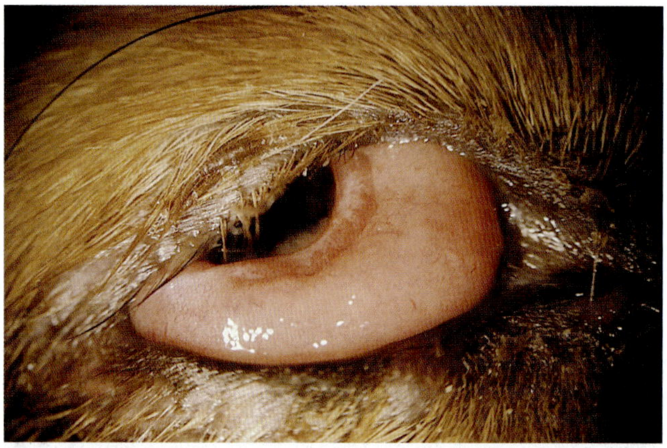

Figure 6-9
Close-up of the right eye of the collie in Figure 6-7.

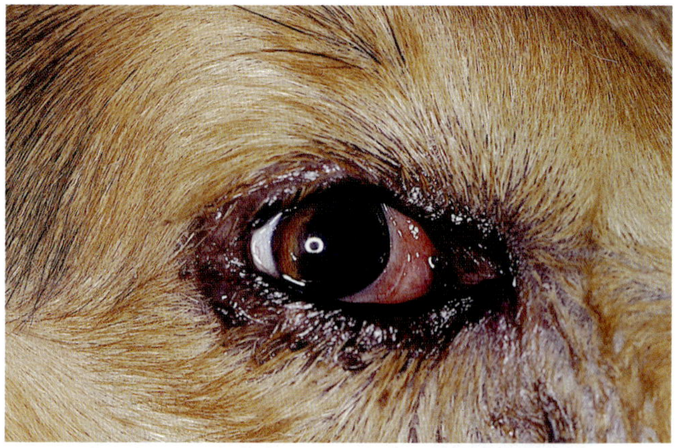

Figure 6-10
Collie in Figures 6-7 to 6-9 after 2 weeks of treatment with Imuran and prednisone.

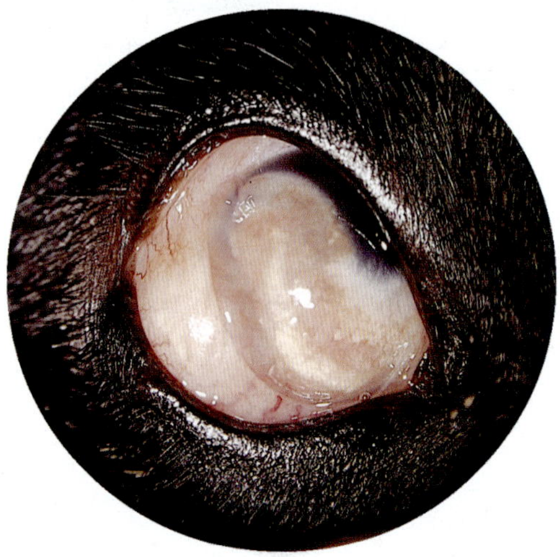

Figure 6-11
Episcleritis and corneal lipid infiltrate in a dog.

Chapter 7

Uvea

INTRODUCTION

The internal vascular layers of the eye—the iris and ciliary body in the anterior segment and the choroid of the posterior segment—make up the uvea. These layers are composed of dense networks of blood vessels of various sizes and have varying degrees of pigmentation. Consequently, the pathology that affects these layers reflects their vascular basis—inflammation, hematogenous spread of infectious agents, and neoplasms. The most significant lesions of the uvea are inflammatory. Various congenital uveal abnormalities, often hereditary, such as colobomas and persistent pupillary membranes, pigmentation variations, uveal cysts, and tumors, are also frequently seen in small animal practice.

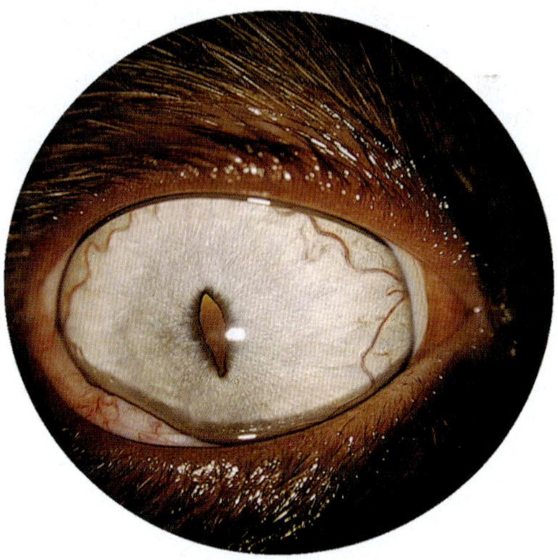

Figure 7-1
Normal cat iris with major arterial circle.

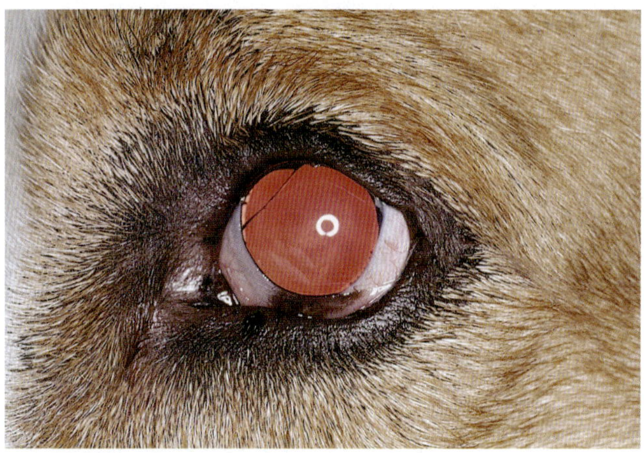

Figure 7-2
Aniridia in a dog.

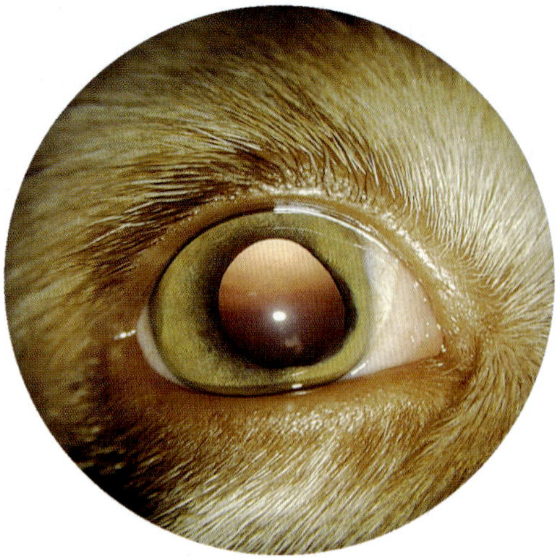

Figure 7-3
Iris coloboma extending nasally in an Australian shepherd. A coloboma is a congenital defect—in this case, in the nasal iris—that involves the sphincter muscle. Iris colobomas are hereditary in this breed and can be associated with multiple ocular anomalies.

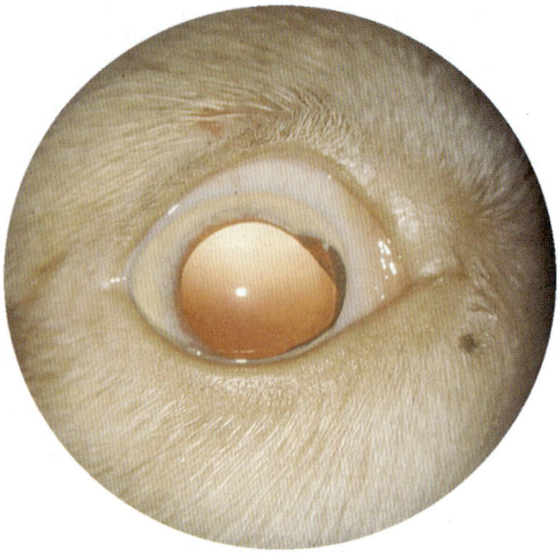

Figure 7-4
Iris coloboma extending nasally in the pupil of an Australian shepherd.

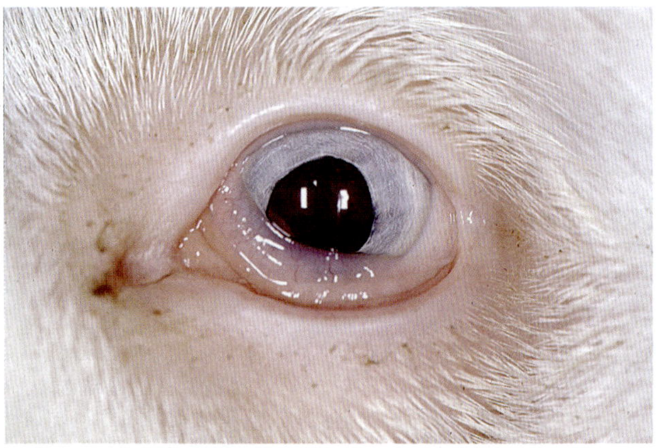

Figure 7-5
Australian shepherd with dyscoria. Dyscoria is abnormally shaped pupil; usually a dyscoric pupil is not round and is eccentric in the iris. The condition is hereditary in Australian shepherds and is associated with multiple ocular anomalies.

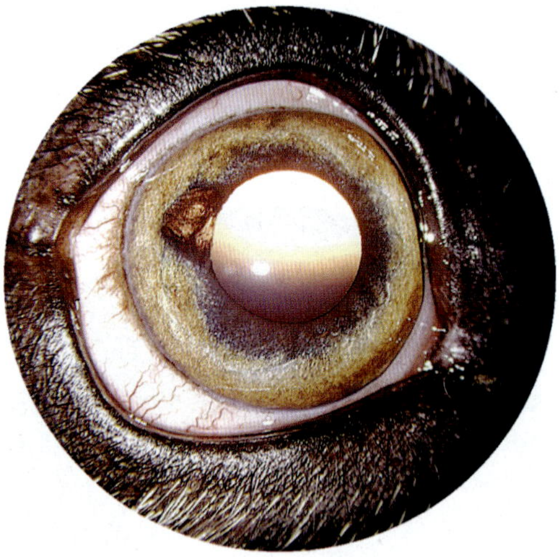

Figure 7-6
Iris coloboma.

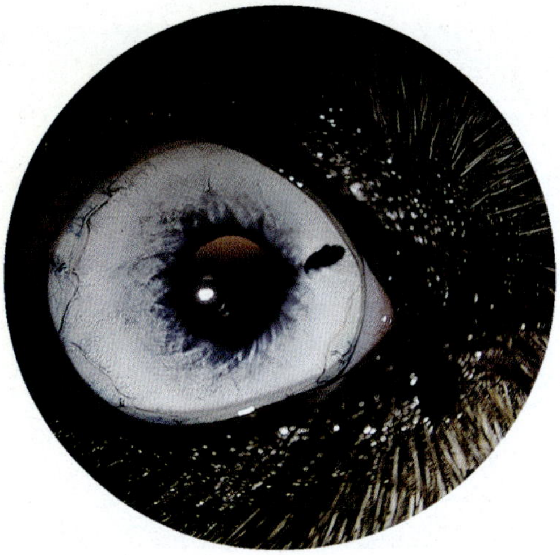

Figure 7-7
Iris coloboma extending nasally and heterochromia iridis in an Australian shepherd. This coloboma involves the iris dilator muscle.

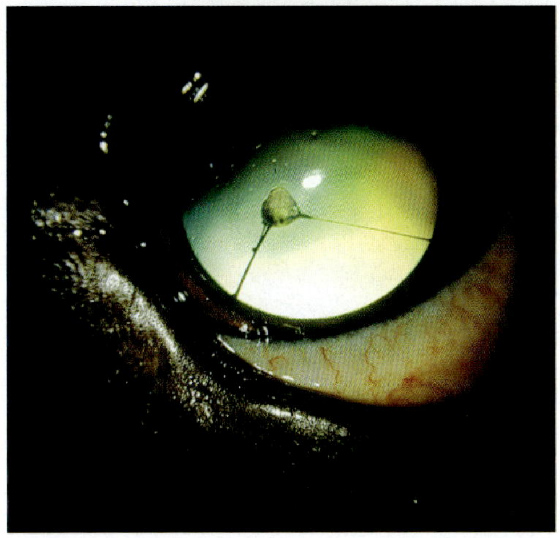

Figure 7-8
Iris-to-lens persistent pupillary membrane (PPM). PPMs are remnants of the vasculature that fills the anterior chamber during fetal development of the eye. Iris-to-lens PPMs are usually associated with cataracts where the PPM touches the lens capsule.

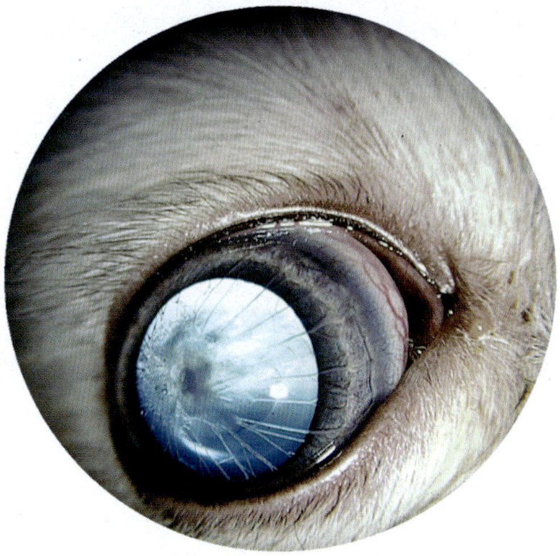

Figure 7-9
Iris-to-lens PPM showing attachment of the PPM to the iris collarette.

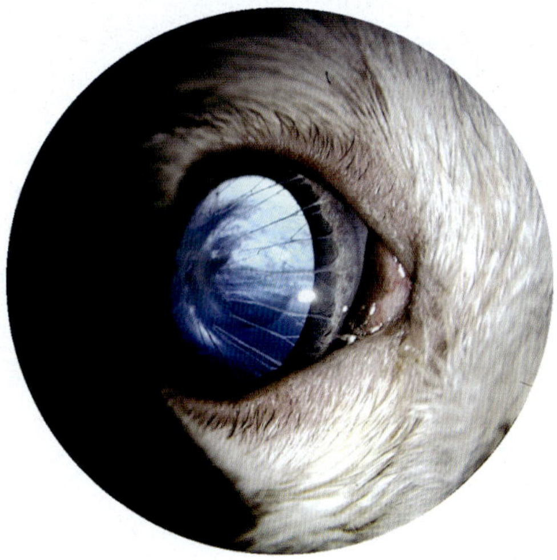

Figure 7-10
Iris-to-lens PPM. Same dog as in Figure 7-9.

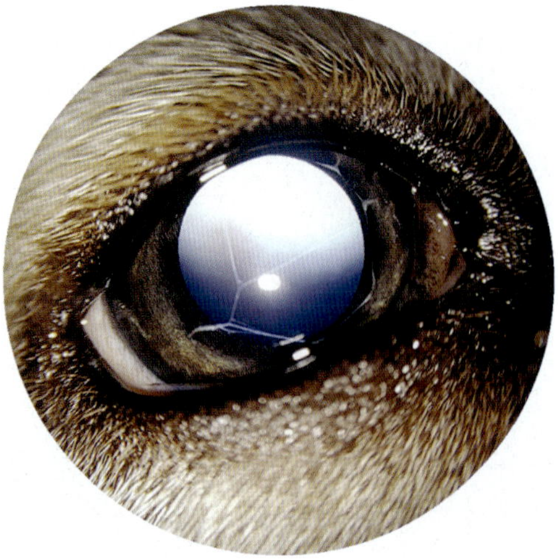

Figure 7-11
PPM: iris to lens and iris to iris.

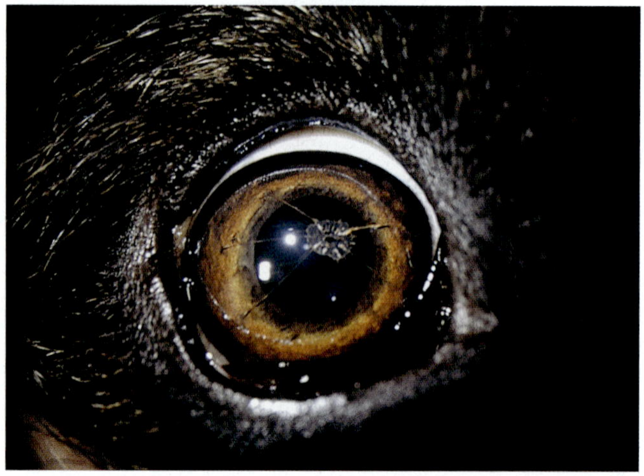

Figure 7-12
Iris-to-lens PPM in a Doberman pinscher.

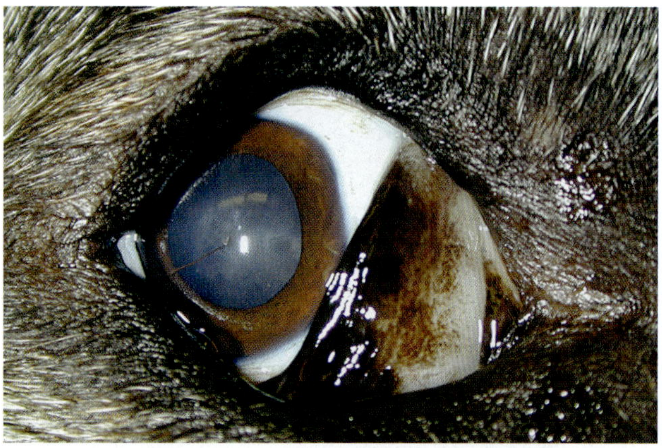

Figure 7-13
PPM: iris to lens capsule.

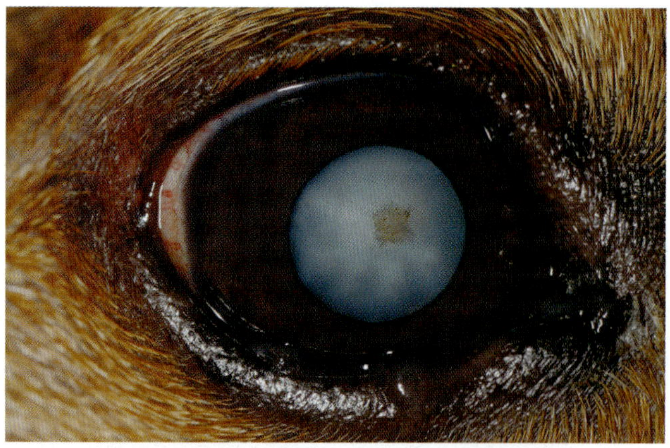

Figure 7-14
PPM remnants on the lens capsule. Linear opacity is a hair on the cornea. These small pigment deposits on the anterior lens capsule are seen in many dogs and rarely cause any vision-related or other problems. The heritability of these types of deposits is unknown.

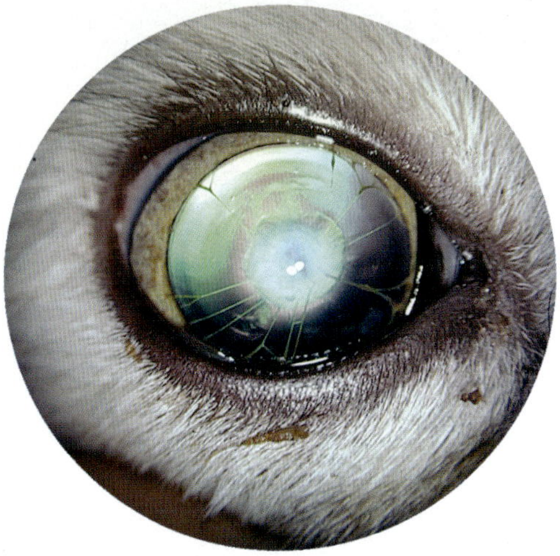

Figure 7-15
Iris-to-lens PPM with associated central cataract in a cat.
(Courtesy Dr. Robert Playter.)

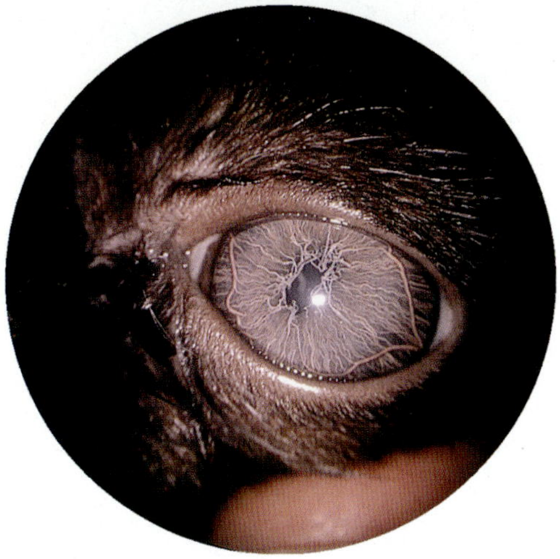

Figure 7-16
Young kitten with lipoprotein lipase deficiency and lipemia with patent PPMs and lipemic iridal vessels.

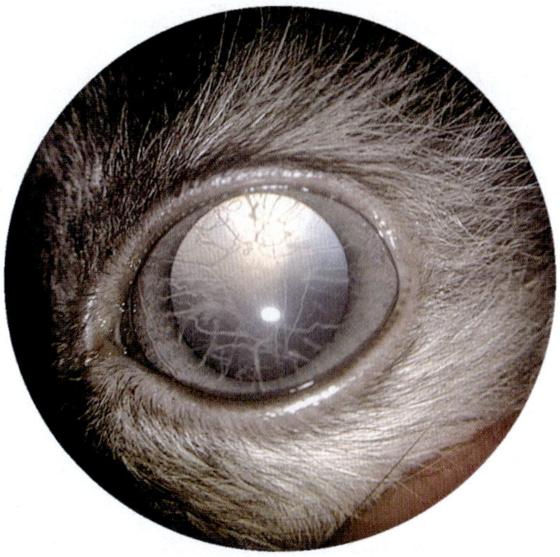

Figure 7-17
Same cat as in Figure 7-16 at a later date. The PPMs have decreased.

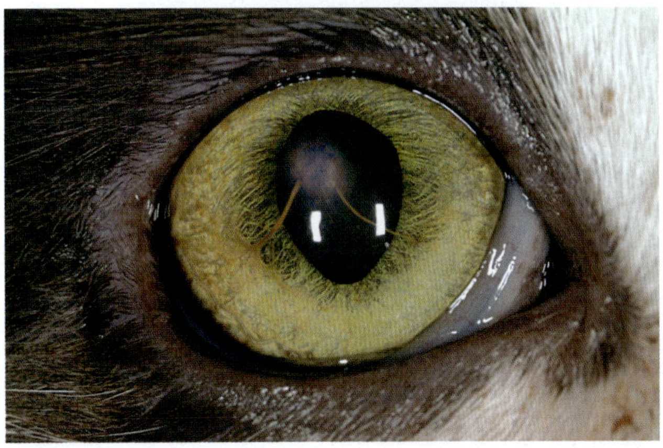

Figure 7-18
Iris-to-cornea PPM in a cat. Corneal edema may be present where the PPM touches the cornea.

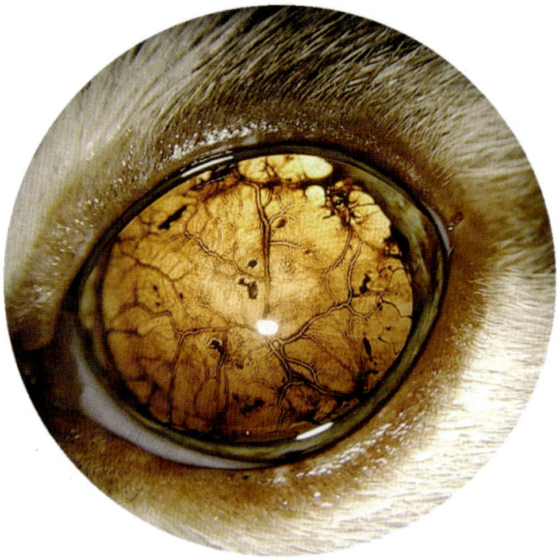

Figure 7-19
PPMs in a cat. Vascular remnants on the anterior lens capsule.

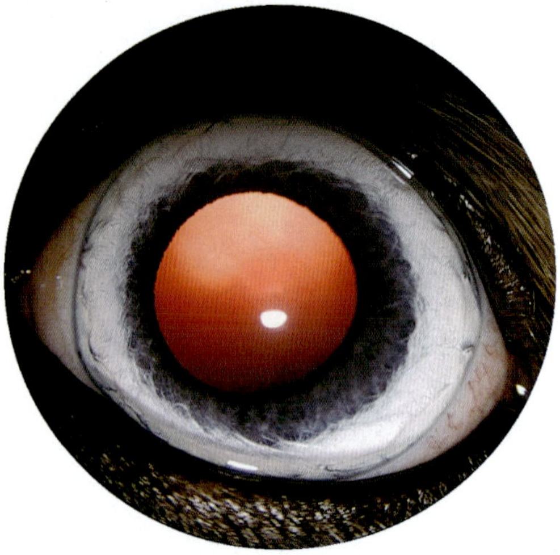

Figure 7-20
Heterochromia iridis. A marked reduction in pigmentation results in a blue color of the iris.

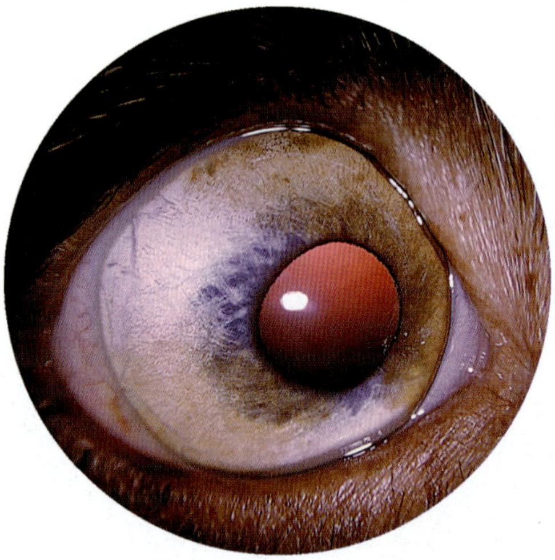

Figure 7-21
Heterochromia iridis. Heterochromia iridis is a condition in which a difference in color between the irides or in different parts of the same iris exists.

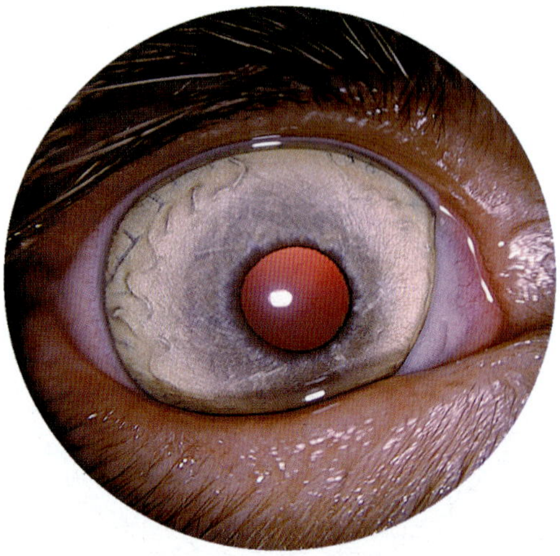

Figure 7-22
Heterochromia iridis in an Australian shepherd.

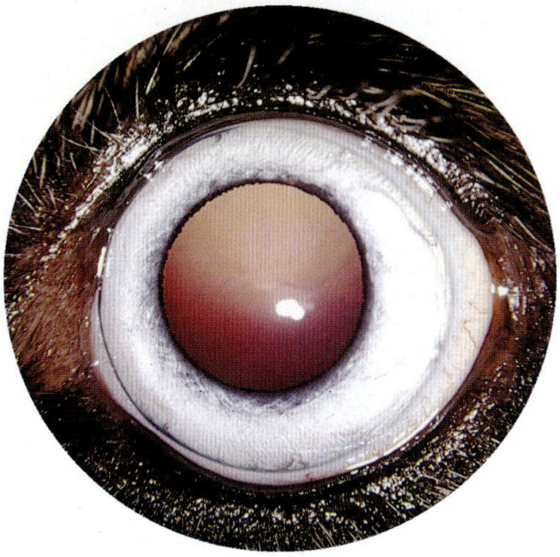

Figure 7-23
Subalbinotic iris.

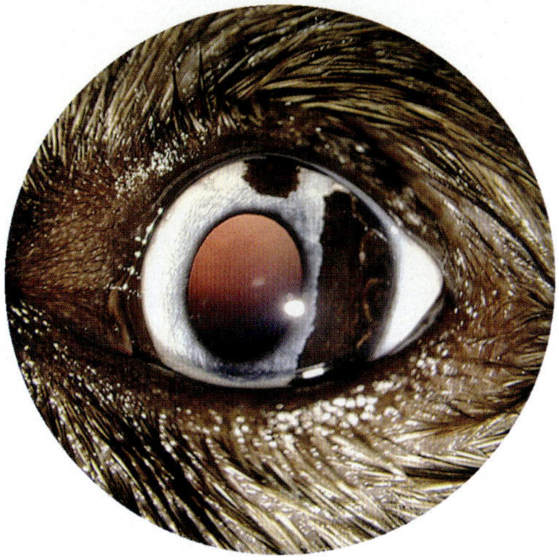

Figure 7-24
Heterochromia iridis.

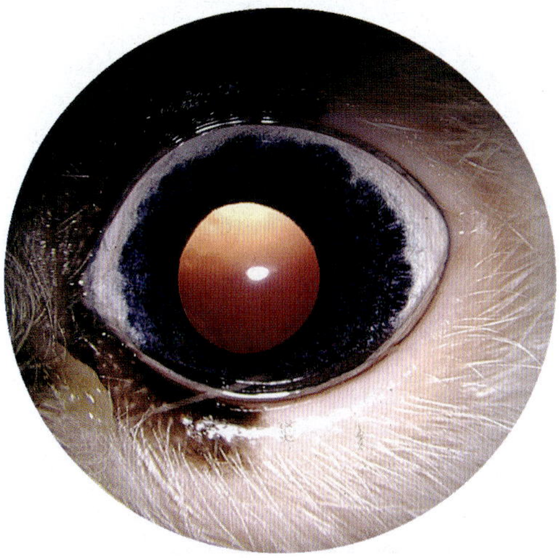

Figure 7-25
Heterochromia iridis.

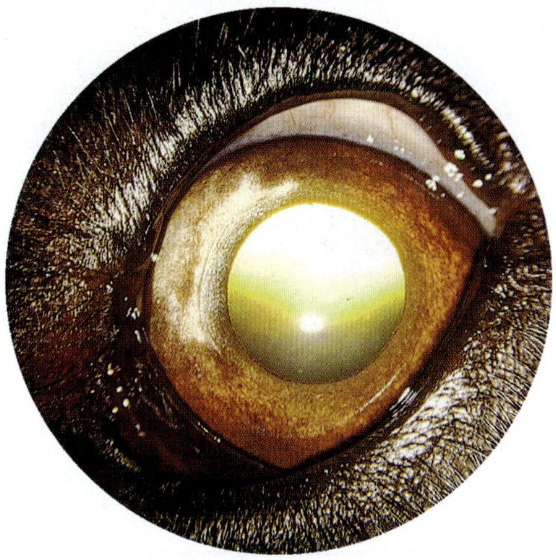

Figure 7-26
Heterochromia iridis.

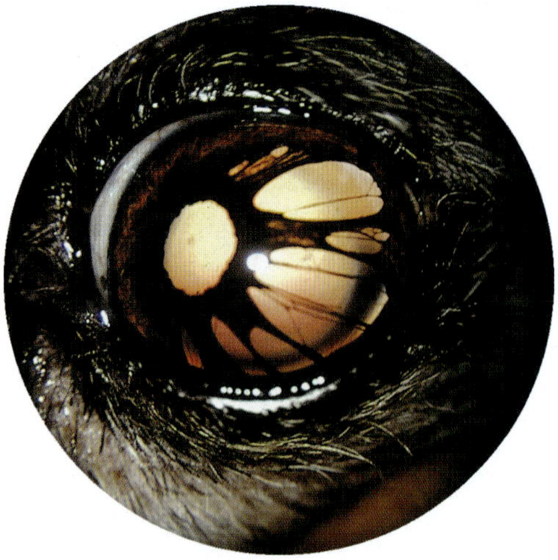

Figure 7-27
Iris dilator muscle atrophy.
(Courtesy Dr. Robert Playter)

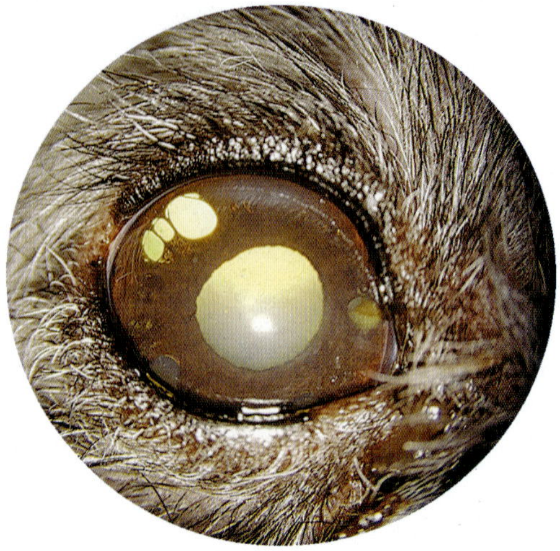

Figure 7-28
Iris dilator muscle atrophy.

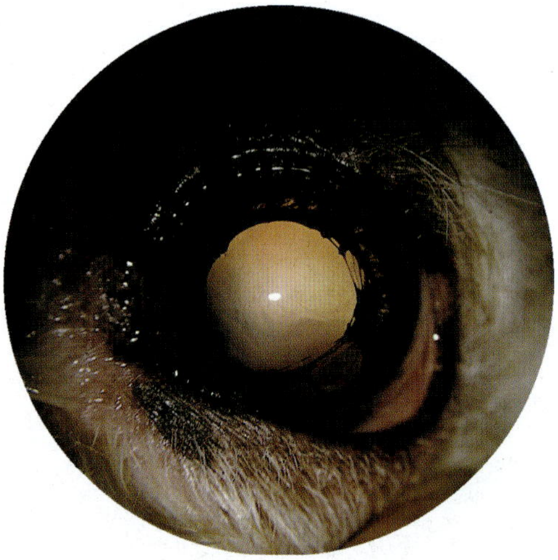

Figure 7-29
Iris sphincter and dilator muscle atrophy; nuclear sclerosis.

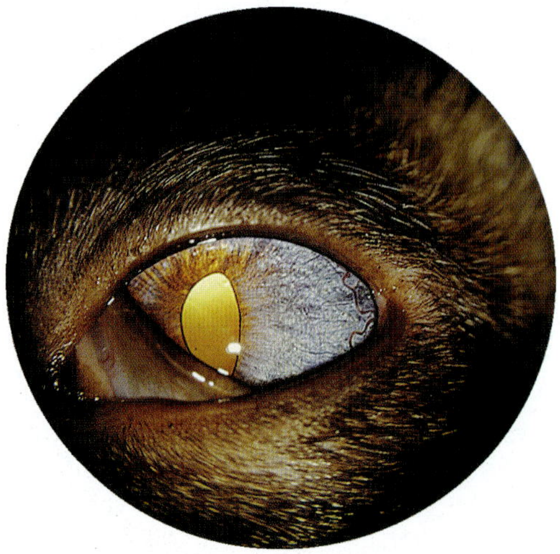

Figure 7-30
Thinned iris stroma (atrophy) in a blue-eyed cat.

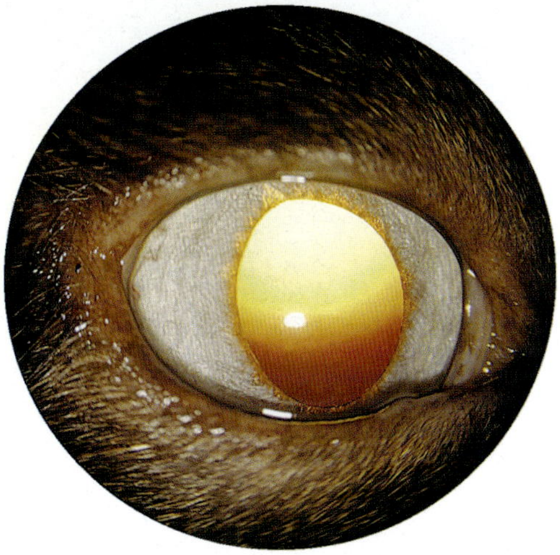

Figure 7-31
Thinned iris (atrophy) near the pupillary margin in a cat.

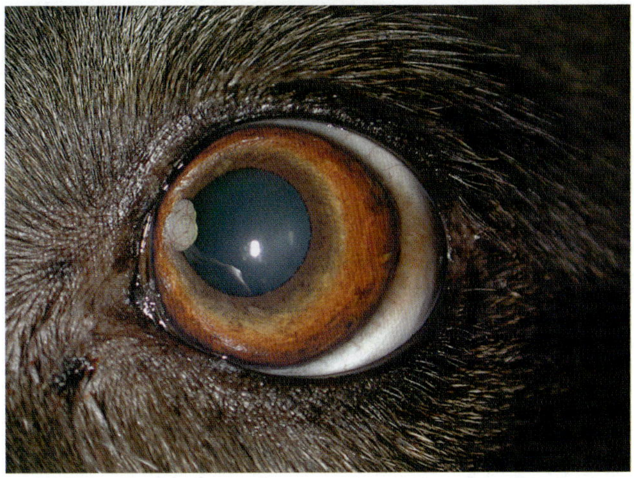

Figure 7-32
Nonpigmented cyst arising from the ciliary epithelium in a dog.

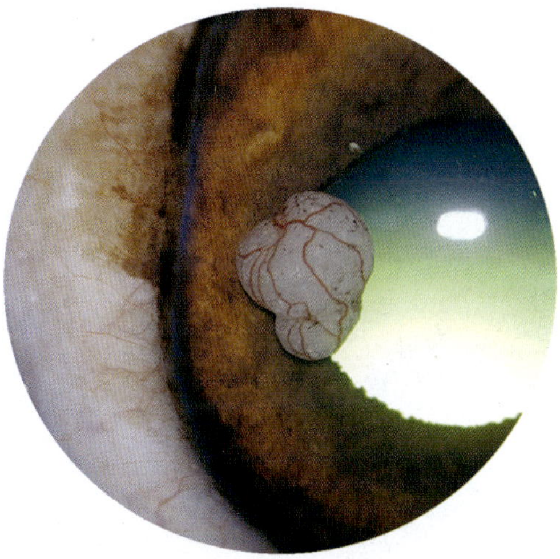

Figure 7-33
Close-up of cyst shown in Figure 7-32.

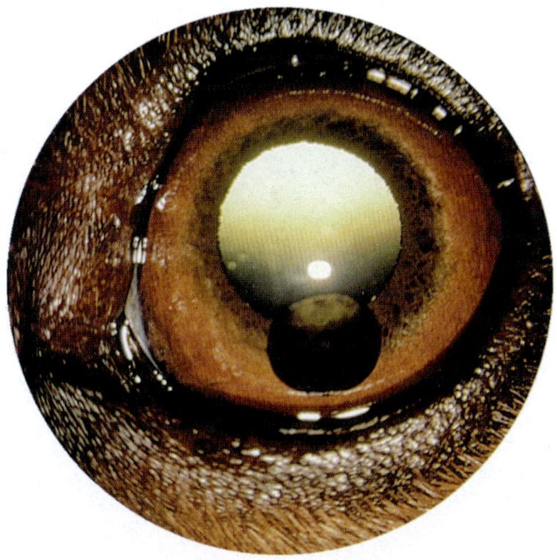

Figure 7-34
Free-floating iris cyst in anterior chamber in a dog; note the transillumination of the tapetal reflex through the cyst. These cysts must be distinguished from iris melanomas and rarely need treatment.

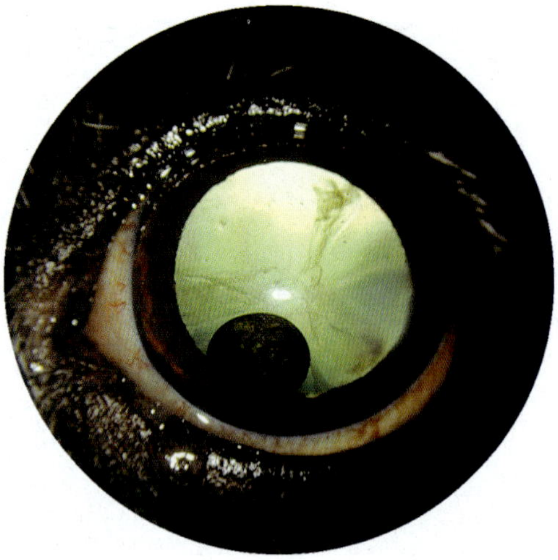

Figure 7-35
Free-floating iris cyst in the anterior chamber of a Boston terrier. Note the transillumination of the tapetal reflex. An immature cataract is incidentally present.

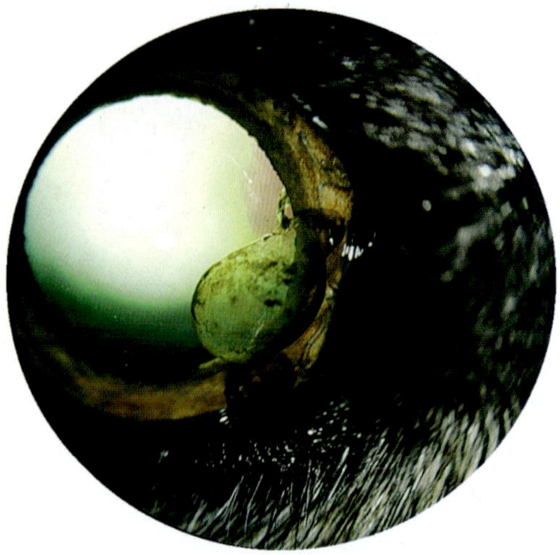

Figure 7-36
Iris cysts at the pupillary margin and in the anterior chamber in a 7-year-old Irish wolfhound.

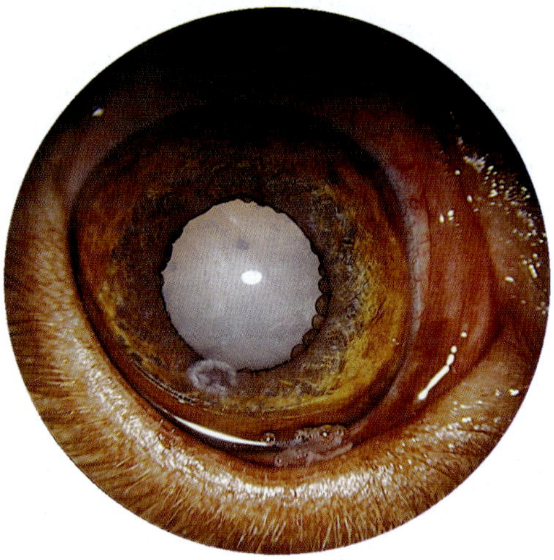

Figure 7-37
Multifocal small iris cysts at pupil margin of a dog with a cataract. Lipid keratopathy also is present.

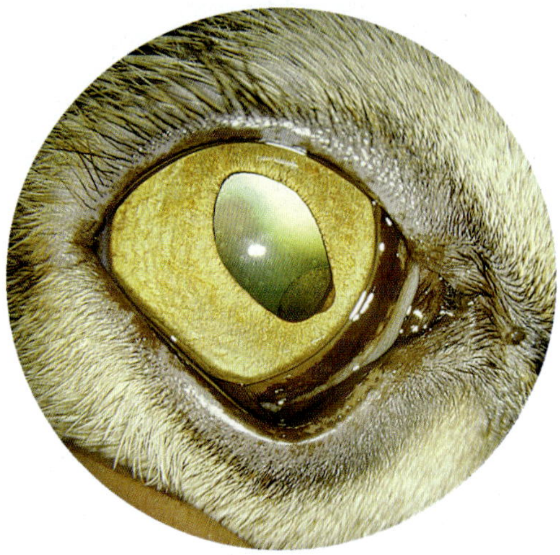

Figure 7-38
Iris cyst in a 4-year-old cat.

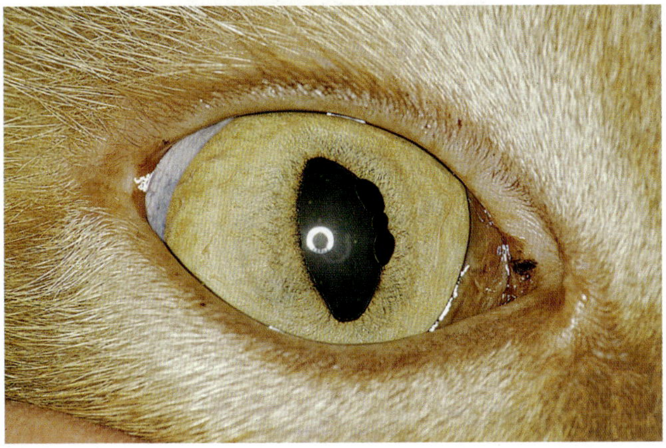

Figure 7-39
Iris cysts at the pupil margin of a cat.

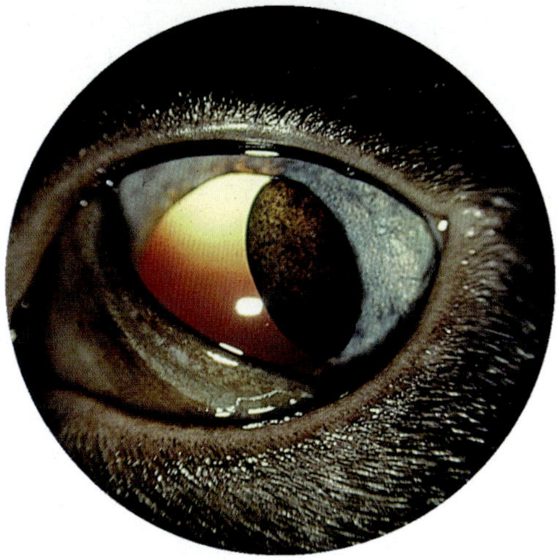

Figure 7-40
Iris and ciliary body cyst visible through the pupil of a cat.

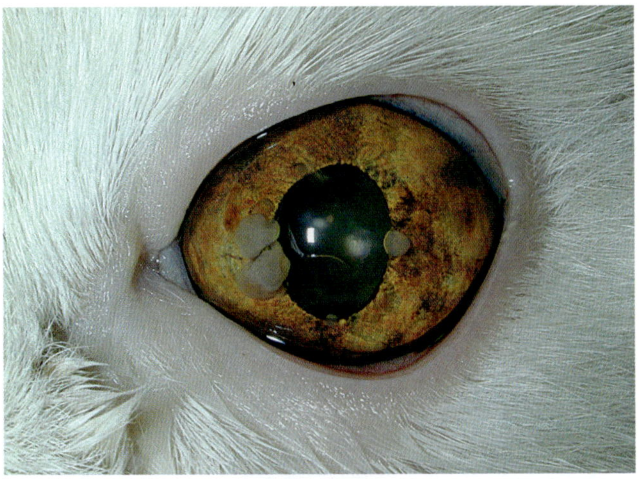

Figure 7-41
Iris cysts in a cat.

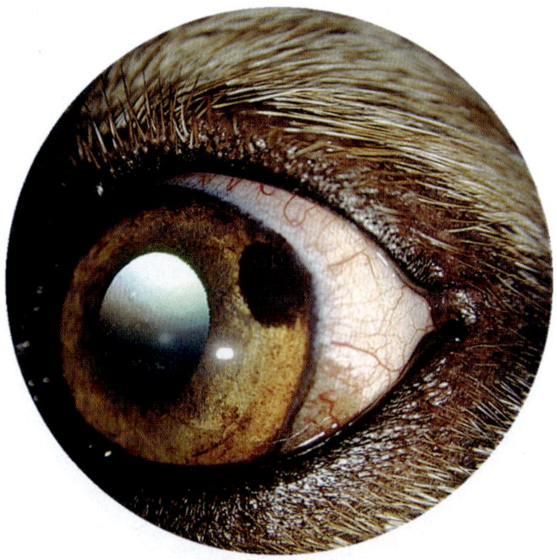

Figure 7-42
Nevus in the iris of a dog; the differential diagnosis is melanoma. A nevus is also called a *freckle.* Nevi are acquired lesions that are usually flat with the iris surface.

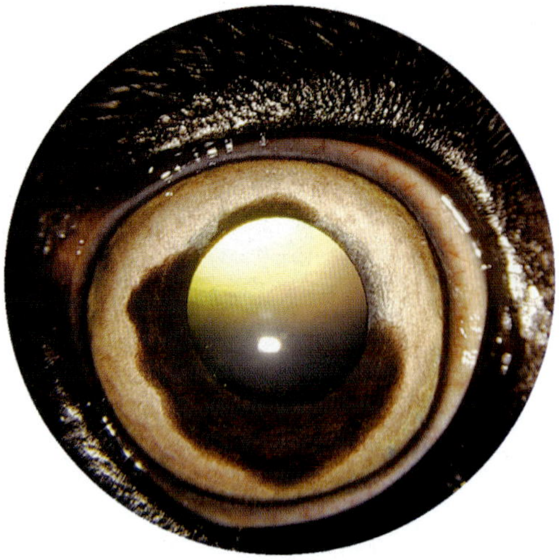

Figure 7-43
Large nevus in a dog's iris.

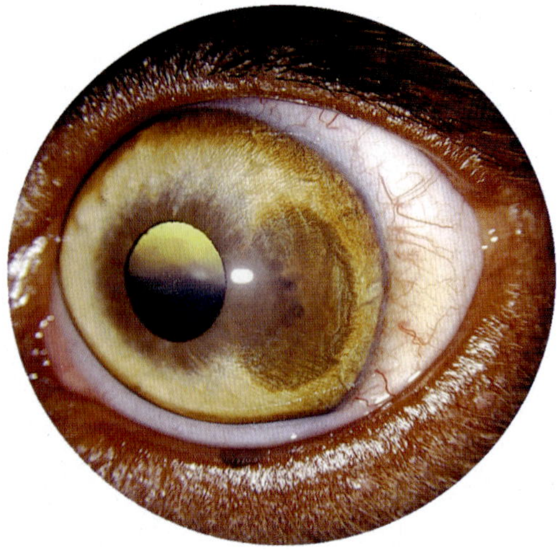

Figure 7-44
Nevus in the iris of a dog.

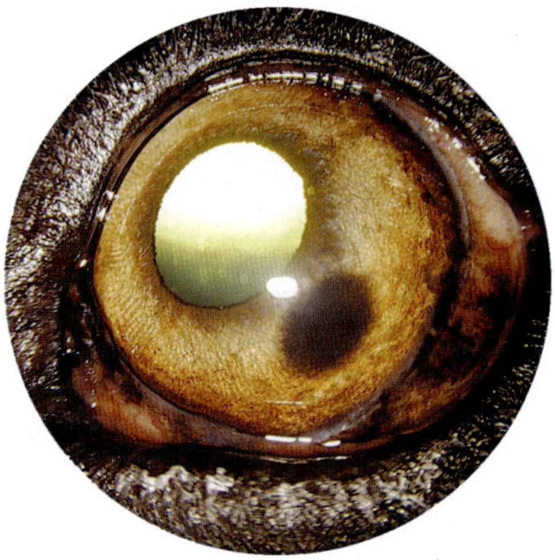

Figure 7-45
Nevus in a dog.

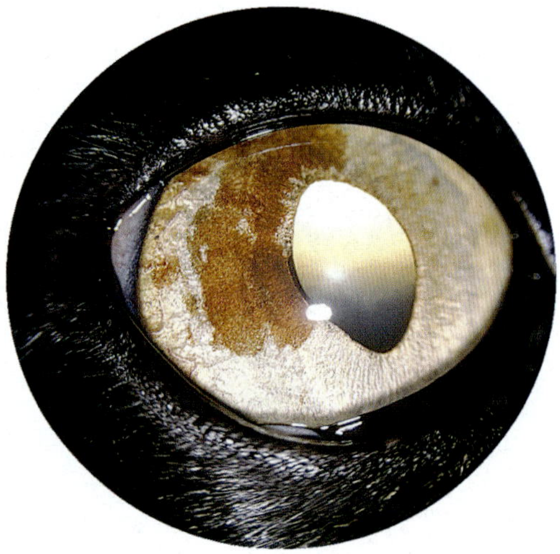

Figure 7-46
Nevus in a cat.

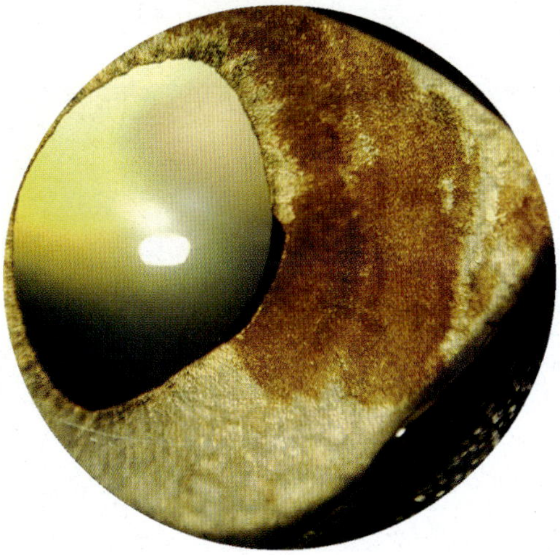

Figure 7-47
Nevus with area of ectropion uveae. Ectropion uveae is a swelling and rolling out of the posterior pigmented layer of the iris and can be seen at the papillary margin in cases of uveitis.

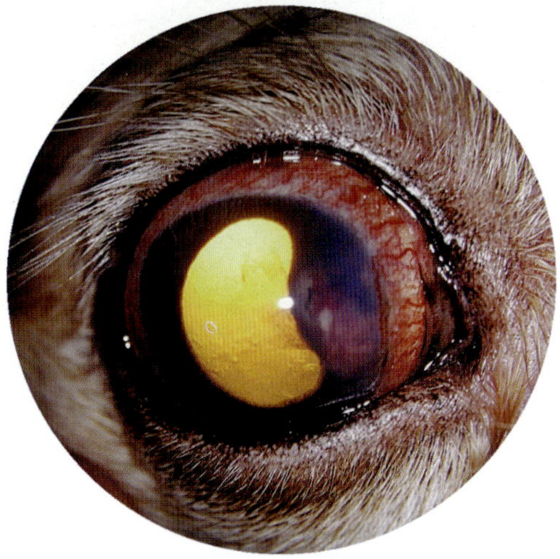

Figure 7-48
Iris mass of unknown cell type in a dog. Note the distortion of the pupil and "red eye" caused by inflammation resulting from the tumor.

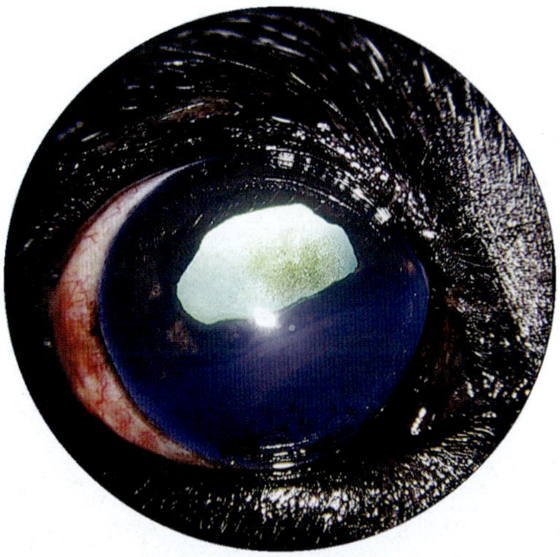

Figure 7-49
Iris melanoma. The majority of the tumor is inferior, but increased pigmentation is present throughout the iris. Pupil distortion extends 360 degrees.

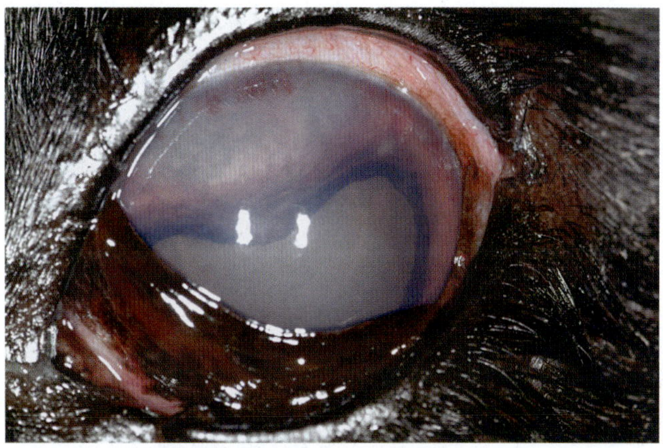

Figure 7-50
Ciliary body adenoma in a dog. Iris distortion and uveitis are present.

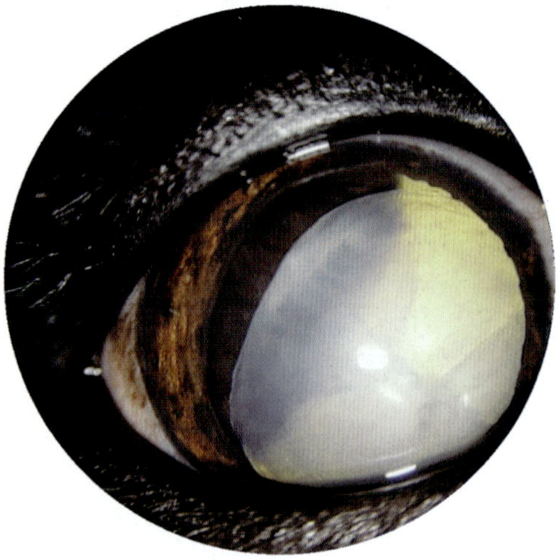

Figure 7-51
Standard poodle with uveal melanoma that is causing lens subluxation (the lens is cataractous).

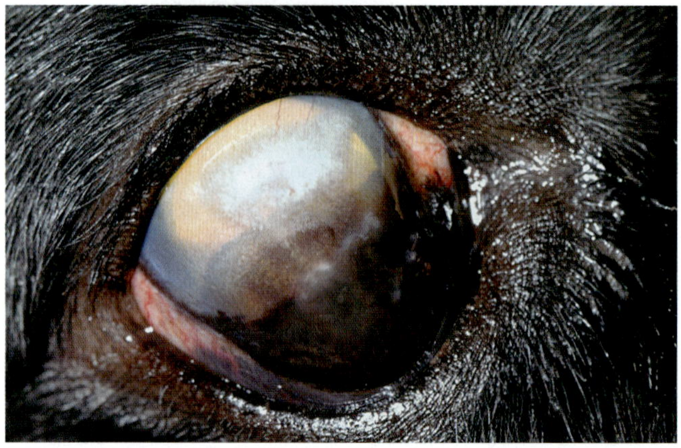

Figure 7-52
Uveal melanoma in a dog. The melanoma has distended and is eroding through the fibrous coats of the globe ventrally and laterally.

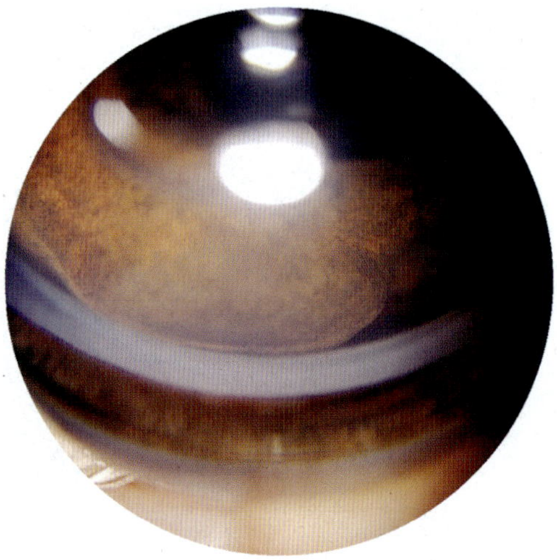

Figure 7-53
Iris melanoma visible on gonioscopy. The drainage angle is distorted by the melanoma.

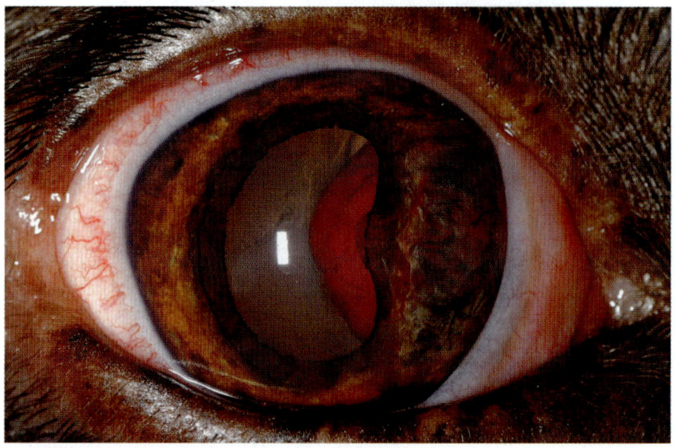

Figure 7-54
Ciliary adenocarcinoma in a Labrador retriever seen through the pupil and causing swelling and distortion of the iris.

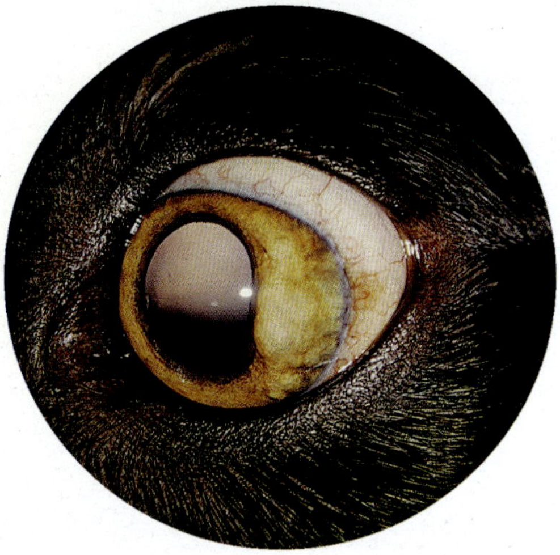

Figure 7-55
Iris tumor of unknown cell type in a dog.

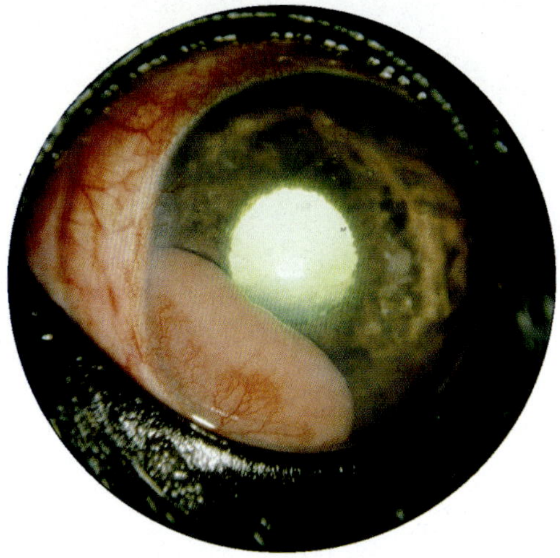

Figure 7-56
Undefined tumor invading the anterior chamber of a dog.
(Courtesy Dr. Robert Playter.)

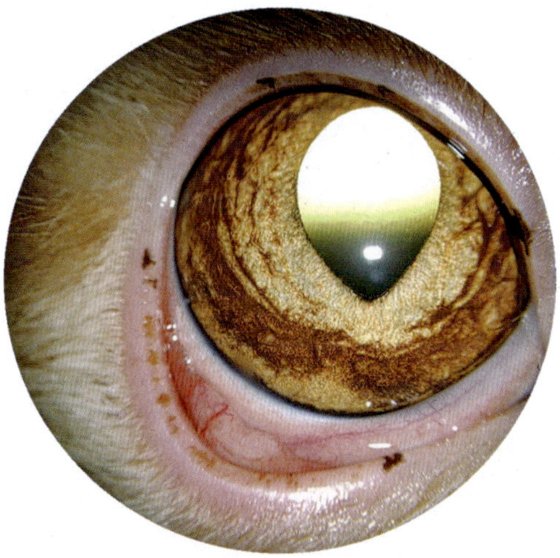

Figure 7-57
Diffuse iris melanoma in a cat. This pupil did not constrict as well as did the opposite pupil. The neoplastic nature of the tumor was confirmed on histopathology of the enucleated eye. Differential diagnosis is nevus. This type of diffuse melanoma, which has been described in the veterinary literature only in the cat eye, metastasizes readily.

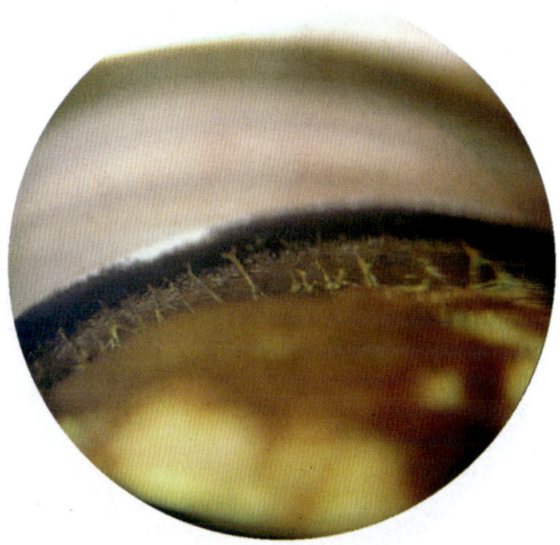

Figure 7-58
Extension of diffuse iris melanoma into the iridocorneal angle of a cat. The pigment in the angle results in a chronic insidious rise of intraocular pressure (glaucoma) if the eye is not enucleated early.

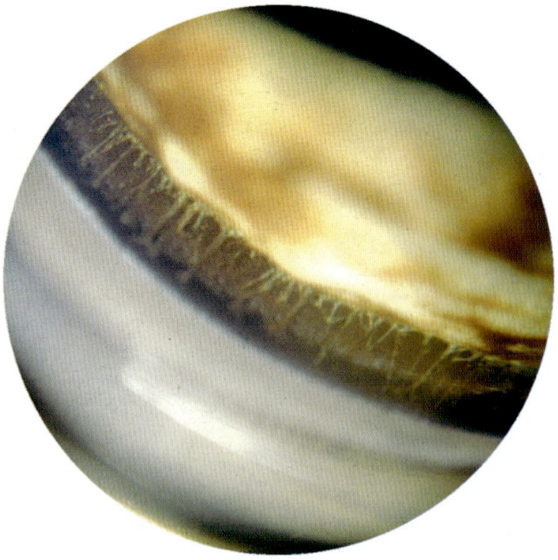

Figure 7-59
Goniophotograph of increased drainage angle pigmentation in a cat with diffuse iris melanoma.

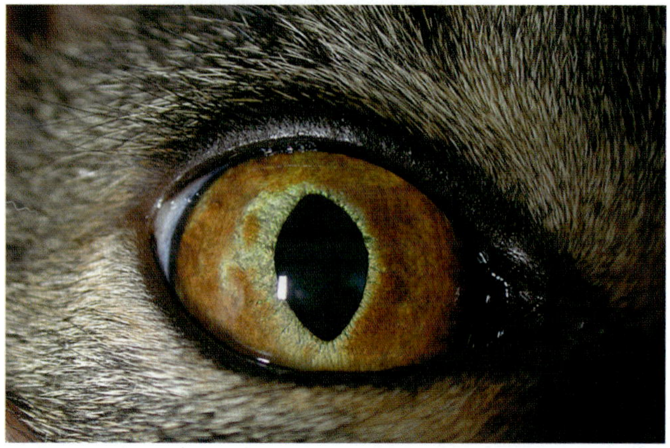

Figure 7-60
Diffuse iris melanoma in a Siamese cat, with an increase in pigmentation and thickening of the iris stroma.

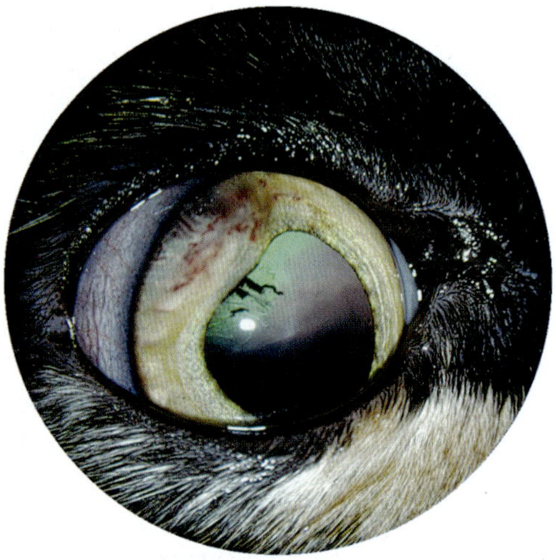

Figure 7-61
Ciliary adenoma in a cat.

UVEITIS

Uveitis is an inflammation of the uveal tract—the iris, ciliary body, and choroid. Uveitis begins with an insult of some sort. Inflammatory mediators such as prostaglandins are released. Just as in other parts of the body, the release of inflammatory mediators leads to increased blood flow ("red eye"); leakage of blood vessels (edema of the iris as well as the choroid and retina) and other tight junctions (anterior chamber flare, hypopyon, hyphema, and keratic precipitates); and muscle spasms (miosis and ciliary muscle spasms that cause pain). Uncontrolled inflammation then leads to posterior synechiae (adhesions of the iris to the lens) and peripheral anterior synechiae (adhesions of the iris to the cornea at the drainage angle), which lead to glaucoma and cataracts. Retinal detachments can be associated with choroidal inflammation. The clinician's job is to determine the cause of the uveitis, treat the cause if possible, and moderate the inflammatory response of the eye in order to maintain vision. In many of the photographs of uveitis, the pupil is large. In all cases this reflects the fact that the pupil was dilated with tropicamide before the photo was taken.

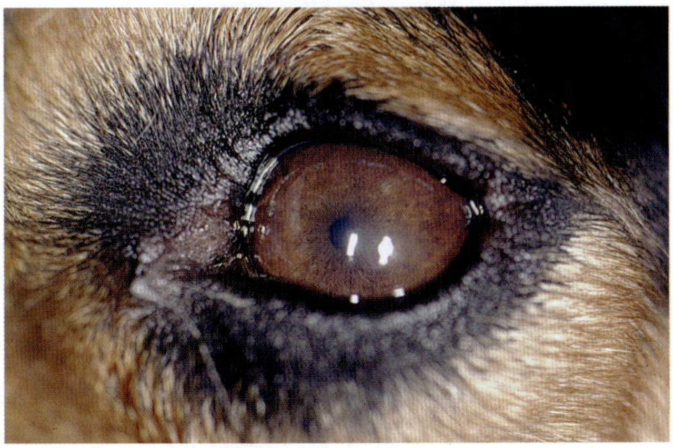

Figure 7-62
Miosis, one of the hallmarks of uveitis. The differential diagnosis in a patient with miosis is Horner's syndrome.

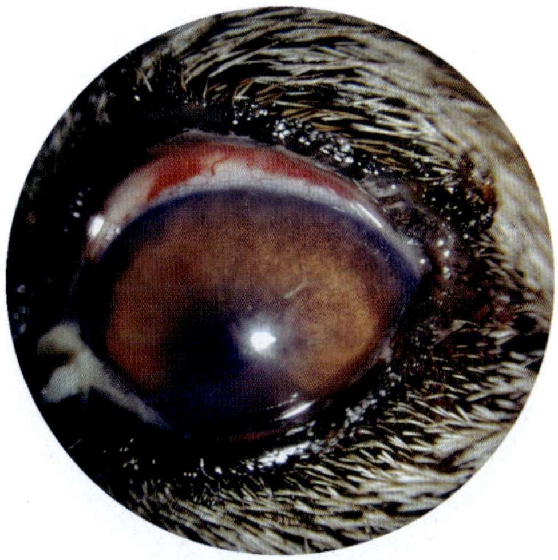

Figure 7-63
Acute uveitis. Miosis, cloudy aqueous, and subconjunctival hemorrhage are present.

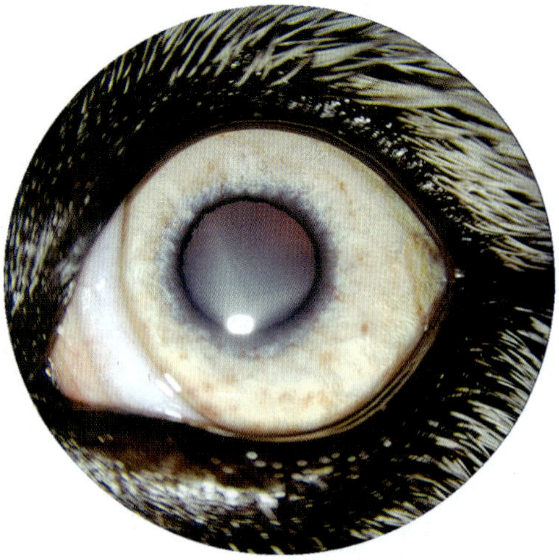

Figure 7-64
Trauma-induced uveitis in a husky. The normally blue iris has become yellowish. Dilation of the iridal blood vessel and inherited cataract are present.

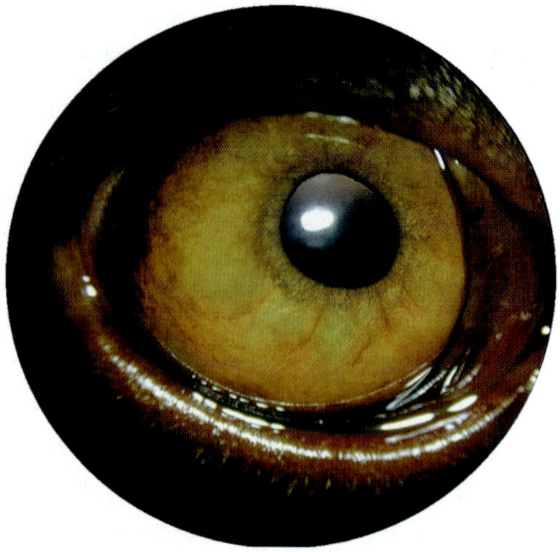

Figure 7-65
Thickened swollen iris (iritis). Surface features are rendered less distinct.

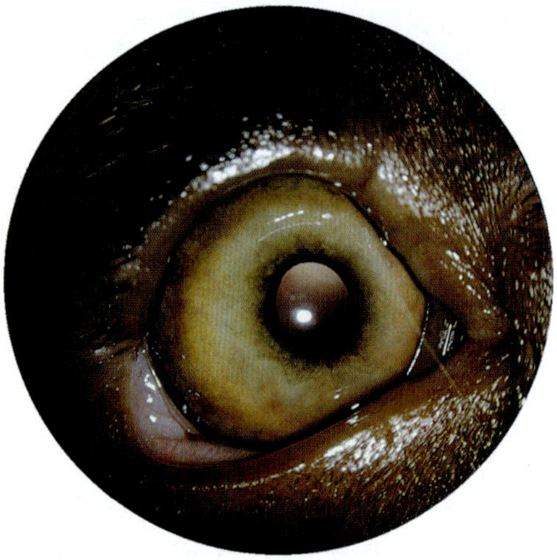

Figure 7-66
Thickened swollen iris in a pit bull with uveitis.

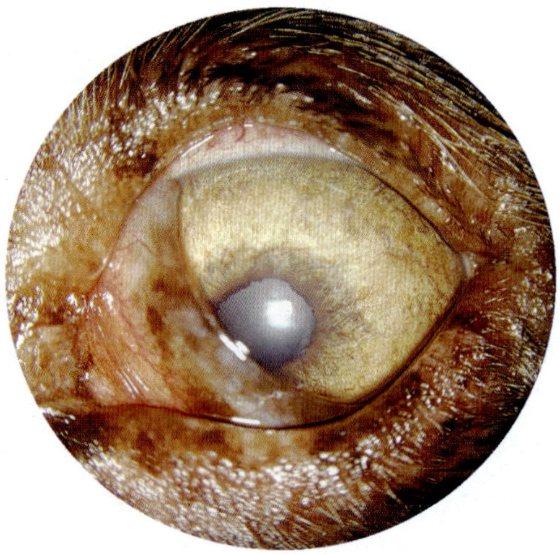

Figure 7-67
Acute uveitis. Miosis and "red eye" can be seen.

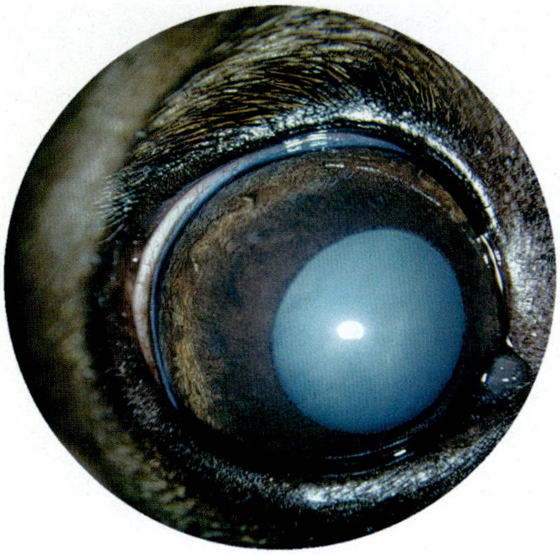

Figure 7-68
Mature cataract and uveitis in a dog with *Brucella canis.*

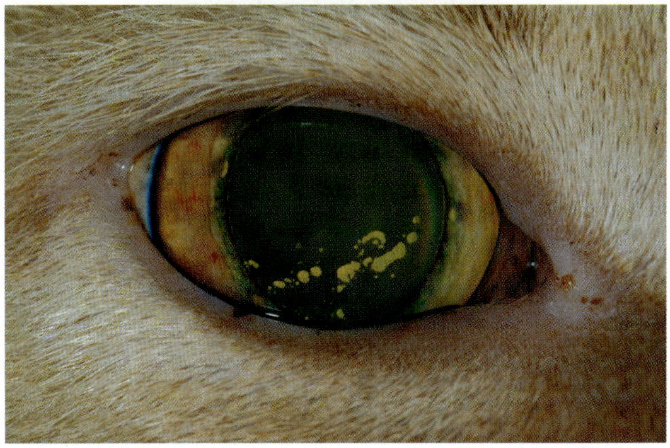

Figure 7-69
Cat with keratic precipitates. Keratic precipitates are inflammatory cells that have settled on the endothelial surface of the cornea; they usually are most obvious on the inferior aspect of the cornea.

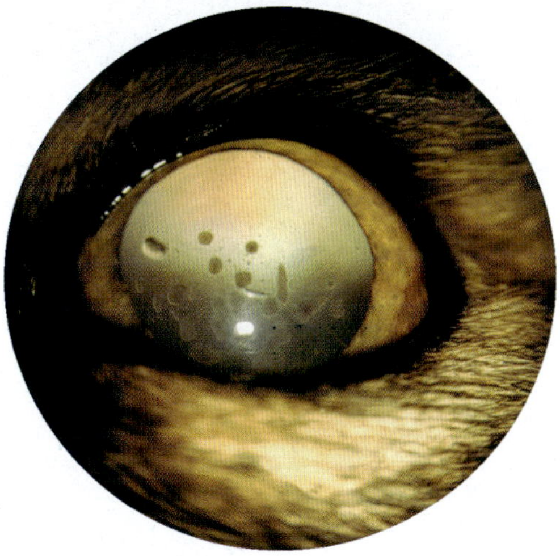

Figure 7-70
Keratic precipitates in a cat.

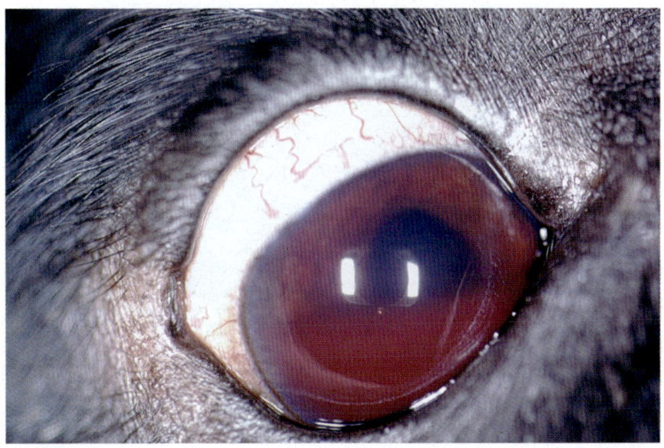

Figure 7-71
Hyphema—the presence of red blood cells in the anterior chamber. Hyphema can result from uveitis, especially with vasculitis, but can also be seen with systemic bleeding disorders, ocular tumors, trauma, and retinal detachments.

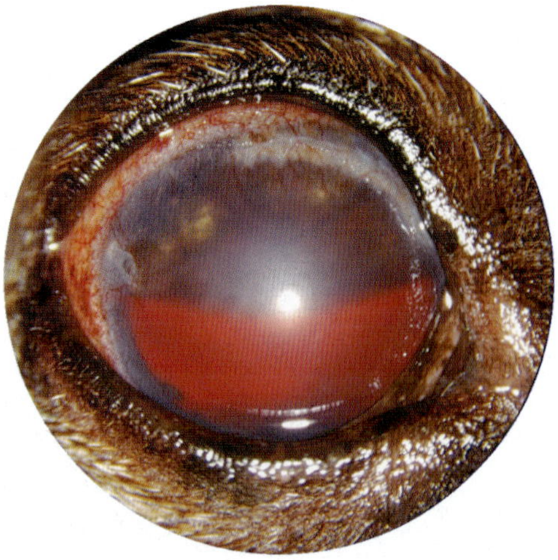

Figure 7-72
Hyphema and iridal swelling in a dog after cataract surgery.

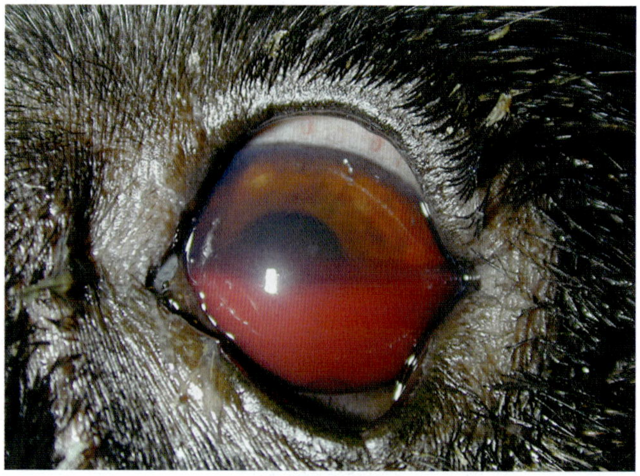

Figure 7-73
Hyphema associated with intraocular neoplasia in a rottweiler.

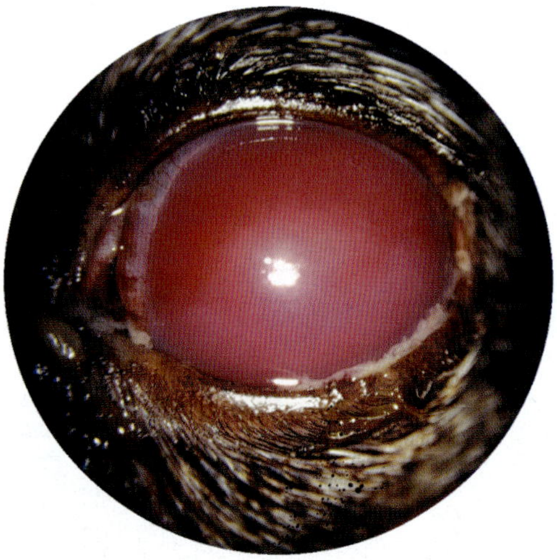

Figure 7-74
Hyphema.

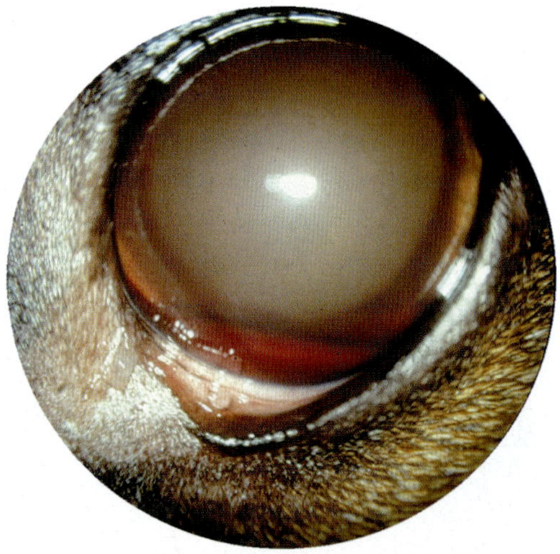

Figure 7-75
Hyphema. There is a red tinge to the aqueous, and a line of red cells has settled out inferiorly.

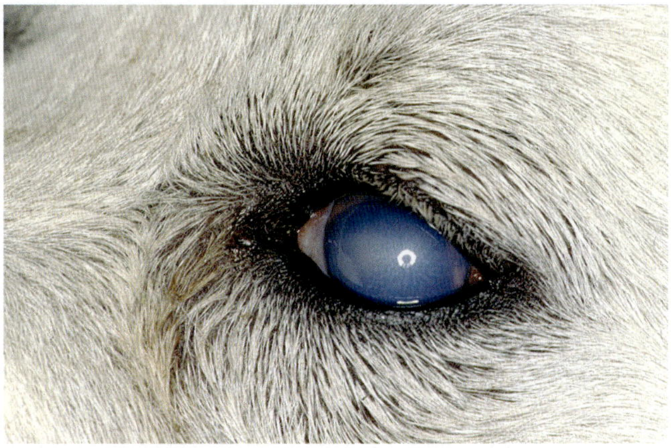

Figure 7-76
Corneal edema resulting from canine adenovirus infection.
(Courtesy Dr. Robert Playter.)

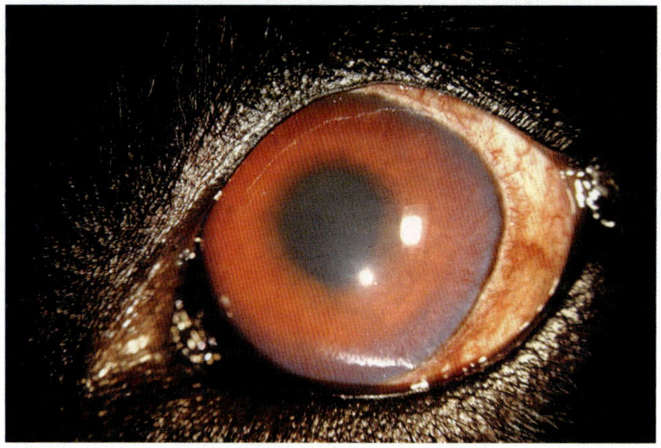

Figure 7-77
Uveitis with a reddened, swollen iris, corneal edema, and neovascularization.

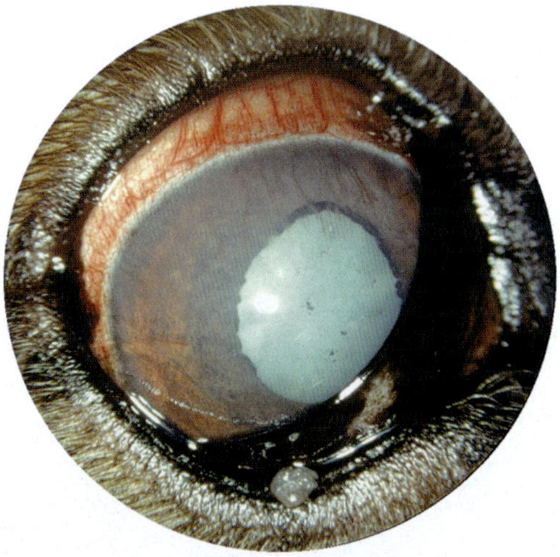

Figure 7-78
Ectropion uveae, corneal neovascularization and edema, and cataract and pigment on the anterior lens capsule. Ectropion uveae is a swelling and rolling out of the posterior pigmented layer of the iris and can be seen at the pupillary margin in cases of uveitis.

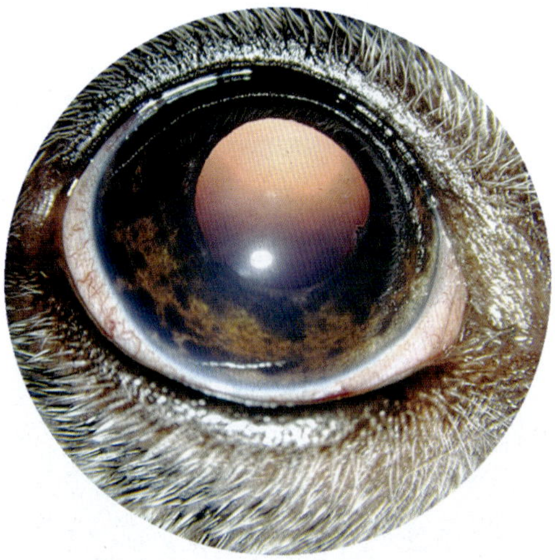

Figure 7-79
Dog with anterior uveitis and glaucoma. Note the increased iris pigmentation, which can be seen in chronic cases of uveitis.

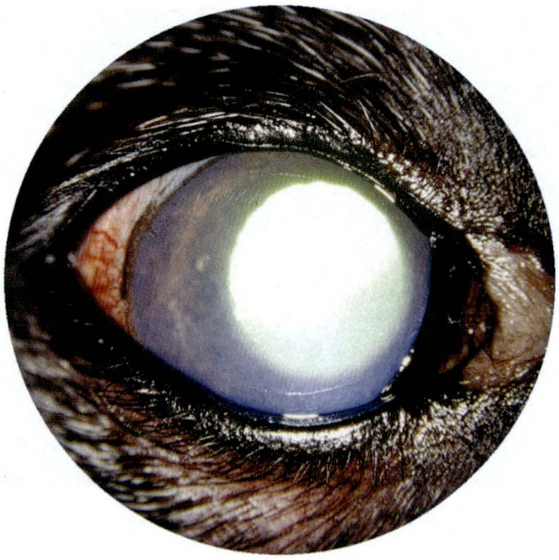

Figure 7-80
Corneal edema in a greyhound with uveitis. Inflammation can interfere with the corneal endothelial pump and lead to diffuse corneal edema.

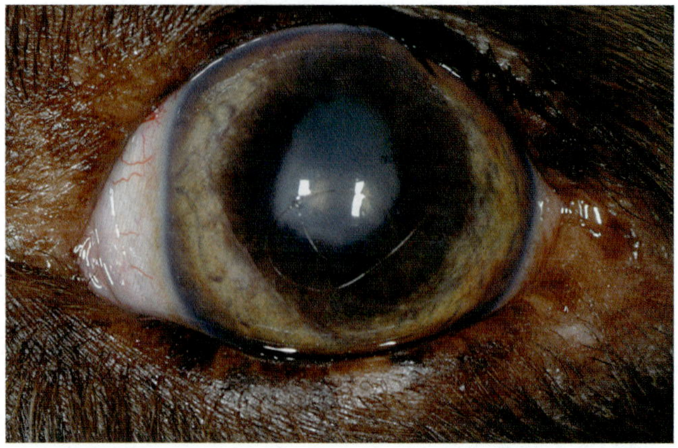

Figure 7-81
Posterior synechiae, iris bombé, and cataract associated with a high enzyme-linked immunosorbent assay titer to *Borrelia burgdorferi* in a mixed-breed dog. (The linear opacity on the cornea is a hair.)

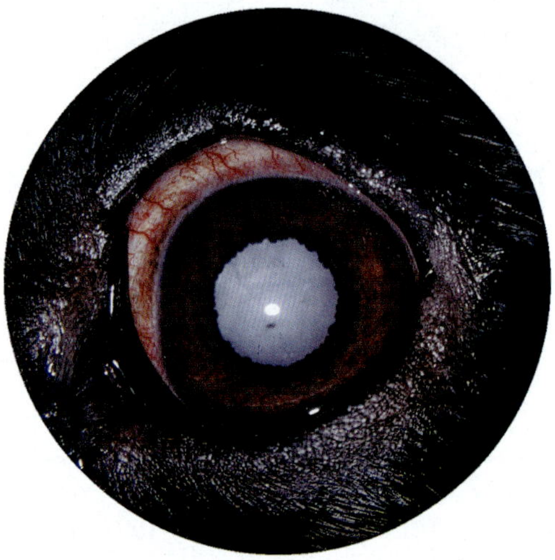

Figure 7-82
Uveitis. "Red eye," ectropion uveae, and cataract are present in this American cocker spaniel.

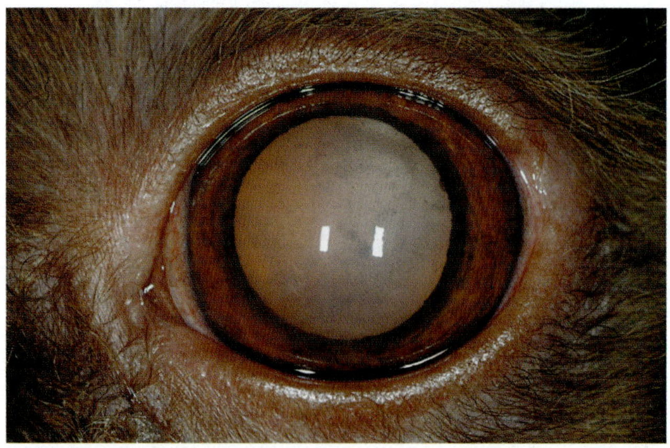

Figure 7-83
Immature cataract and uveitis can be seen in this miniature poodle that was hit in the eye with a tennis ball.

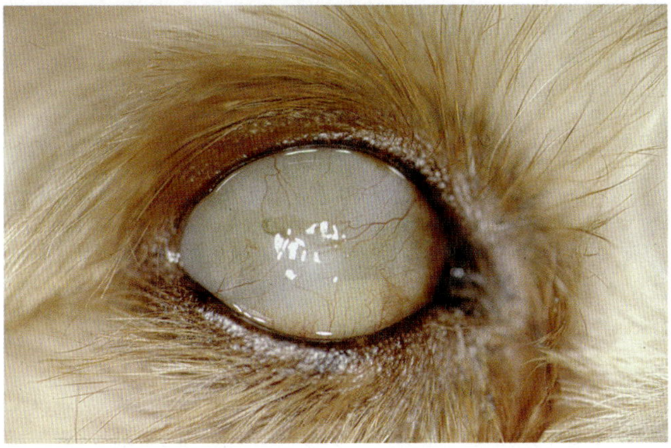

Figure 7-84
Opaque, vascularized cornea and hypopyon (white cells in the aqueous, which have settled out inferiorly) resulting from uveitis.

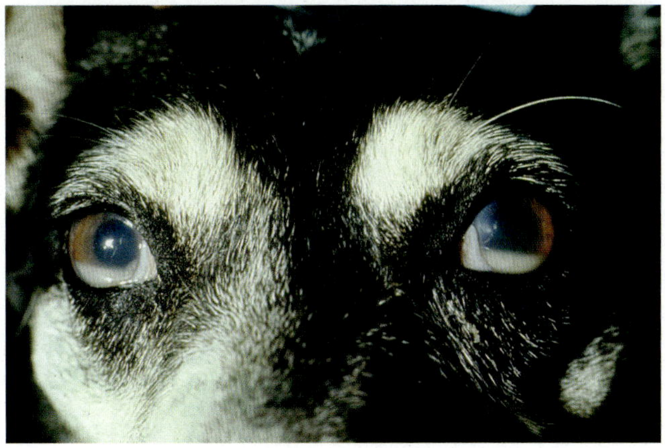

Figure 7-85
Bilateral hypopyon in a dog with lymphosarcoma and leukemia.

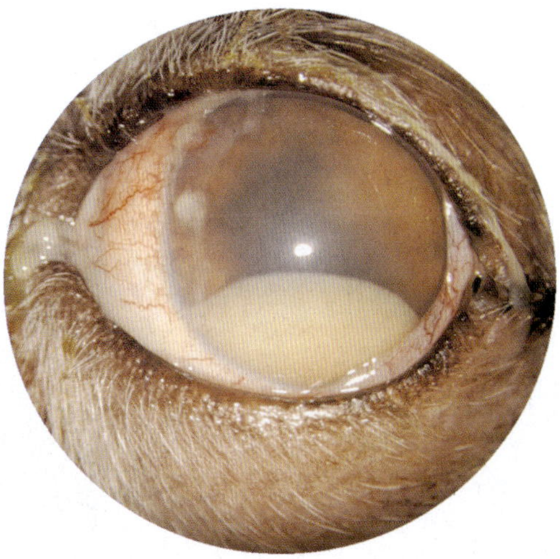

Figure 7-86
Hypopyon in a dog after cataract surgery.

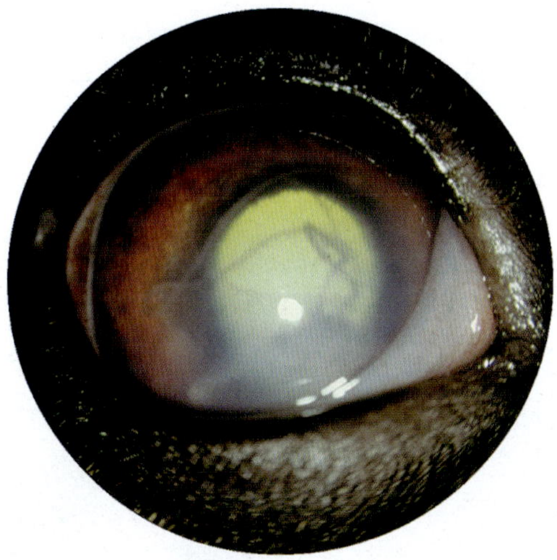

Figure 7-87
Subadult *Dirofilaria* organism in the eye is causing corneal edema and uveitis.

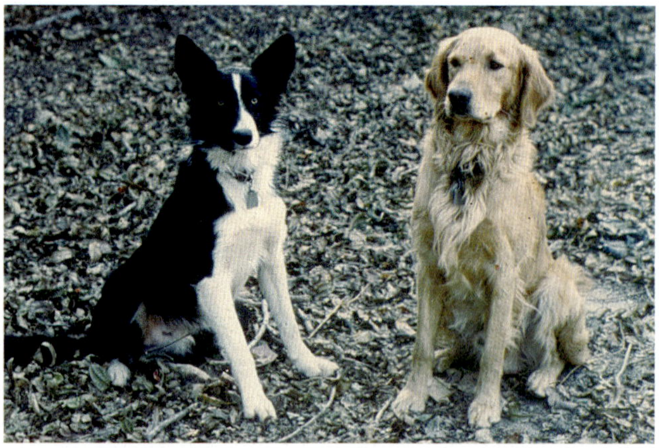

Figure 7-88
Dog on the left is an adult border collie crossbreed, shown before the onset of Vogt-Koyanagi-Harada syndrome (VKH). VKH is an immune-mediated disease of dogs and humans in which melanin is perceived as foreign. Patients develop vitiligo (depigmentation of skin, especially the planum nasale, lip, and eyelid margins); poliosis (whitening of dark hairs); and bilateral, severe uveitis.

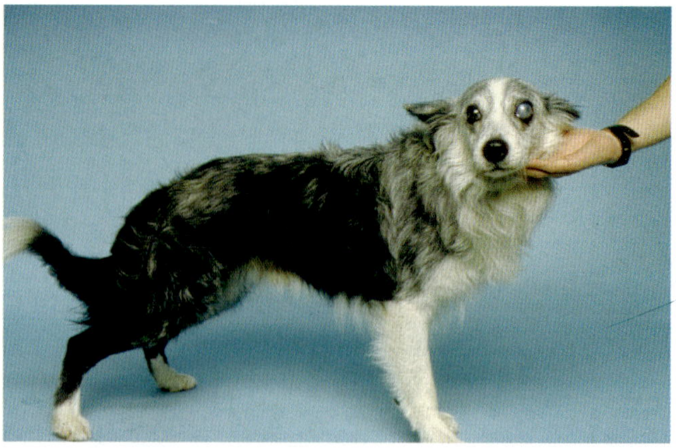

Figure 7-89
The dog shown in Figure 7-88 after the onset of VKH. Poliosis, bilateral uveitis, and secondary glaucoma in the left eye are present.

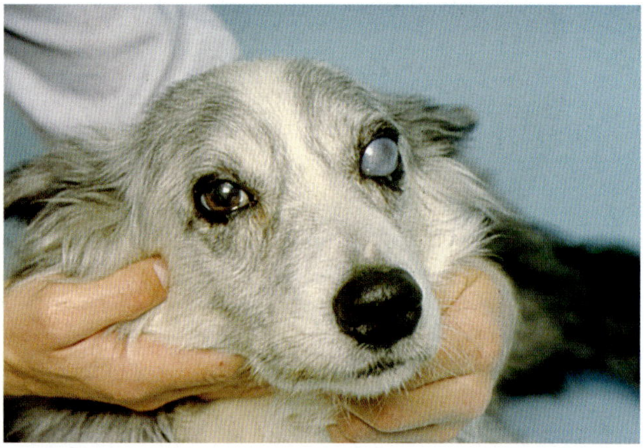

Figure 7-90
Close-up of the dog shown in Figures 7-88 and 7-89. Poliosis, bilateral uveitis, and secondary glaucoma in the left eye are present.

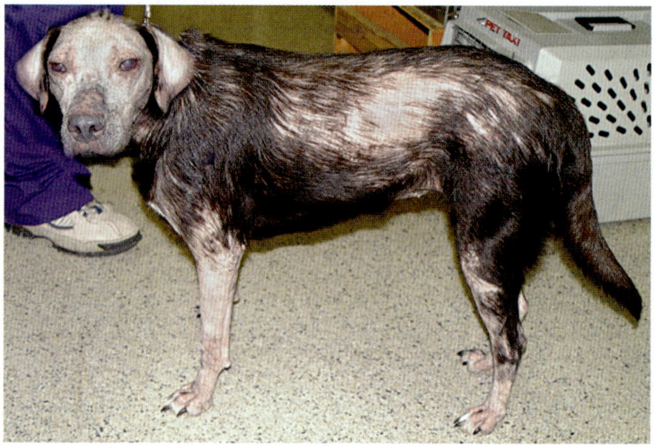

Figure 7-91
Dog with VKH. Vitiligo, alopecia, and bilateral uveitis with secondary glaucoma are present.

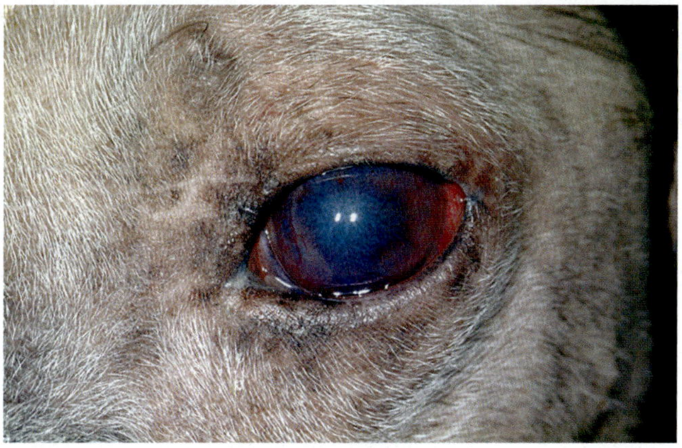

Figure 7-92
Close-up of dog shown in Figure 7-91 that shows uveitis and secondary glaucoma in the left eye. The eye is buphthalmic, corneal edema and neovascularization are present, and the pupil is mid-dilated. Poliosis and vitiligo are also present.

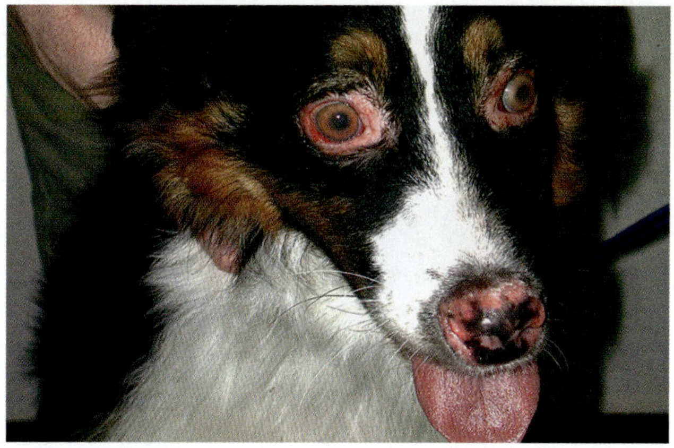

Figure 7-93
VKH in an Australian shepherd. Mucocutaneous junction depigmentation (vitiligo) and erythema around the eyelids and the external nares, anterior uveitis with corneal edema and vascularization, and aqueous flare and miosis are present.

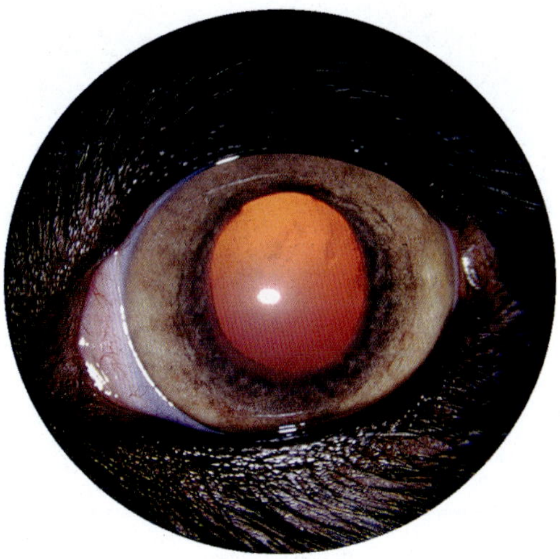

Figure 7-94
Corneal edema and uveitis in an Akita with possible VKH (swollen iris, posterior synechiae, and pigment on the anterior lens capsule).

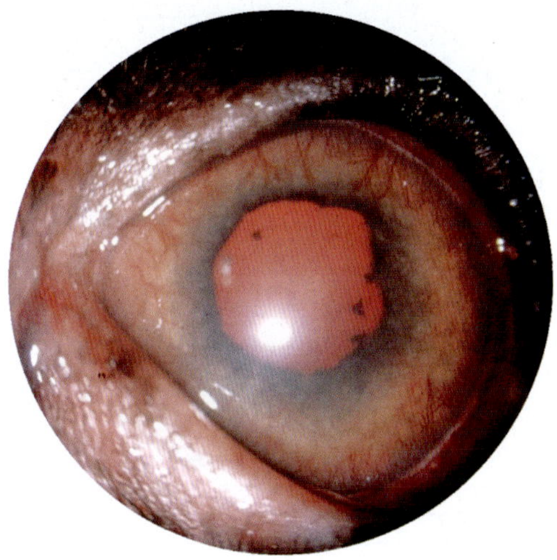

Figure 7-95
Chronic uveitis and secondary glaucoma in a golden retriever with VKH. Posterior synechiae, corneal neovascularization, corneal edema, and "red eye" are present.

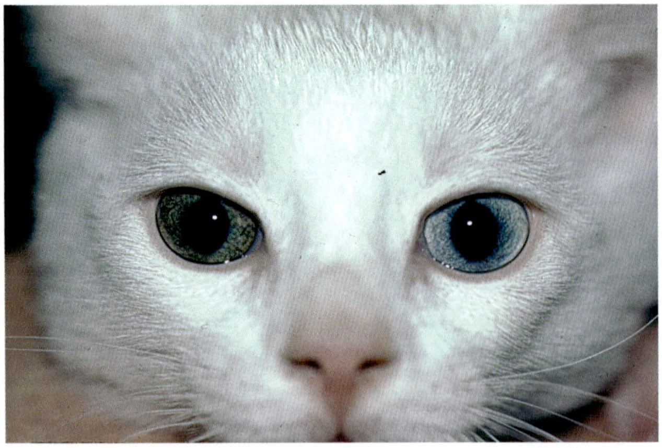

Figure 7-96
Iris color change in the right eye resulting from uveitis.

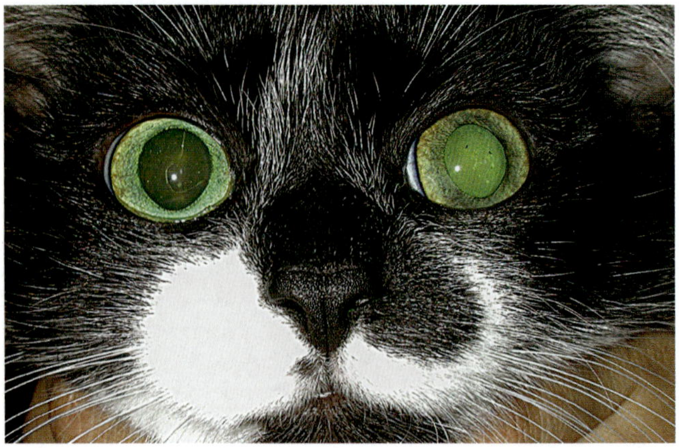

Figure 7-97
Change in color of the left iris in a cat with anterior uveitis. Endothelial keratic precipitates and mild corneal edema are also present.

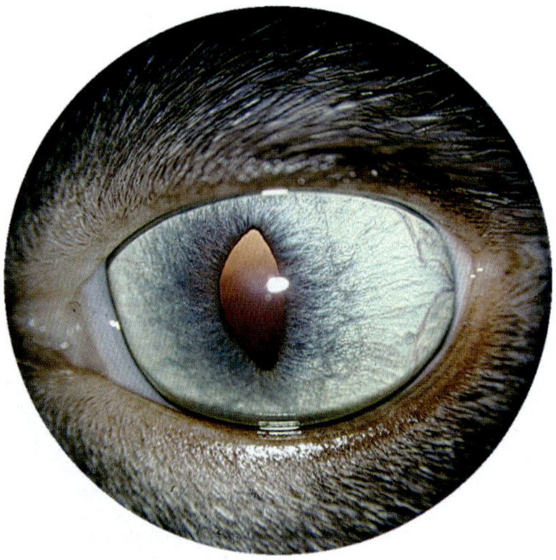

Figure 7-98
Normal iris the left eye in a cat that tested positive for feline leukemia virus.

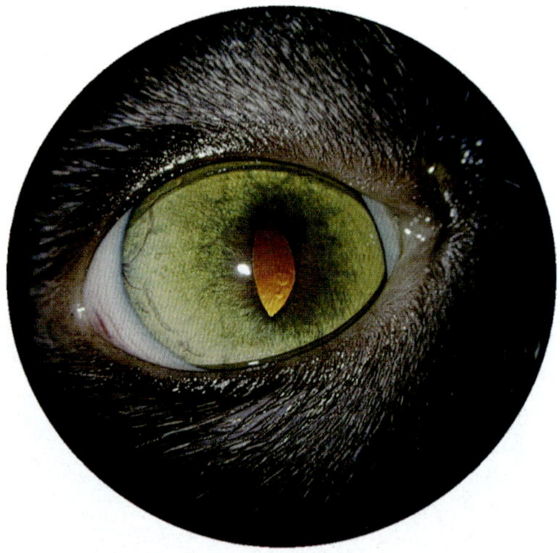

Figure 7-99
Iris color change resulting from uveitis in the right eye of the cat shown in Figure 7-98.

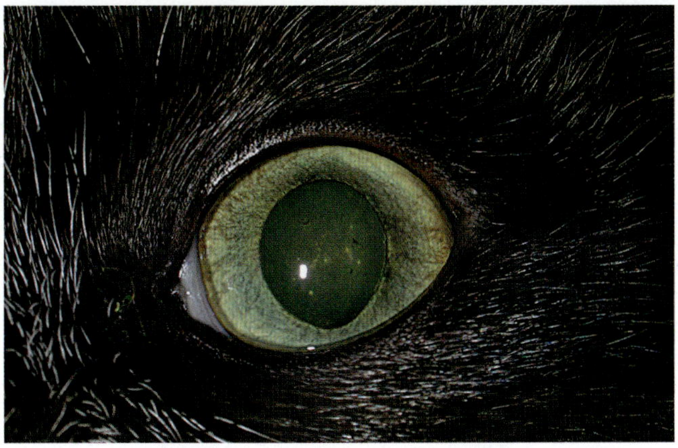

Figure 7-100
Rubeosis iridis and pigment deposits on the anterior lens capsule in a cat with chronic low-grade anterior uveitis.

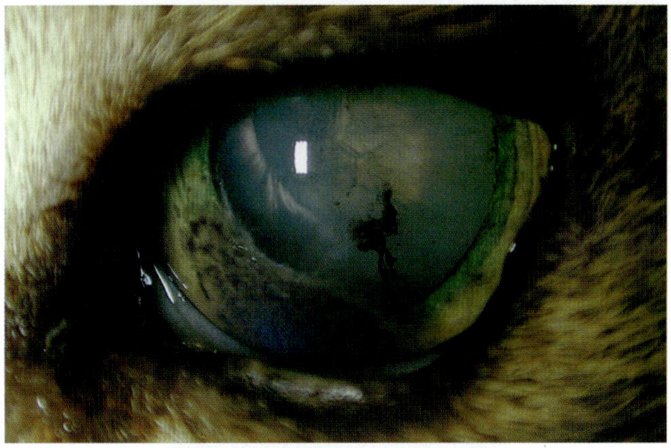

Figure 7-101
Cat with chronic uveitis. Corneal edema extends inferonasally over the area with endothelial keratic precipitates. Pigment from the posterior iris epithelium is present on the anterior lens capsule, and an immature cataract with anterior sutures is visible.

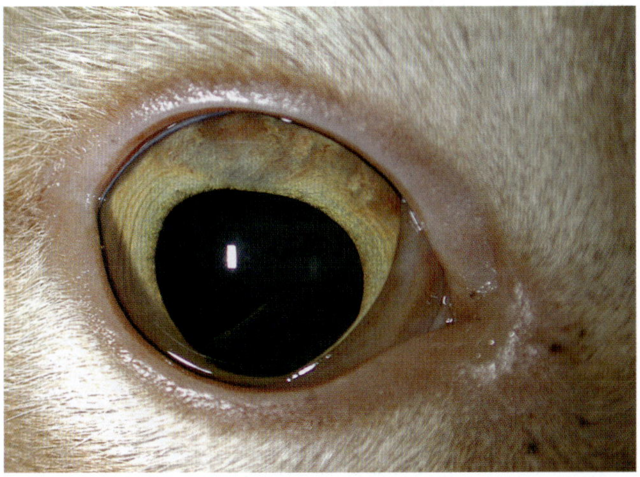

Figure 7-102
Focal idiopathic iritis in a cat.

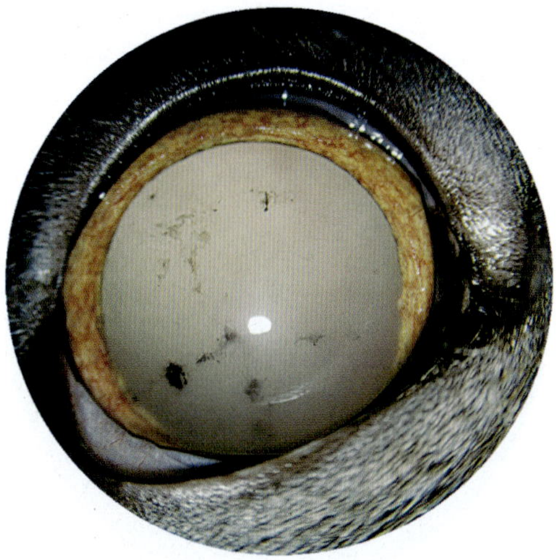

Figure 7-103
Cat with iritis, pigment deposits on the anterior lens capsule, and vitreal exudate secondary to chorioretinitis resulting from lymphosarcoma.

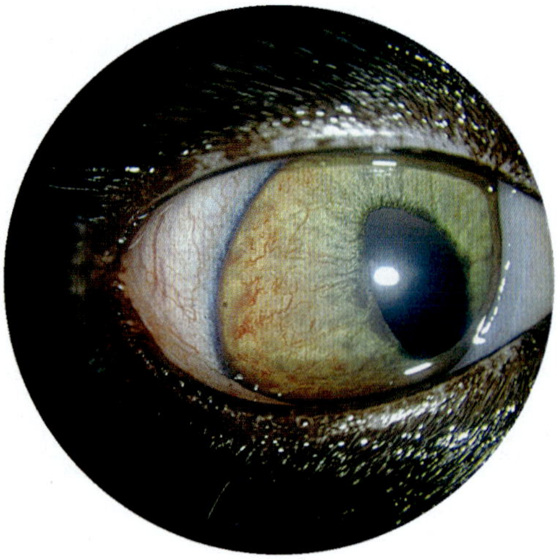

Figure 7-104
Rubeosis iridis in a cat with lymphosarcoma and feline leukemia virus infection.

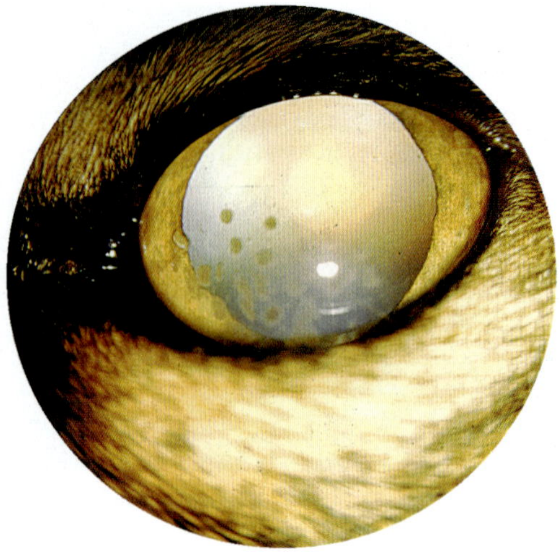

Figure 7-105
Keratic precipitates in a cat with uveitis.

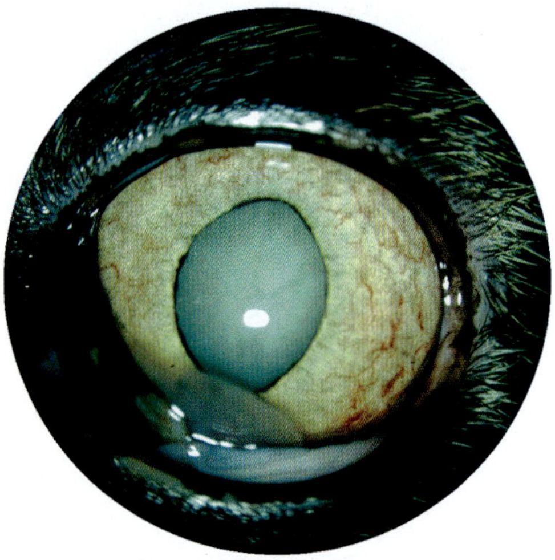

Figure 7-106
Cat with rubeosis iridis, cataract, and fibrin clot positioned inferiorly in the anterior chamber. The cat had lymphosarcoma and had tested positive for feline leukemia virus.

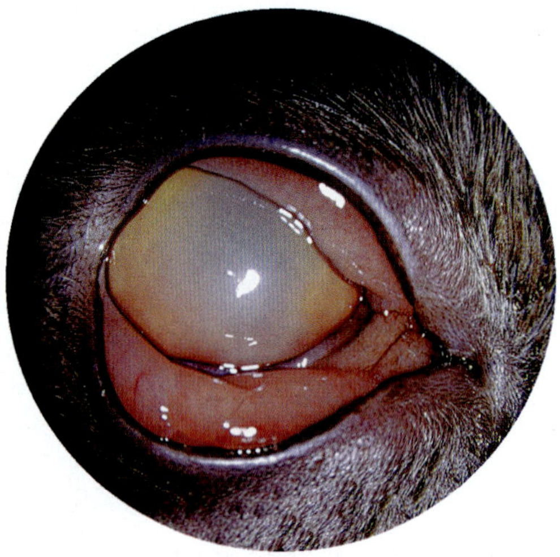

Figure 7-107
Cat with lymphosarcoma. Conjunctival infiltrates and uveitis with secondary corneal edema.

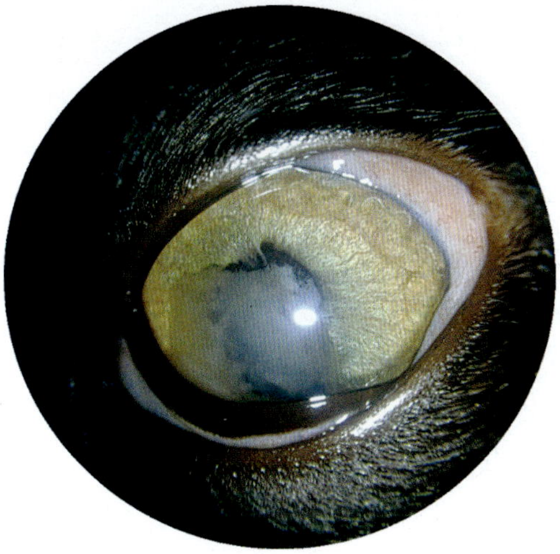

Figure 7-108
Uveitis in a cat that tested positive for feline leukemia virus. Posterior synechiae are present, as is a fibrin clot in the anterior chamber.

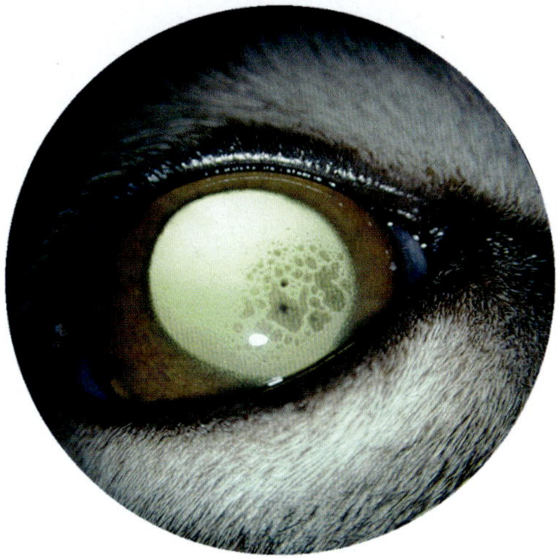

Figure 7-109
Keratic precipitates in a cat with uveitis caused by feline infectious peritonitis (FIP).

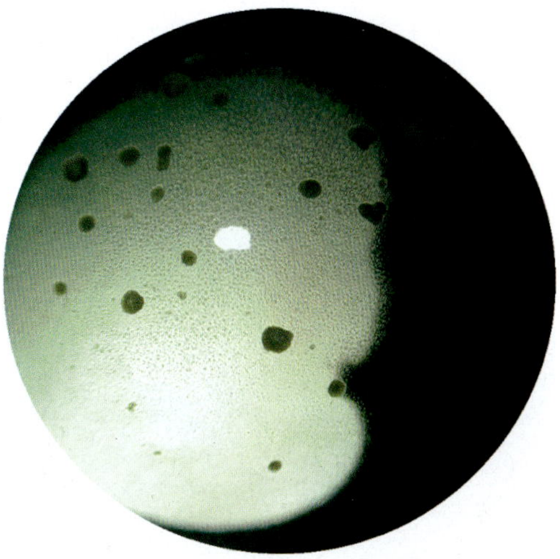

Figure 7-110
Keratic precipitates in a cat with FIP uveitis. Posterior synechiae are causing dyscoria.

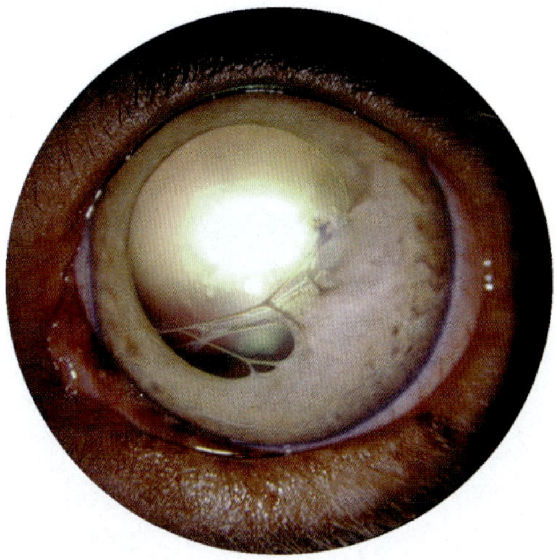

Figure 7-111
Posterior synechiae secondary to trauma in a cat.

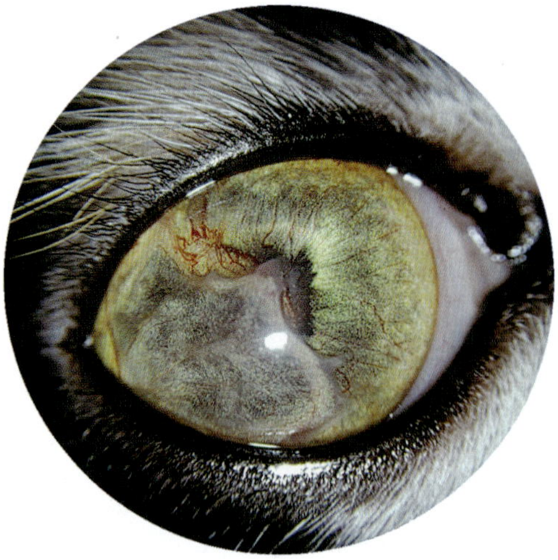

Figure 7-112
Cat with uveitis. Iris bombé, a fibrovascular membrane that extends across the iris temporally, and posterior synechiae are present. Iris bombé is the result of 360-degree posterior synechiae. Aqueous, which is formed in the posterior chamber, no longer has access through the pupil to the drainage angle. Aqueous pushes the iris forward so that it bulges into the anterior chamber.

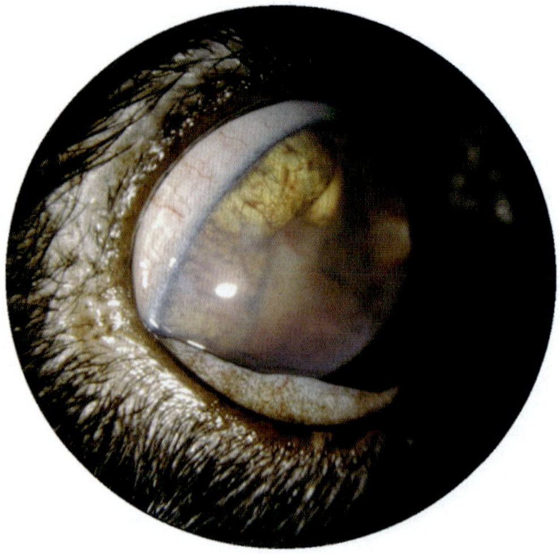

Figure 7-113
Chronic uveitis, iris bombé, fibrovascular iridal membranes, and secondary glaucoma are present in the left eye of a cat. Both eyes had chronic uveitis as a result of iatrogenic lens capsular rupture. Traumatic sarcoma was diagnosed on evisceration.

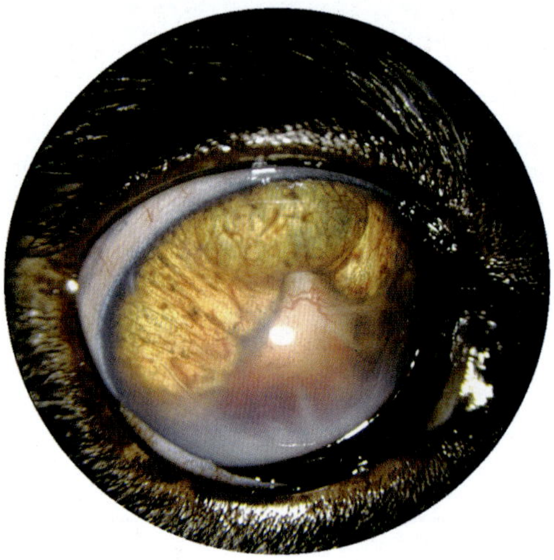

Figure 7-114
Another view of the left eye in Figure 7-113, showing chronic uveitis, iris bombé, fibrovascular iridal membranes that have grown across the pupil, and secondary glaucoma. Traumatic sarcoma was diagnosed on evisceration.

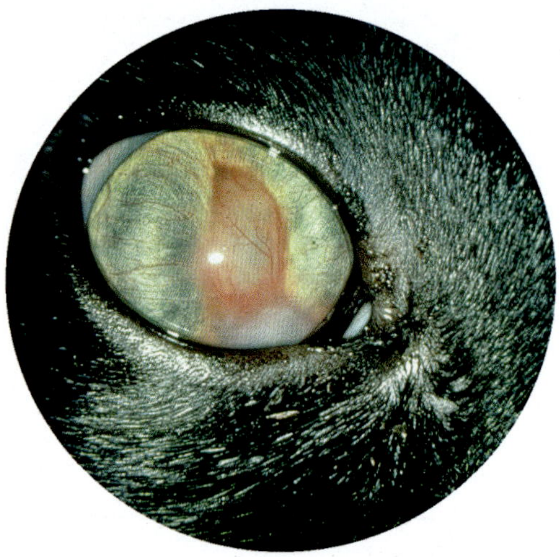

Figure 7-115
Iris bombé with vascularization of the anterior lens capsule in a cat.

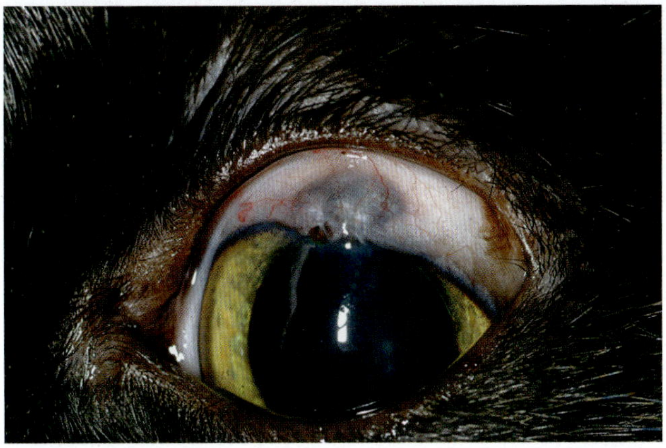

Figure 7-116
Limbal (scleral) staphyloma secondary to ocular trauma in a 3-year-old cat.

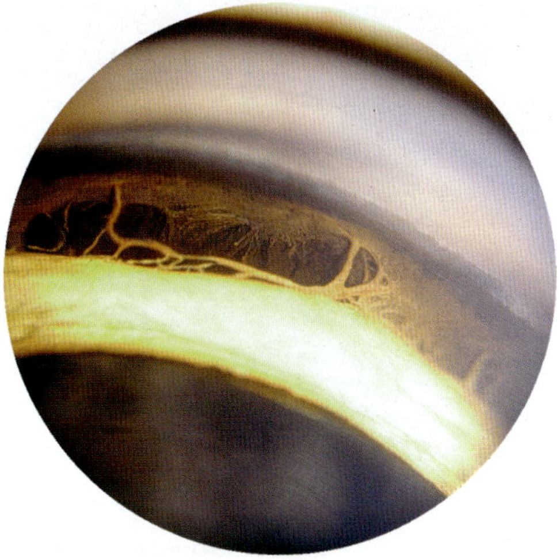

Figure 7-117
Iridodialysis—traumatic separation of the iris from the sclera at the level of the ciliary cleft—in a cat.

Chapter 8

Lens

INTRODUCTION

Most pathology that affects the lens, aside from rare congenital defects, is described as a *cataract.* A cataract is an opacity in the lens that can vary from a small defect visible only under magnification to an opacity that affects the entire lens and causes blindness. Most cataracts in dogs of any age are hereditary. Diabetic cataracts are also fairly common. Most cataracts in cats are secondary to uveitis.

Descriptions of cataracts include the location of the cataract, the causes of the cataract, and the stage of cataract development. Early, small opacities that do not interfere with vision and may not progress are referred to as *incipient.* Cataracts that are *immature* involve more of the lens and, depending on their size and location, may affect vision. When the entire lens is involved and no tapetal reflex is seen through the lens, the cataract is called *mature.* Immature and mature cataracts can liquefy, and lens proteins can leak out of the lens capsule, leading to shrinkage of the lens. At this stage the cataract is called *hypermature.*

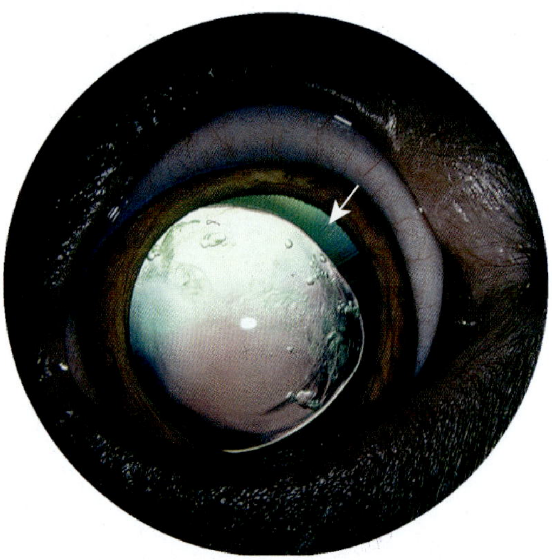

Figure 8-1
Microphakia and cataract in a Labrador retriever. Zonules are seen nasally.

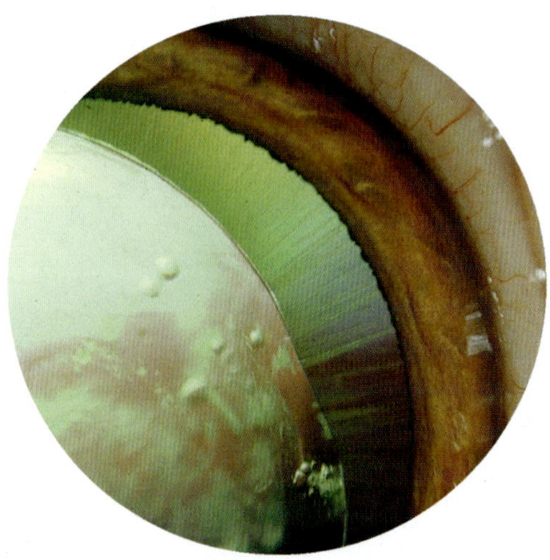

Figure 8-2
Close-up of Figure 8-1 that shows intact zonules nasally in a Labrador retriever.

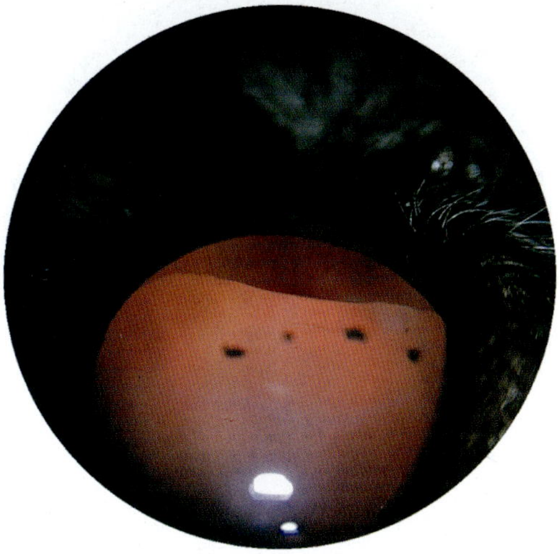

Figure 8-3
Lens coloboma and microphakia. A lens coloboma is a congenitally missing section of lens and often zonules. Here the coloboma is visible as a malformed lens equator in the superior sector.

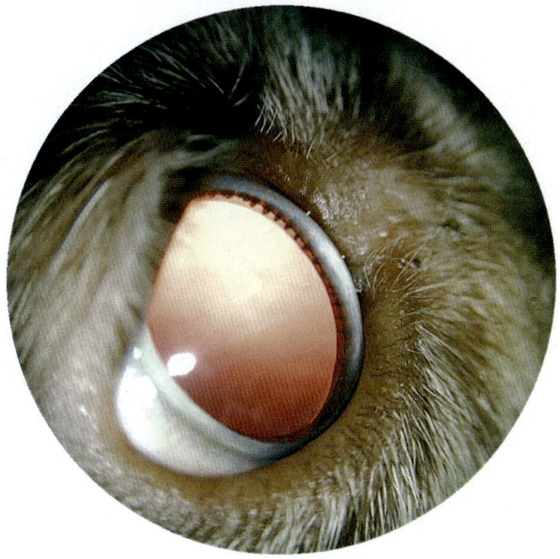

Figure 8-4
Microphakia in an Australian shepherd. Stretched ciliary processes can be seen.

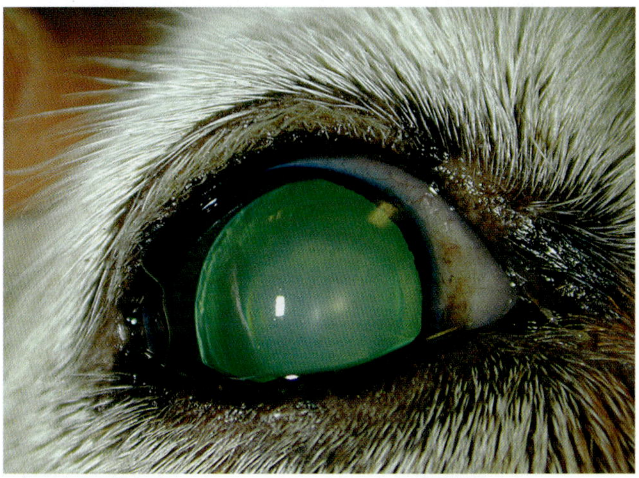

Figure 8-5
Nuclear sclerosis. The nucleus of the lens becomes sclerotic with age and is visible as a circular area of "frosted glass" inside the "clear glass" of the lens equator. No visual impairment occurs in animals.

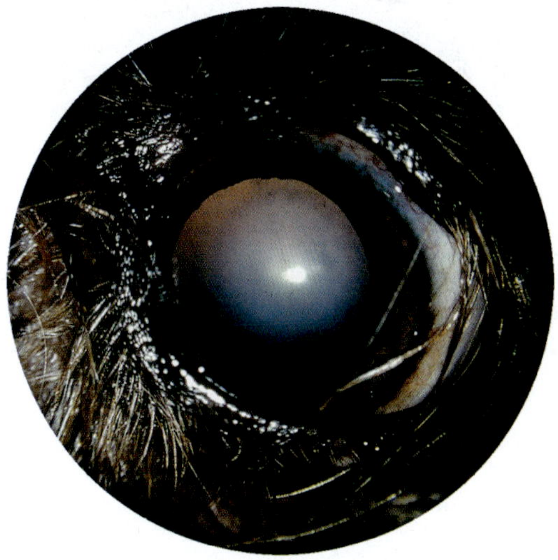

Figure 8-6
Nuclear sclerosis.

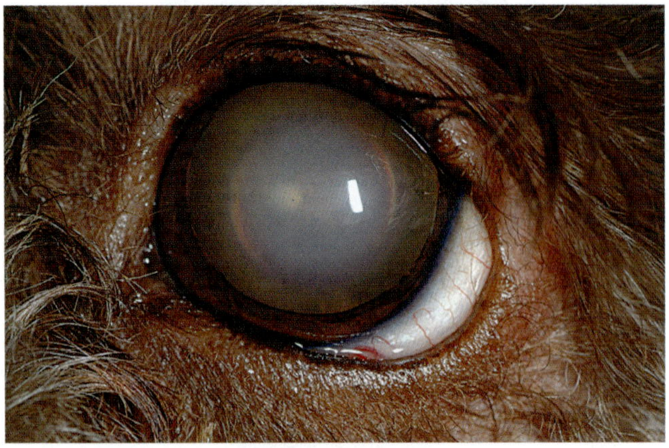

Figure 8-7
Nuclear sclerosis.

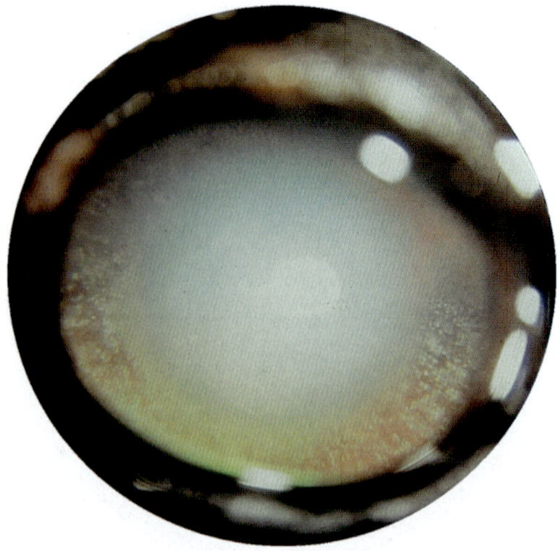

Figure 8-8
Nuclear sclerosis and asteroid hyalosis. Asteroid hyalosis produces "stars" in the vitreous—calcium-lipid complexes that do not interfere with vision.

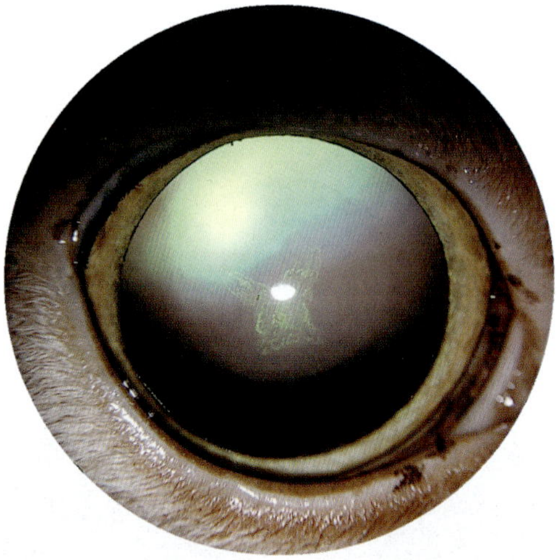

Figure 8-9
Incipient posterior cortical cataract in a cat.

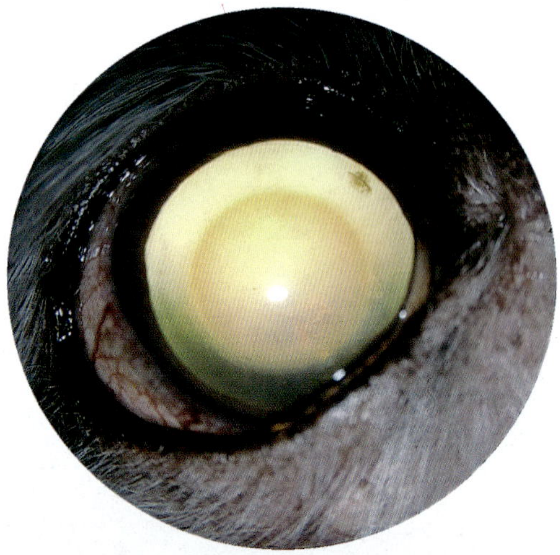

Figure 8-10
Nuclear sclerosis with focal anterior cortical cataracts.

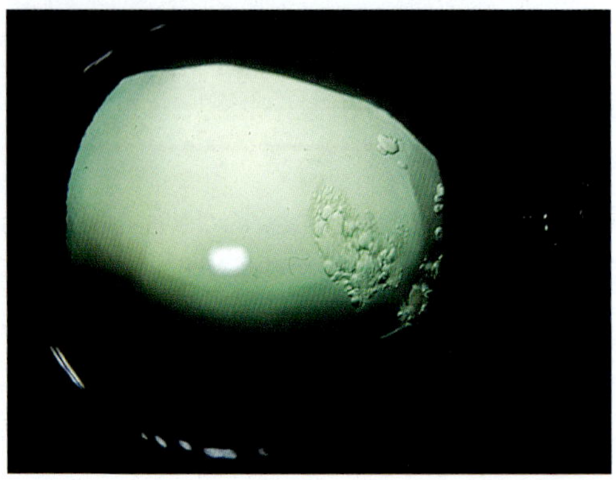

Figure 8-11
Peripheral vacuolar cataracts.

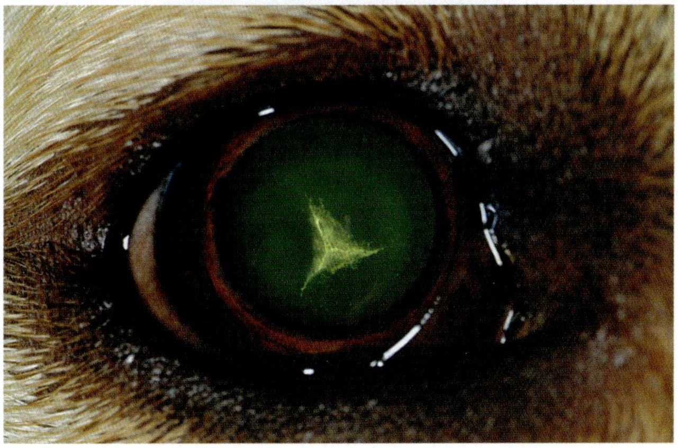

Figure 8-12
Posterior Y-suture cataract in a golden retriever.

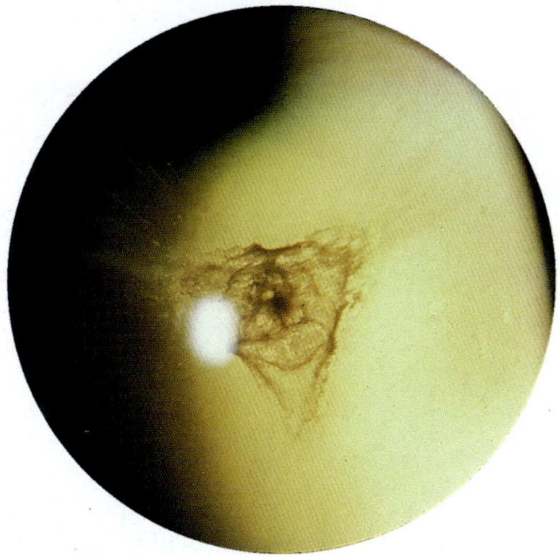

Figure 8-13
Posterior polar Y-suture cataract in a retriever.

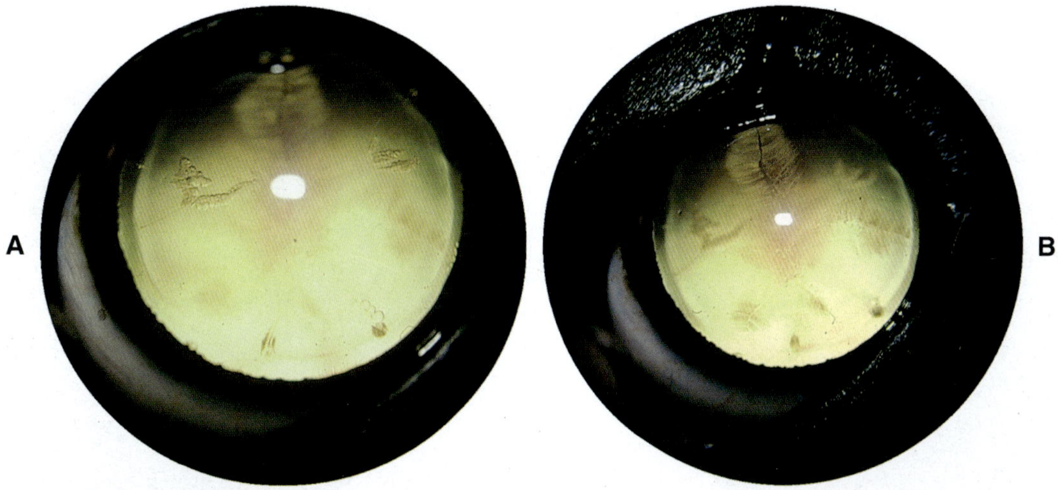

Figure 8-14 A-B
Incipient anterior and posterior cortical cataracts in a standard poodle. **A,** The anterior cataracts in focus. **B,** Feathering of the posterior Y sutures in focus.

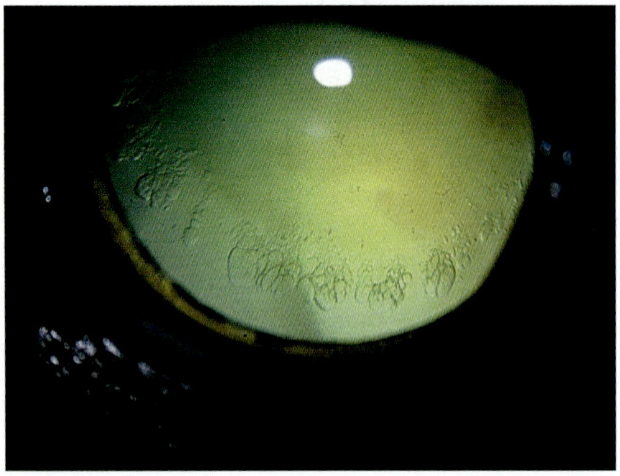

Figure 8-15
Incipient cataracts (vacuoles) positioned equatorially in a dog with hypertensive retinopathy.

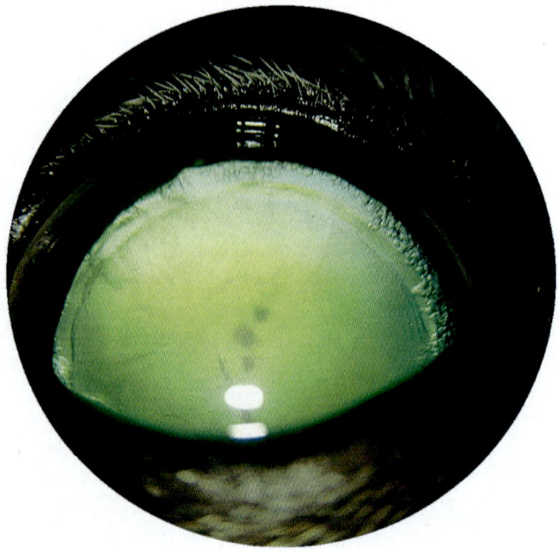

Figure 8-16
Diffuse posterior cataracts with peripheral equatorial vacuoles in a dog with diabetes mellitus.

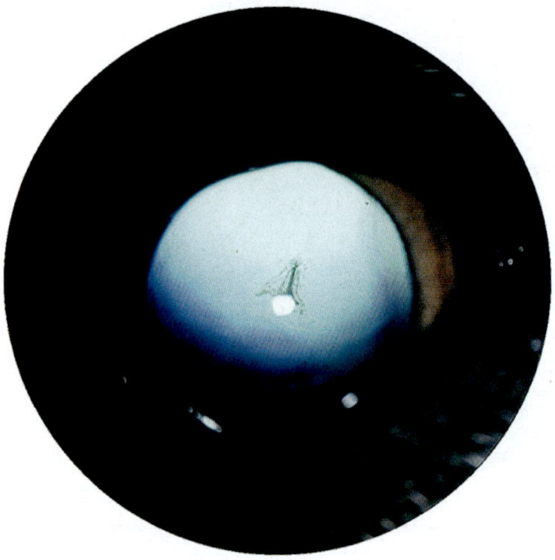

Figure 8-17
Incipient posterior polar, Y-suture cataract in a rottweiler.

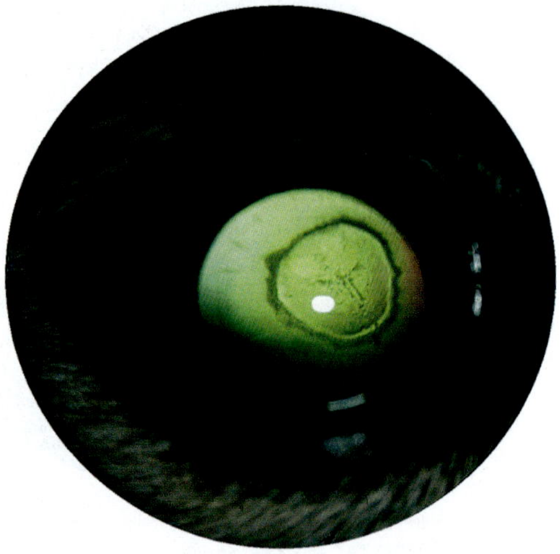

Figure 8-18
Nuclear cataract caused by a milk supplement that was given when this dog was a puppy.

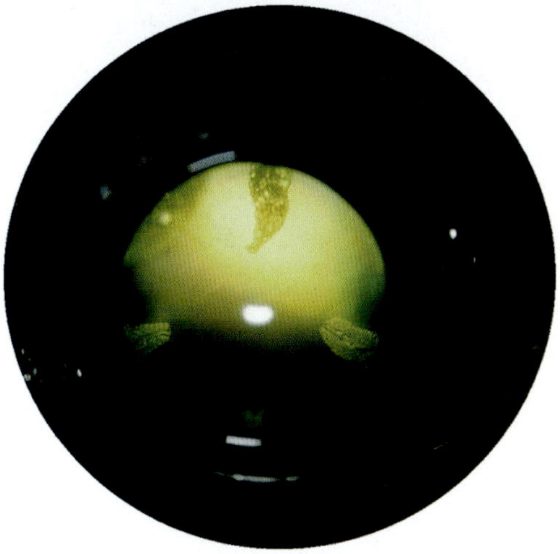

Figure 8-19
Incipient cataract in the lens periphery associated with progressive retinal atrophy (PRA) in a dog.

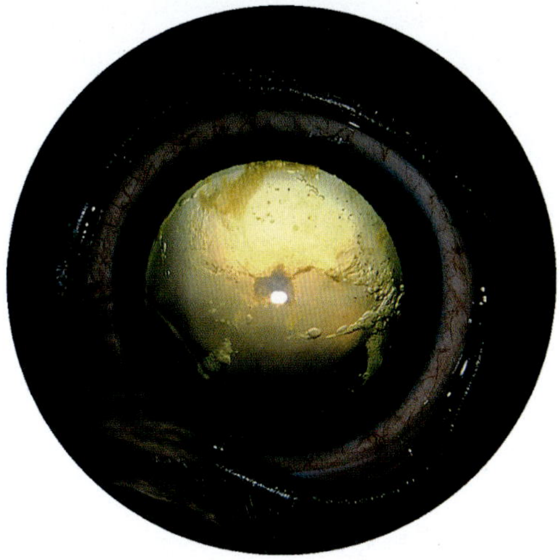

Figure 8-20
Incipient cortical cataract associated with PRA in a dog.

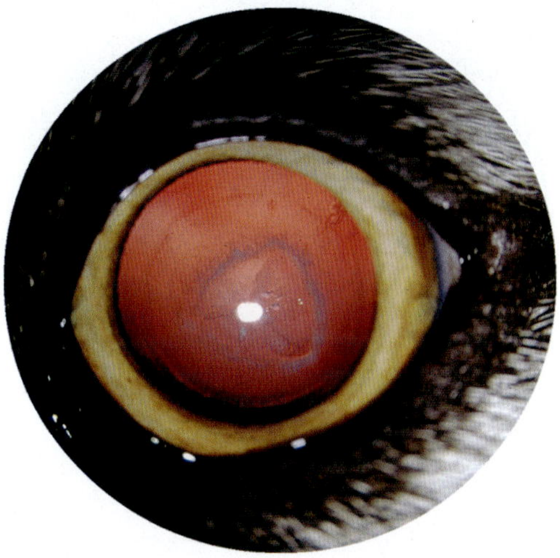

Figure 8-21
Posterior axial cortical cataract in a Siberian husky.

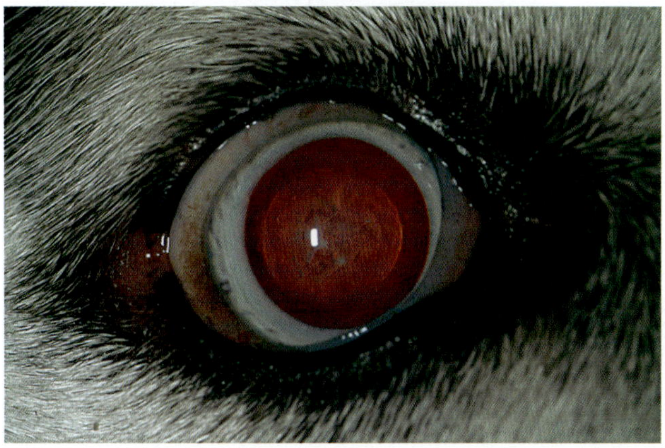

Figure 8-22
Nuclear and posterior subcapsular cataract in a 7-year-old Siberian husky.

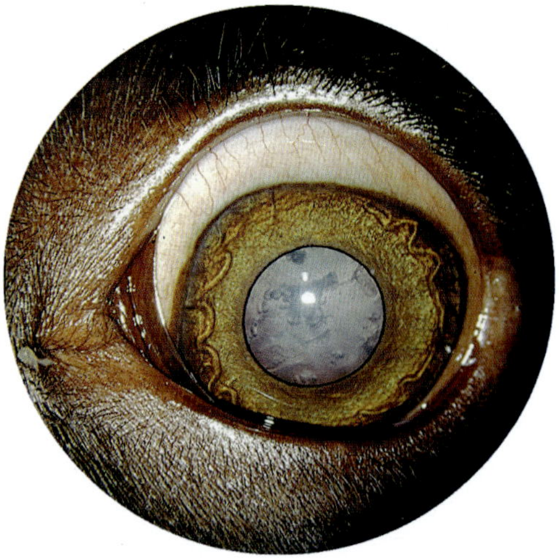

Figure 8-23
Immature cataract.

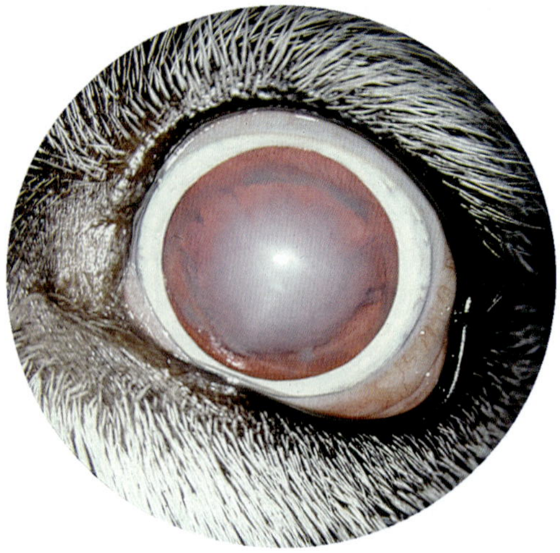

Figure 8-24
Immature cataract in a Siberian husky.

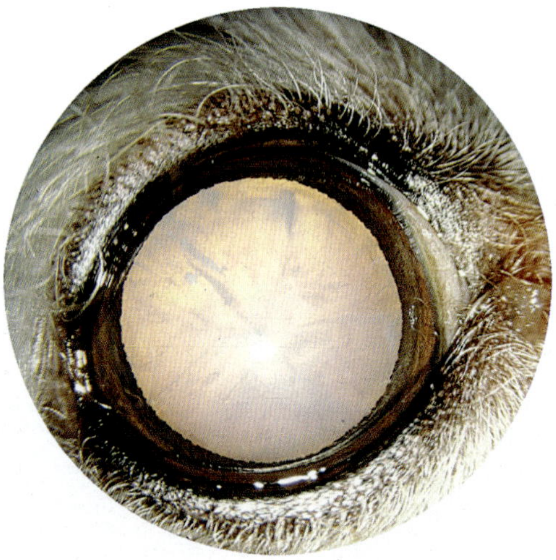

Figure 8-25
Immature cataract in a miniature poodle.

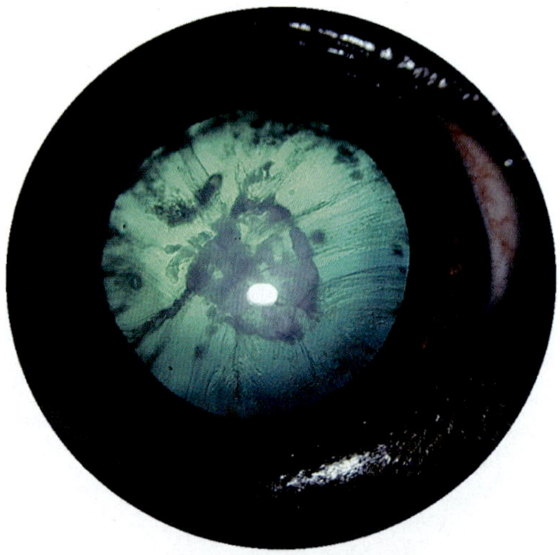

Figure 8-26
Immature cataract in a 2-year-old Boston terrier.

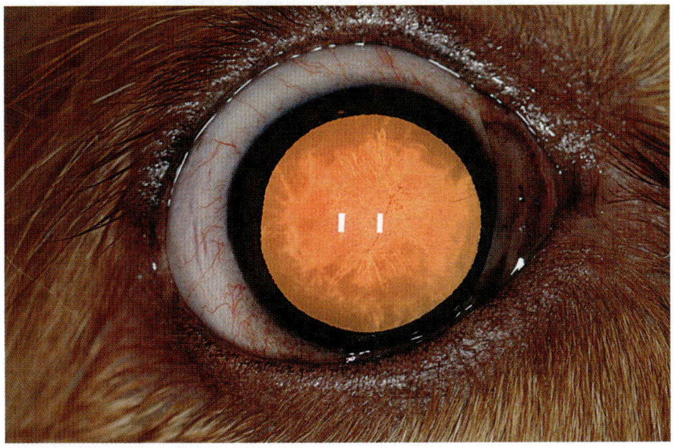

Figure 8-27
Immature anterior and posterior cortical opacities in a 4-year-old cocker spaniel.

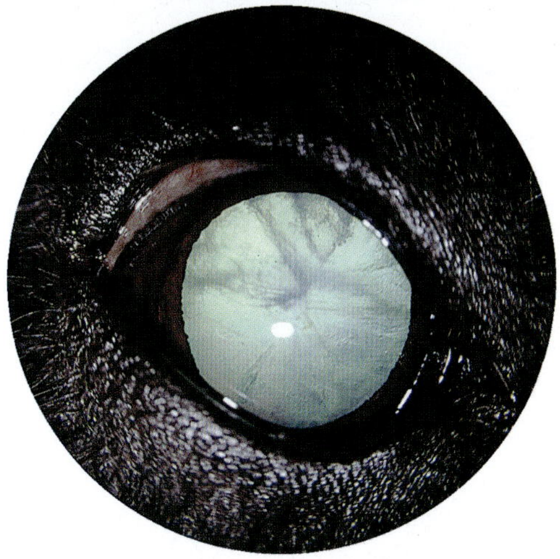

Figure 8-28
Immature cataract in a miniature schnauzer.

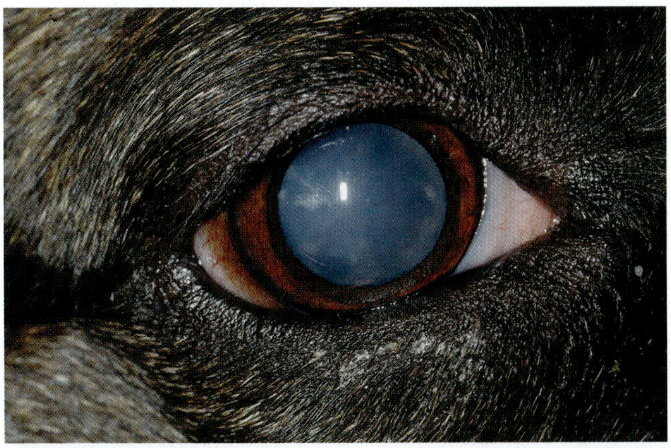

Figure 8-29
Immature cataract in a 6-year-old Boston terrier.

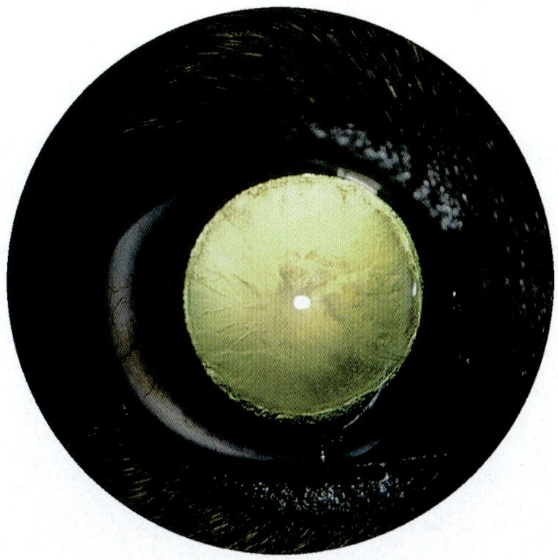

Figure 8-30
Immature cataract in a 3-year-old Afghan hound.

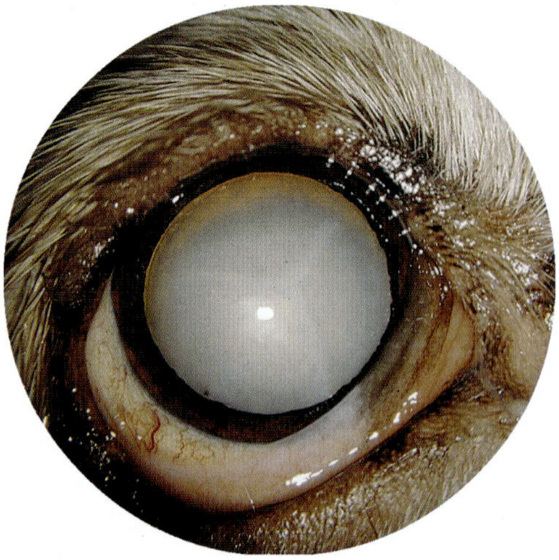

Figure 8-31
Immature cataract and nuclear sclerosis in a poodle. Note the prominent anterior suture lines.

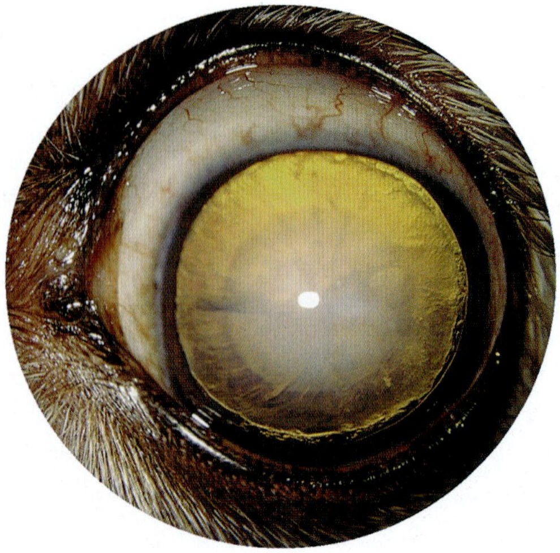

Figure 8-32
Immature cataract and nuclear sclerosis.

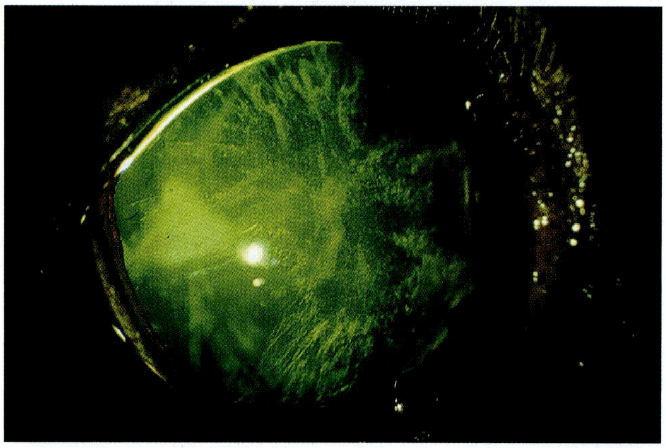

Figure 8-33
Incipient-to-immature cataract in a miniature poodle with PRA.

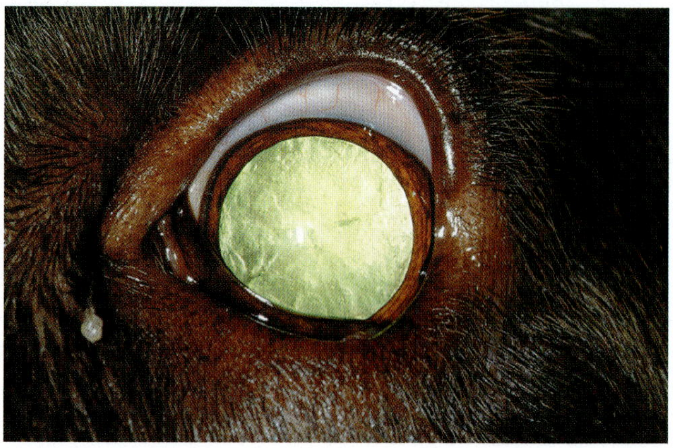

Figure 8-34
Incipient cortical cataract associated with PRA in a 5-year-old Labrador retriever. Note the brightness of the tapetal reflex—the result of retinal thinning.

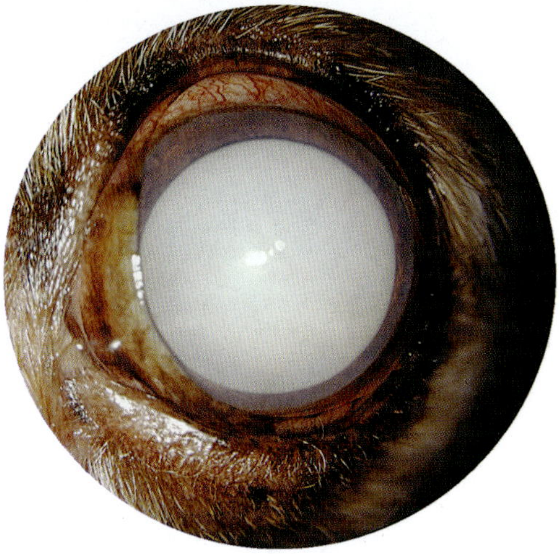

Figure 8-35
Mature cataract, "red eye," and corneal edema. Leakage of lens protein from a cataractous lens can cause lens-induced uveitis, because lens proteins are perceived as foreign substances.

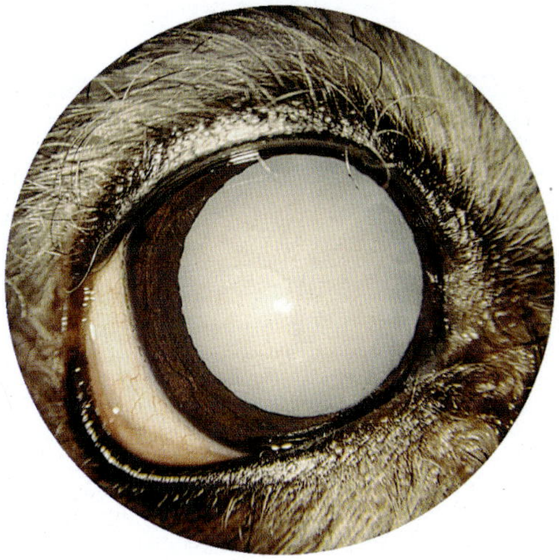

Figure 8-36
Mature cataract.

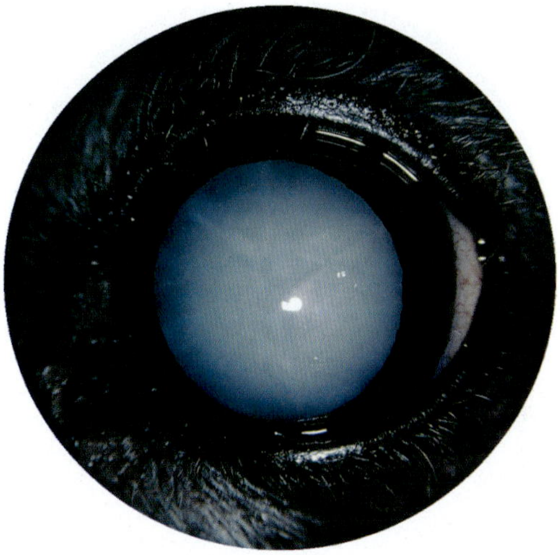

Figure 8-37
Mature cataract.

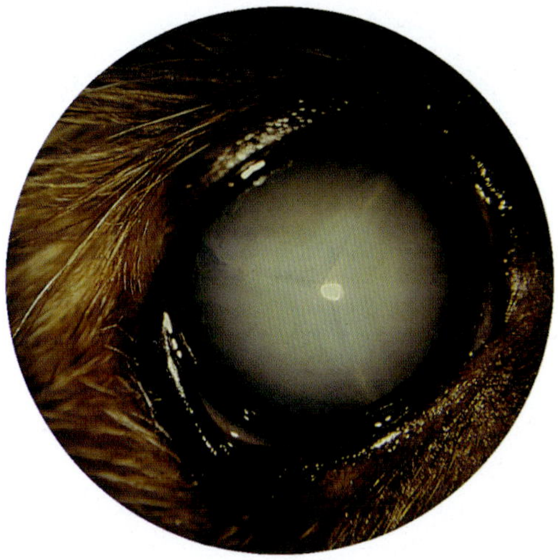

Figure 8-38
Mature cataract with prominent anterior Y sutures. Suture lines are formed where rows of lens fibers meet.

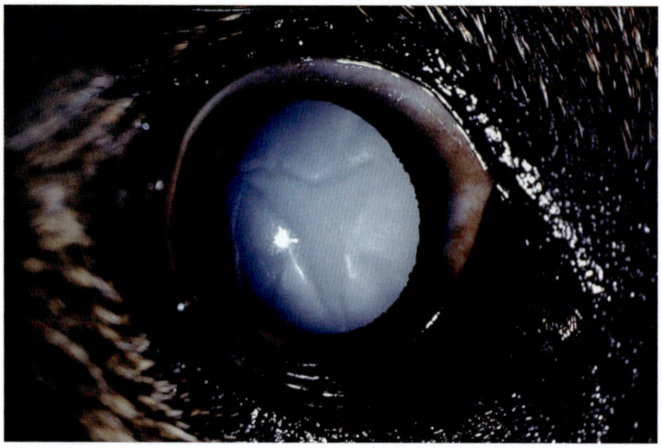

Figure 8-39
Intumescent diabetic cataract. Lens fibers separate at the anterior Y sutures.

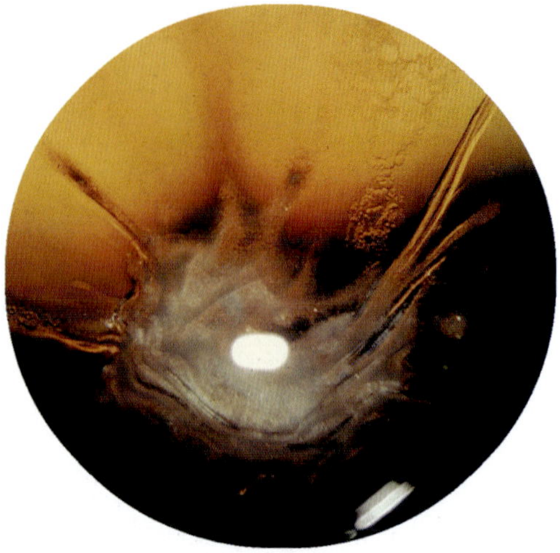

Figure 8-40
Hypermature cataract. The lens capsule is wrinkling, and most of the lens has disappeared.

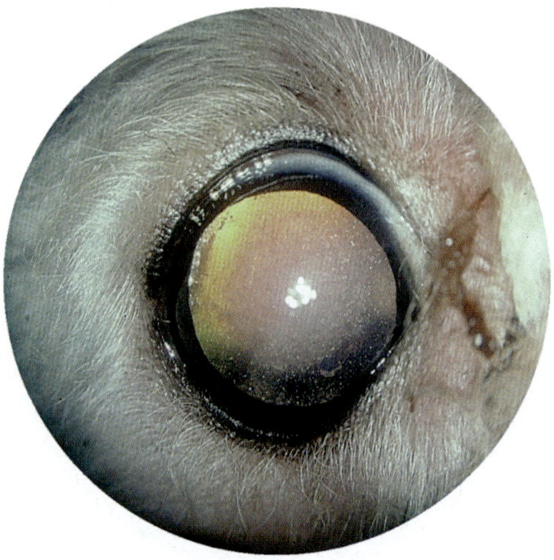

Figure 8-41
Hypermature cataract with liquefaction of much of the lens.

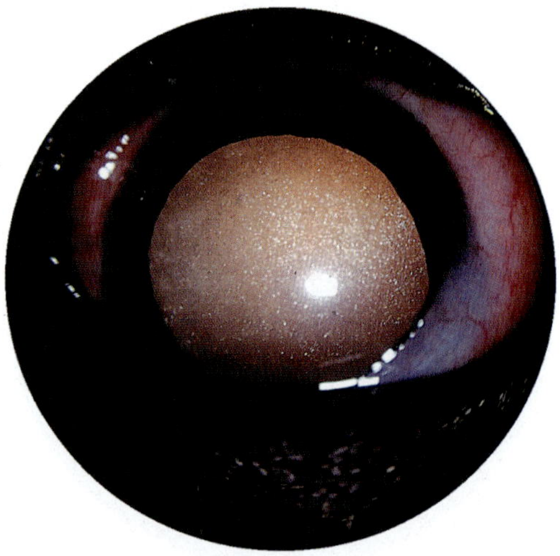

Figure 8-42
Hypermature cataract with liquefaction of much of the lens.

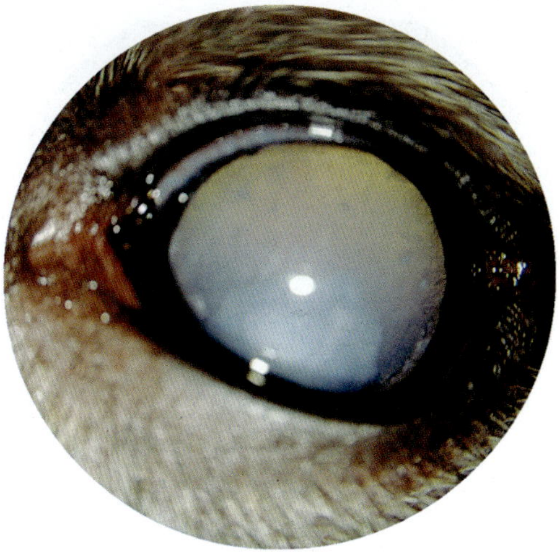

Figure 8-43
Morgagnian cataract in a keeshond. Much of the lens has been resorbed, the remaining cortex is liquefied, and the nucleus has dropped inferiorly in the lens. Pigment is present on the anterior lens capsule.

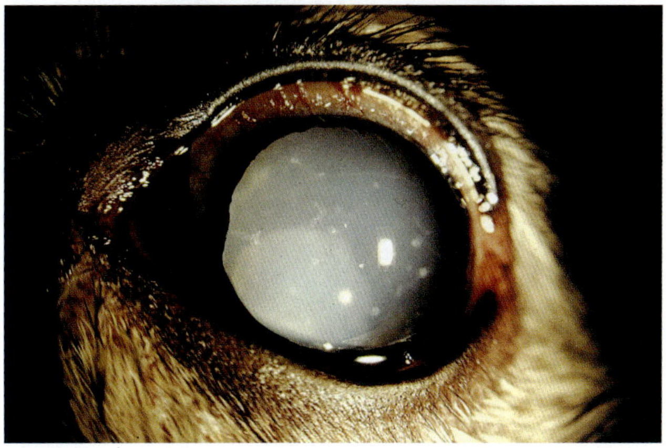

Figure 8-44
Morgagnian cataract.

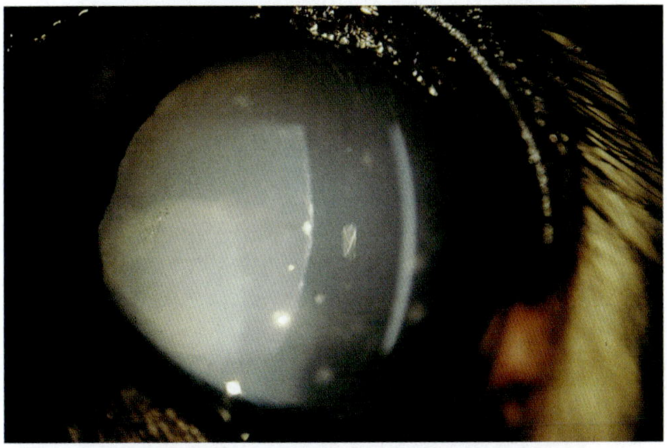

Figure 8-45
Slit lamp photograph of a Morgagnian cataract.

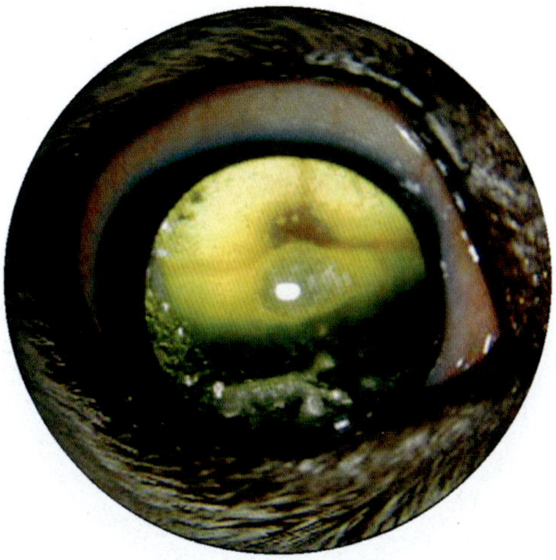

Figure 8-46
Hypermature cataract with wrinkling of the capsule in a poodle.

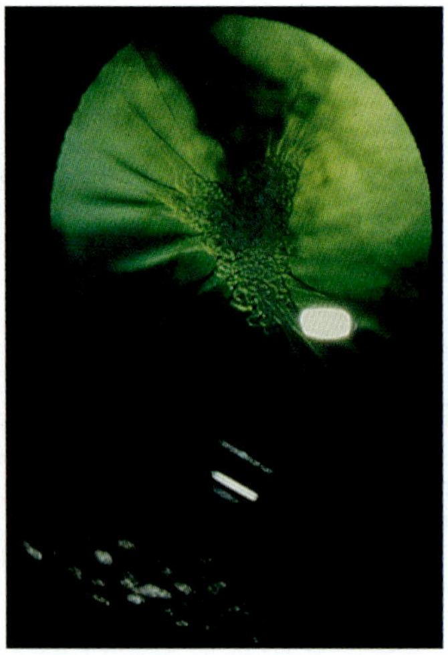

Figure 8-47
Hypermature cataract with wrinkling of the capsule.

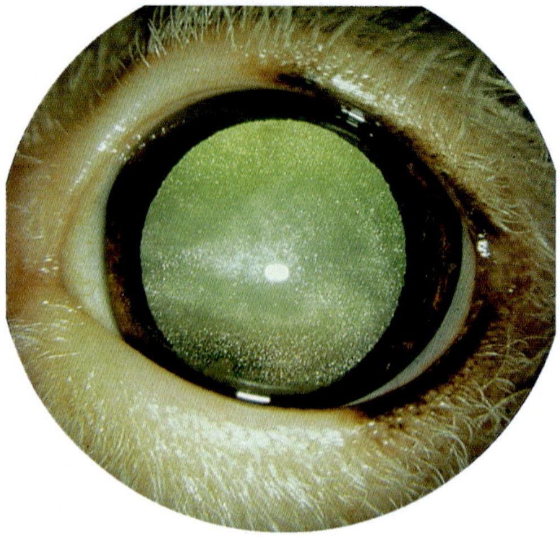

Figure 8-48
Hypermature cataract with liquefaction of the cortex.
(Courtesy Dr. Robert Playter.)

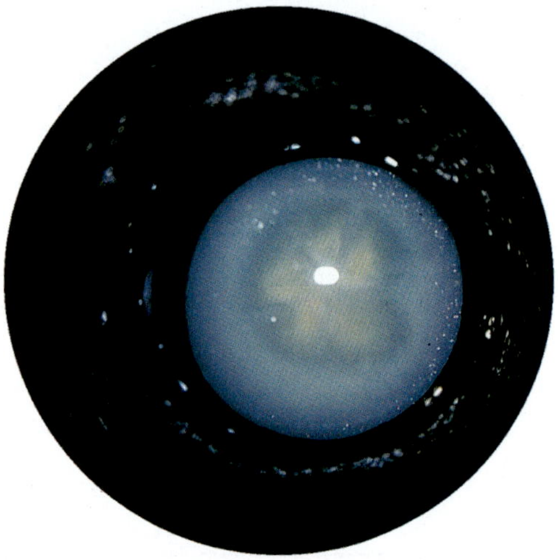

Figure 8-49
Hypermature cataract. The nucleus is visible in the center of the liquefied cortex.

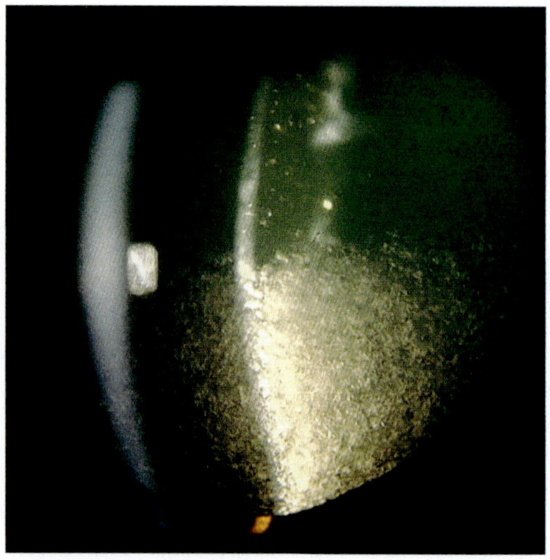

Figure 8-50
Slit lamp photograph of a liquefied, hypermature cataract.

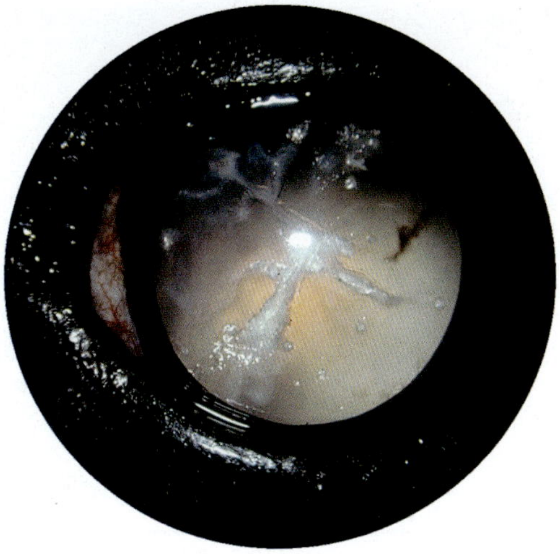

Figure 8-51
Hypermature cataract, glaucoma, and retinal detachment in a poodle. Lens-induced uveitis can lead to secondary glaucoma, especially in a predisposed animal. As the lens shrinks, vitreous moves anteriorly, possibly resulting in a retinal tear and detachment.

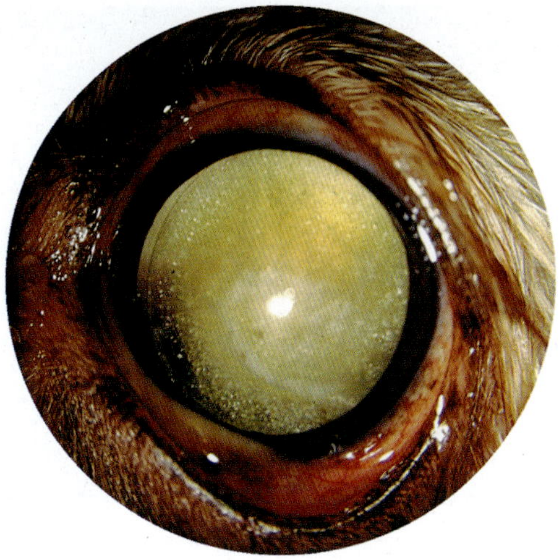

Figure 8-52
Hypermature cataract in a dog.

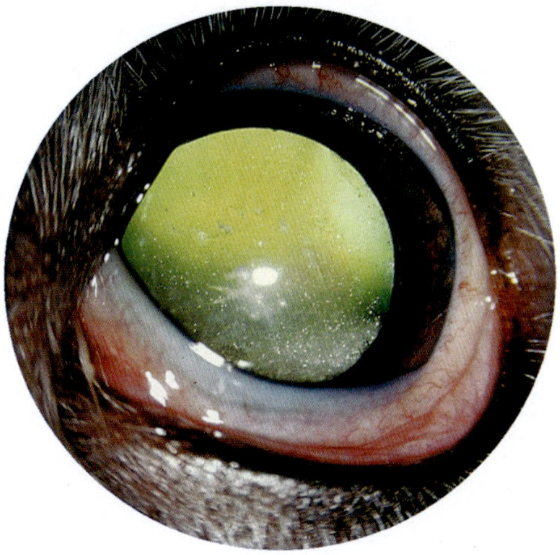

Figure 8-53
Hypermature cataract in a dog.

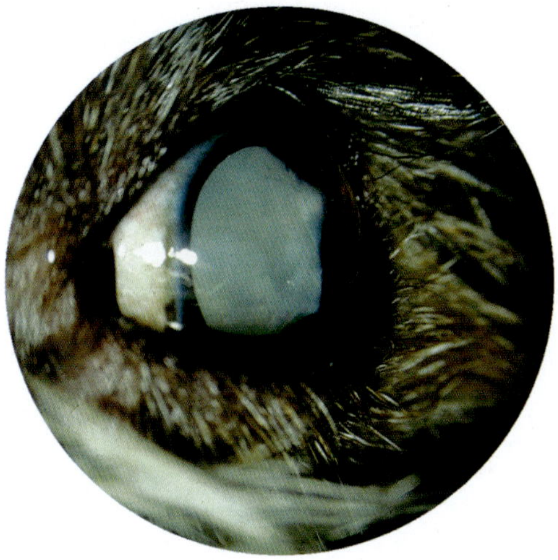

Figure 8-54
Hypermature cataract with a change in the smooth contour of the anterior lens capsule associated with leakage of lens protein into the surrounding media.

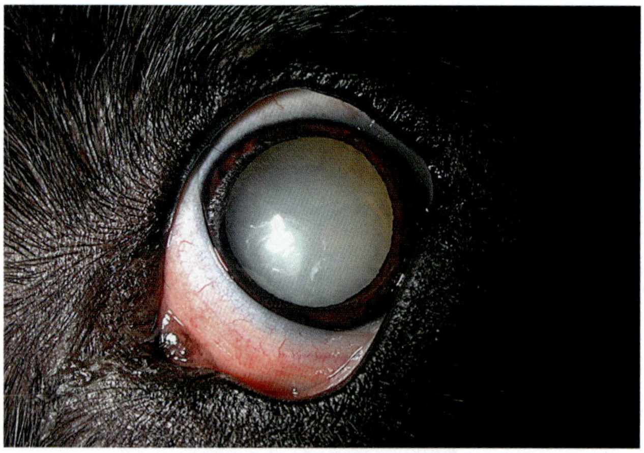

Figure 8-55
Distichia, ectropion, and a mature cataract in a Saint Bernard.

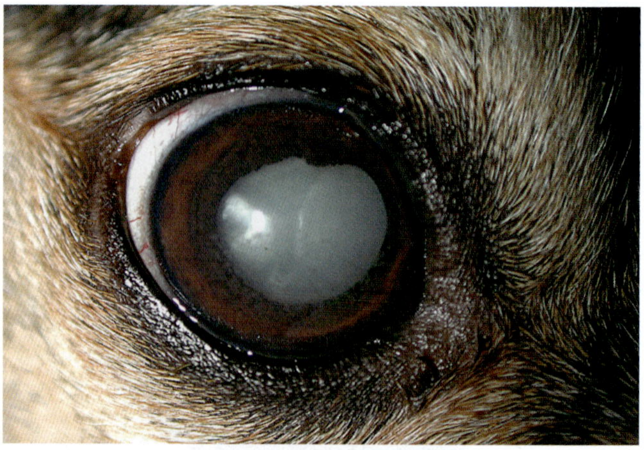

Figure 8-56
Cataract and lens-induced uveitis in a German shepherd dog. Note the mature cataract, keratic precipitates on the corneal endothelium, and posterior synechiae.

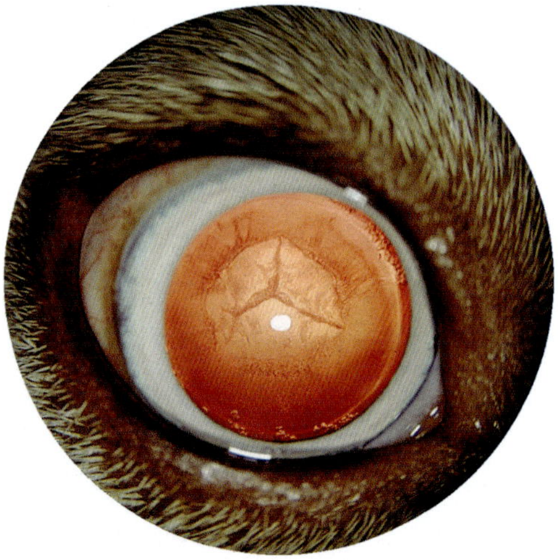

Figure 8-57
Incipient cataract in a cat. The red reflex is from a subalbinotic fundus.

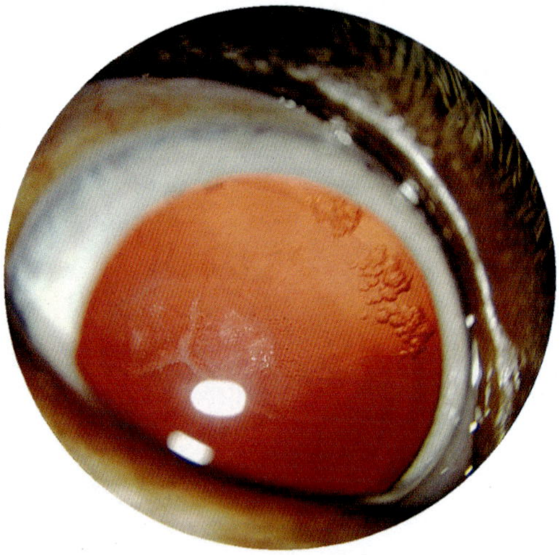

Figure 8-58
Incipient suture line cataract and equatorial vacuoles in the cat shown in Figure 8-57.

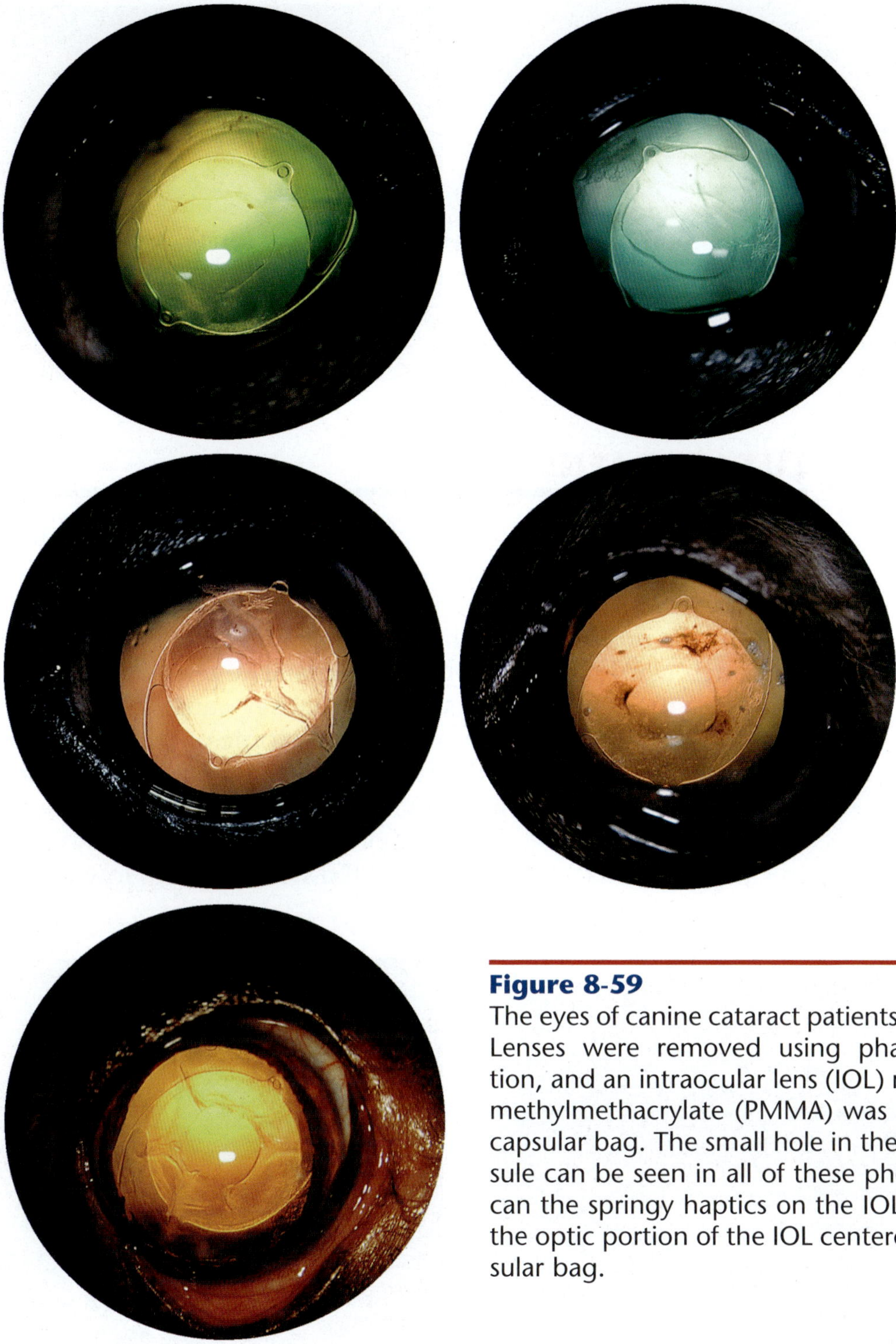

Figure 8-59
The eyes of canine cataract patients after surgery. Lenses were removed using phacoemulsification, and an intraocular lens (IOL) made of polymethylmethacrylate (PMMA) was placed in the capsular bag. The small hole in the anterior capsule can be seen in all of these photographs, as can the springy haptics on the IOL, which keep the optic portion of the IOL centered in the capsular bag.

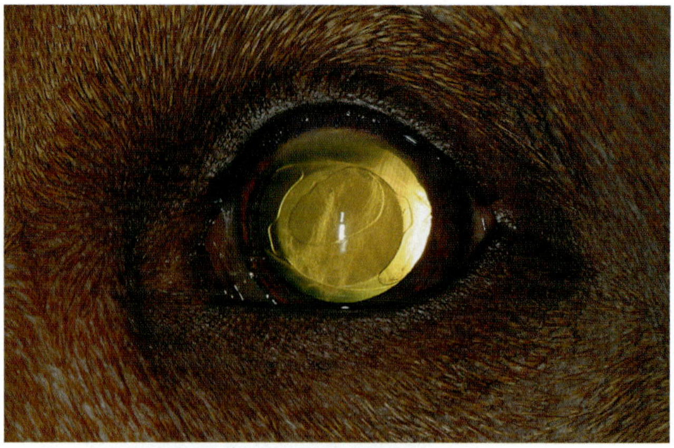

Figure 8-60
Close-up of an IOL 1 week after surgery in a dog.

LUXATED LENS

Luxated lenses occur when the zonules, which hold the lens in place, break down and allow the lens to move from its normal position. The lens can move anteriorly to the iris; this is called an *anterior luxation*. With the lens in this position, pupillary block glaucoma can occur and endothelial touch causes central corneal edema. The lens can luxate posteriorly into the vitreous and, if it stays there, may cause minimal problems or could lead to retinal detachment. If only some of the zonules break down, the lens shifts slightly and vitreous can be seen in the anterior chamber. Many luxations seen in dogs are hereditary. Luxation secondary to buphthalmia and stretching and breaking of the zonules is also common. In cats, luxations are often associated with chronic low-grade uveitis.

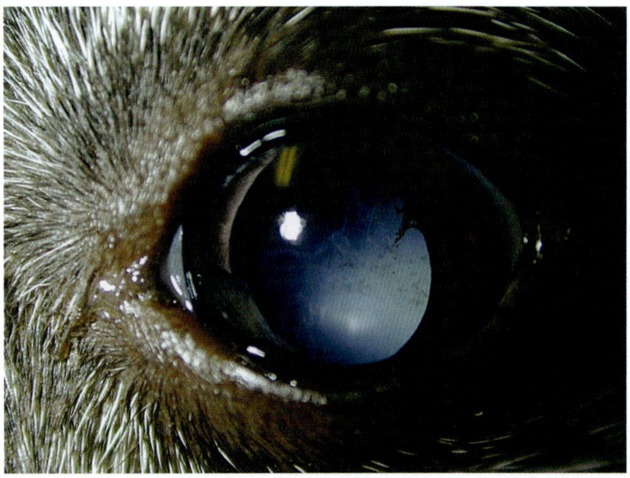

Figure 8-61
Lens subluxation in a fox terrier. White wisps of vitreous are present in the anterior chamber. A focal posterior synechia adheres to the anterior lens capsule at the 2 o'clock position.

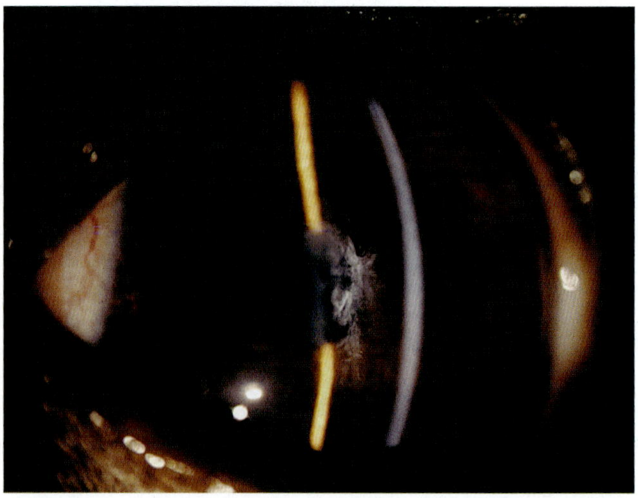

Figure 8-62
Slit lamp photograph of vitreous in the anterior chamber because of a subluxated lens. The vitreous is visible as white fibrils in the anterior chamber.

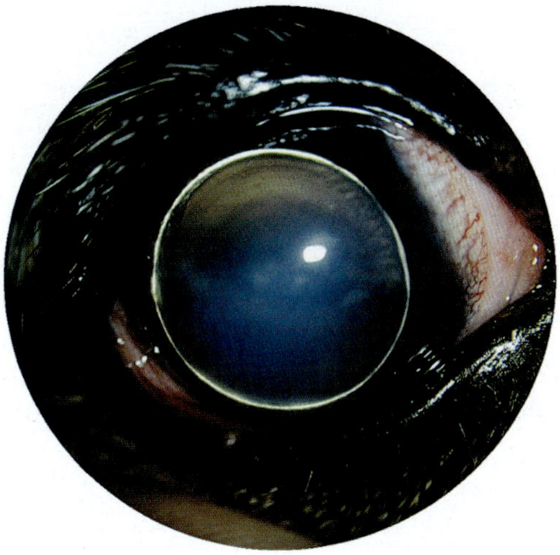

Figure 8-63
Anteriorly luxated lens.

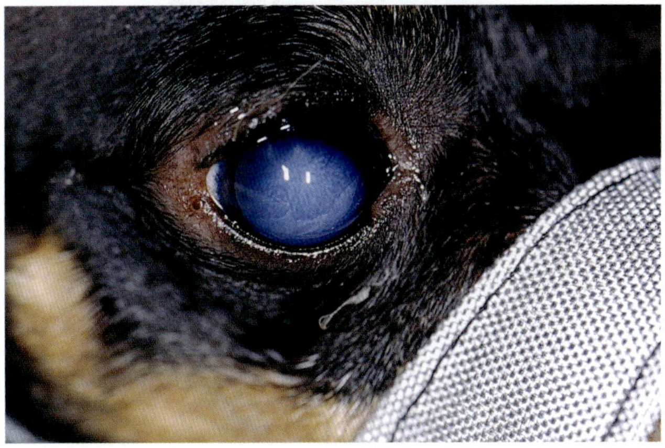

Figure 8-64
Anteriorly luxated lens. The edge of the lens appears temporally. Focal corneal edema is the result of endothelial touch by the lens.

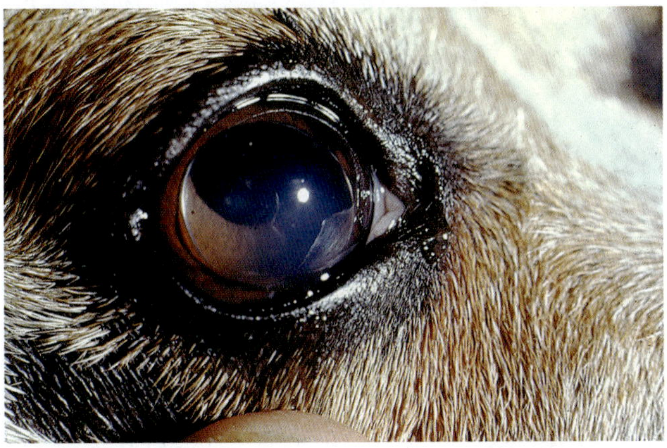

Figure 8-65
Anteriorly luxated lens.
(Courtesy Dr. Robert Playter.)

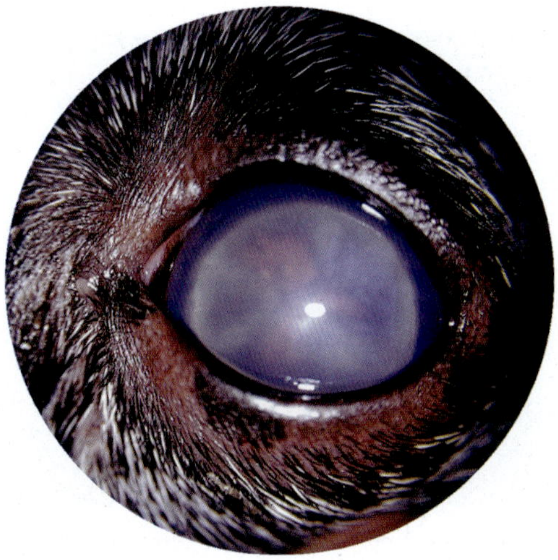

Figure 8-66
Anteriorly luxated, cataractous lens.

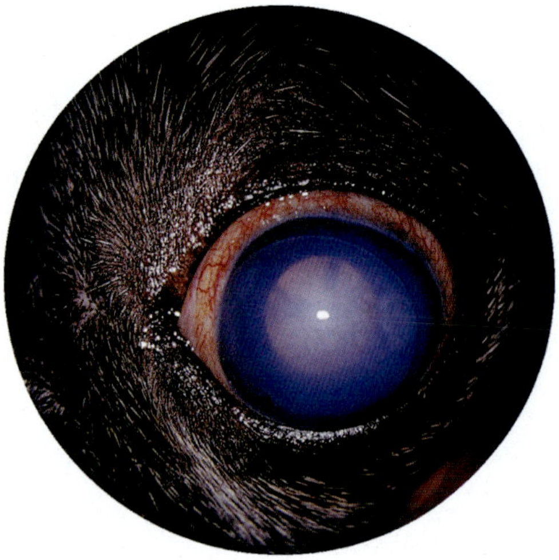

Figure 8-67
Anteriorly luxated, cataractous lens. "Red" eye is the result of glaucoma.

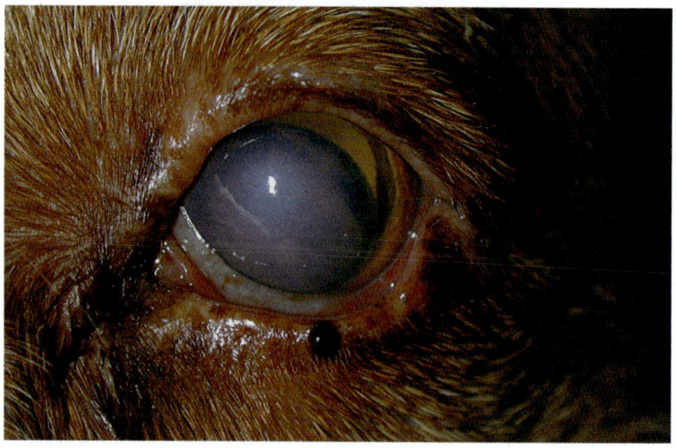

Figure 8-68
Anteriorly luxated lens with central corneal edema in a golden retriever.

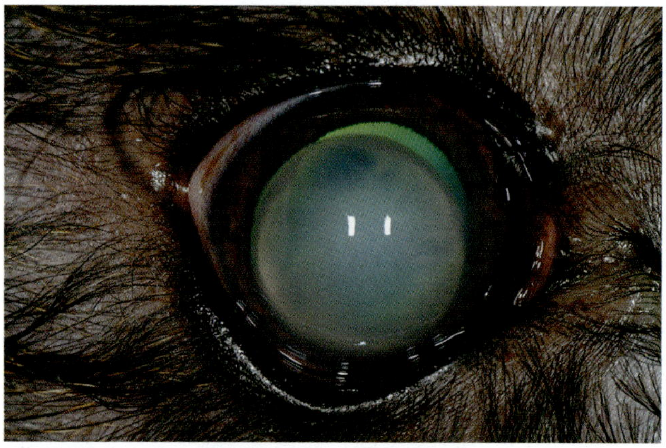

Figure 8-69
Lens luxation with secondary glaucoma in a mixed-breed dog.

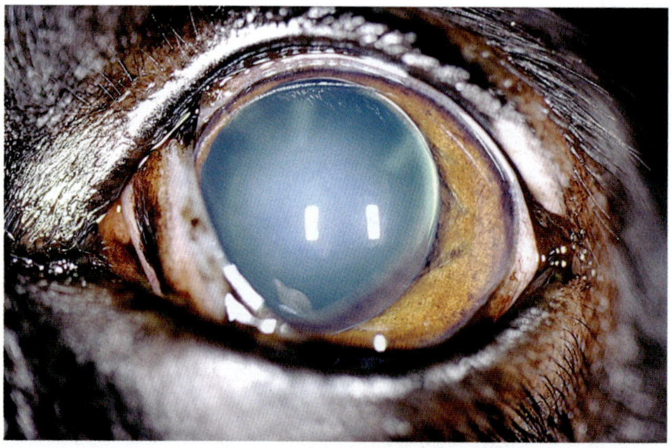

Figure 8-70
Anterior lens luxation and mild corneal edema occurring centrally in a dog.

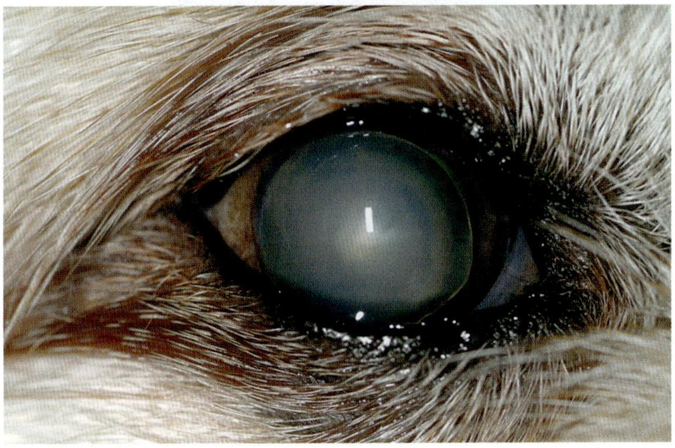

Figure 8-71
Anterior lens luxation in a 4-year-old fox terrier.

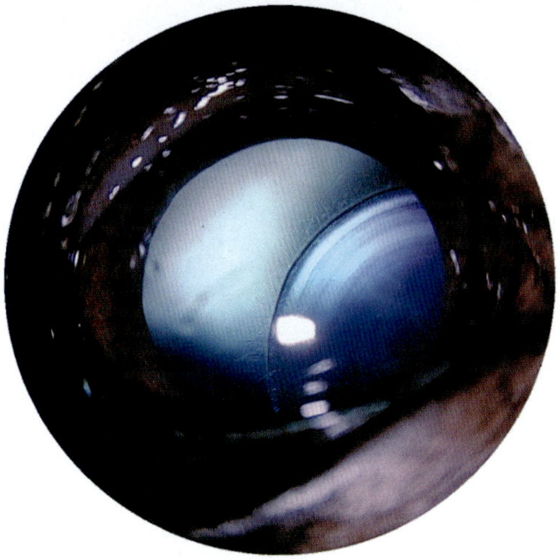

Figure 8-72
Posteriorly luxated lens in a shar-pei. Note the broken zonules on the lens equator.

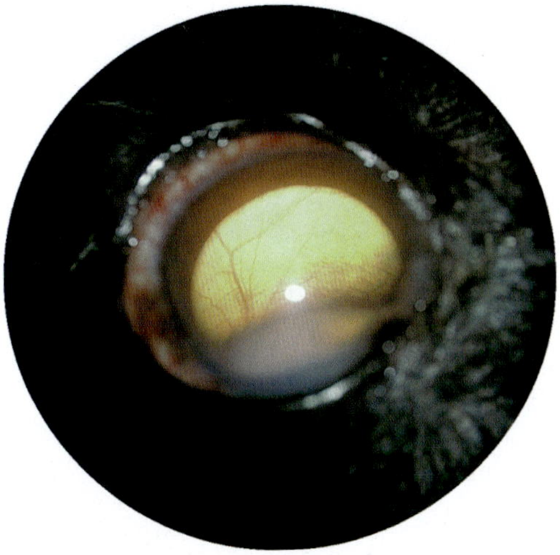

Figure 8-73
Posteriorly luxated lens visible just behind the pupil. The fundus is clearly visible without an indirect lens.

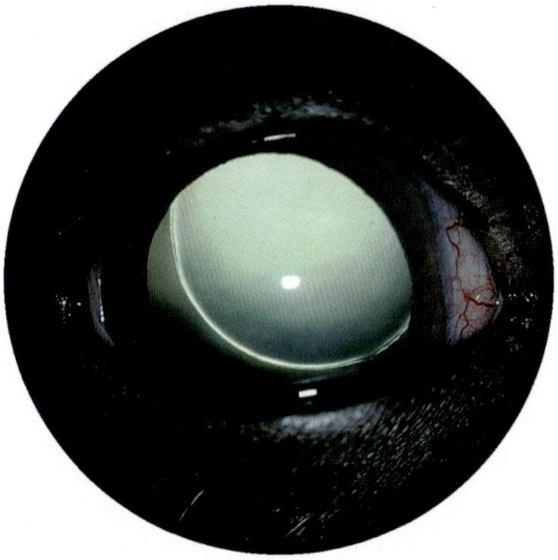

Figure 8-74
Posteriorly luxated lens; aphakic crescent is visible temporally. Aphakic crescent is the crescent-shaped space between the pupil margin and the lens equator.

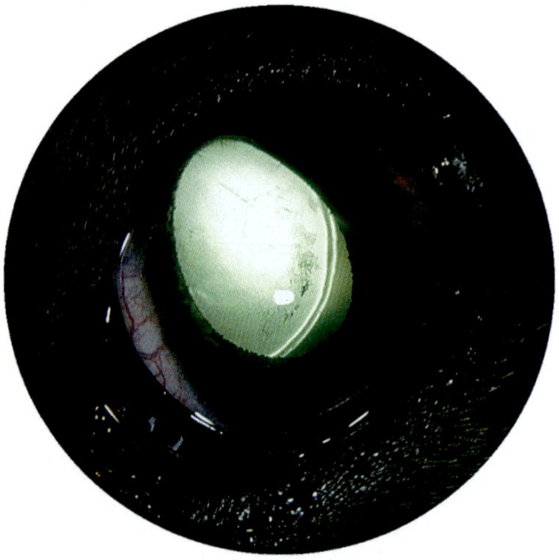

Figure 8-75
Posteriorly luxated lens; aphakic crescent is visible inferiorly. Secondary glaucoma is present.

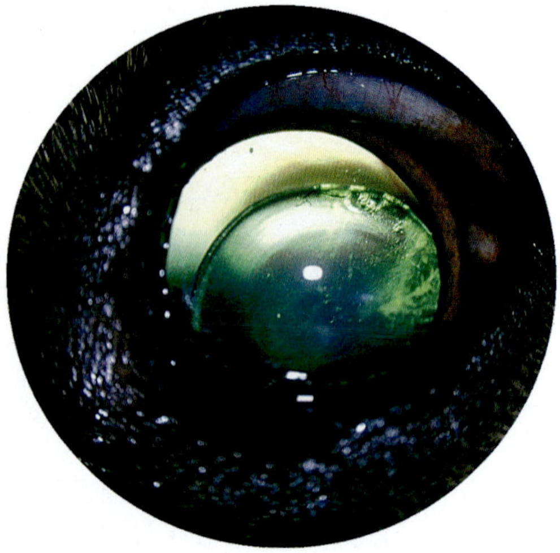

Figure 8-76
Posteriorly luxated lens with incipient cataracts.

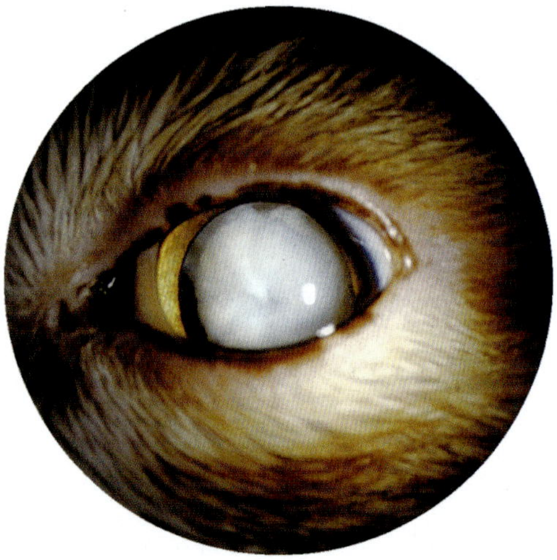

Figure 8-77
Cat with subluxated lens. The lens is displaced temporally.

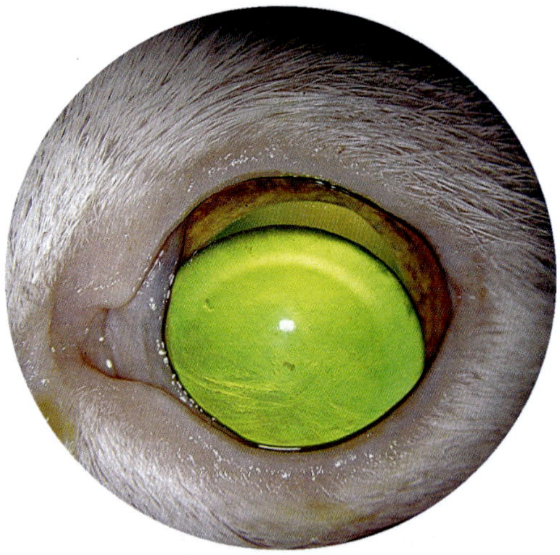

Figure 8-78
Anteriorly luxated lens with incipient cataracts in a cat.

Chapter 9

Glaucoma

INTRODUCTION

Glaucoma, a disease that affects the optic nerve, is characterized by the death of ganglion cells and is associated with a pathologic elevation of the intraocular pressure. Little doubt exists that some of the clinical signs of the disease (e.g., corneal edema and posterior cupping of the optic nerve) are directly related to the increased pressure in the eye. The cause of the elevated pressure is poorly understood in many cases. A reduction of the outflow of aqueous humor from the eye in the face of continued secretion appears to be involved. It is presumed that the major obstruction to aqueous outflow from the eye is the result of either an anatomic or a physiologic abnormality in the outflow mechanism through the iridocorneal angle—the site of the bulk of the aqueous drainage in most mammalian species. Glaucoma can be a primary (and eventually bilateral) inherited disease (certainly the case in dogs), or it can develop secondarily to other ocular conditions in which the flow of aqueous in the eye is impeded or the outflow pathways are obstructed. Obstruction may occur if the lens is abnormally positioned (lens luxation) and when cells or inflammatory debris blocks the drainage angle (as is the case with uveitis, neoplasia, and hemorrhage). Many cases of glaucoma in cats are associated with uveitis. Glaucoma is often a painful, blinding disease in small animals. It is essential that the clinical features of glaucoma are recognized, because therapy for other causes of a red, painful eye may be contraindicated in patients with glaucoma. Only in cases in which the diagnosis is made and treatment started early does any hope exist that the disease may be controlled even remotely for any length of time.

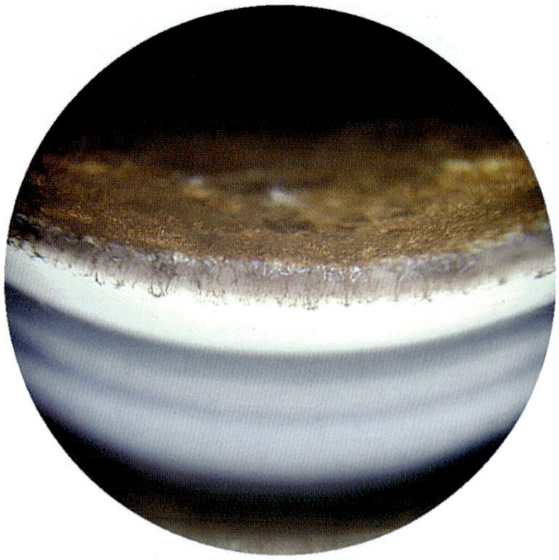

Figure 9-1
Normal iridocorneal angle in a dog.

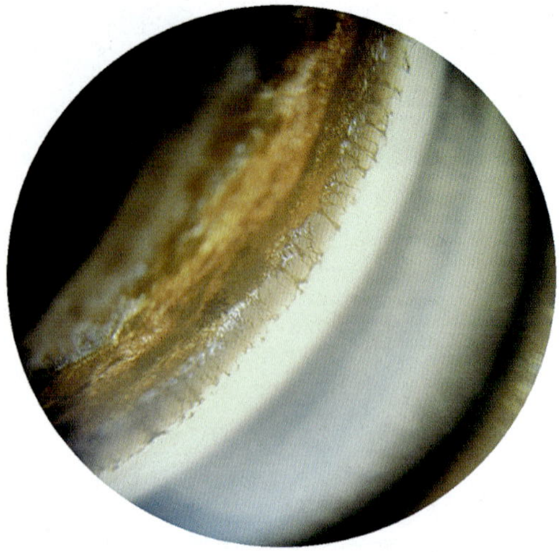

Figure 9-2
Normal iridocorneal angle in a dog.

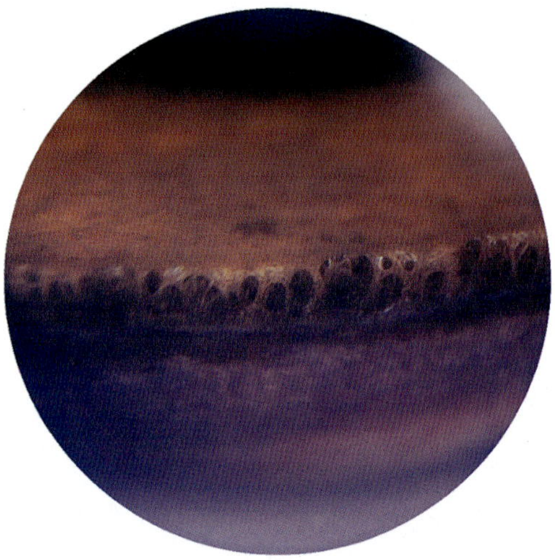

Figure 9-3
Normal iridocorneal angle in a dog.

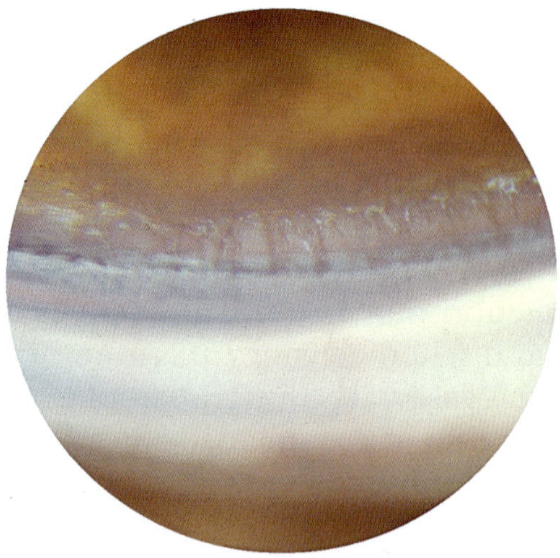

Figure 9-4
Normal iridocorneal angle in a dog.

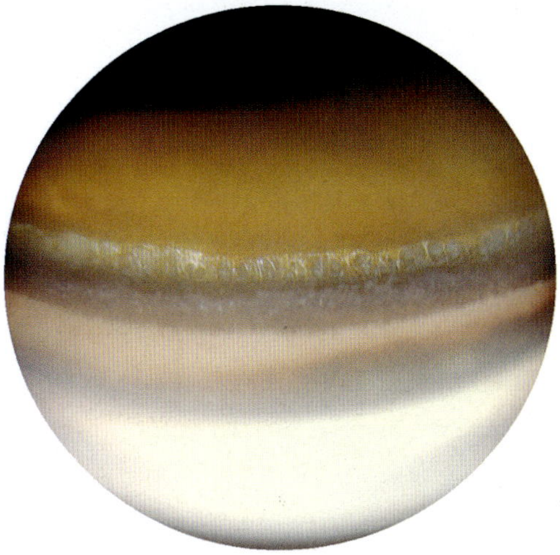

Figure 9-5
Normal iridocorneal angle in a dog.

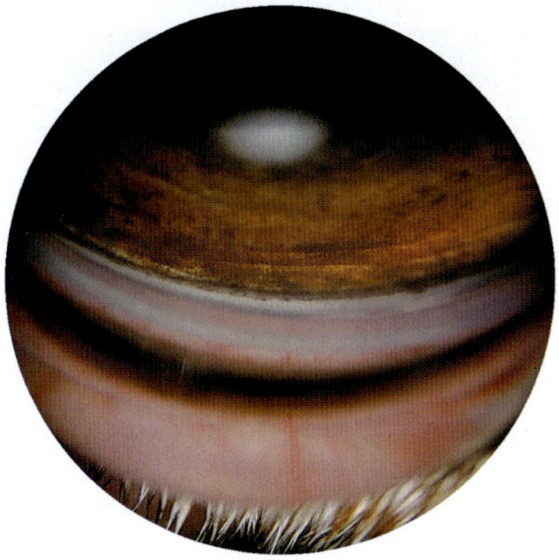

Figure 9-6
Closed iridocorneal angle.

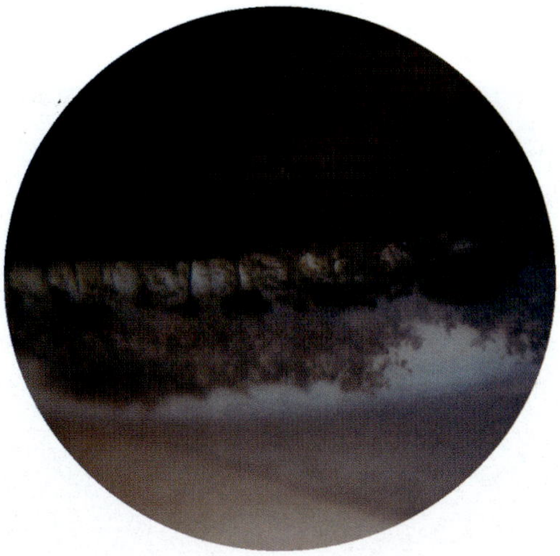

Figure 9-7
Primary open-angle glaucoma in a beagle. The iridocorneal angle is open.

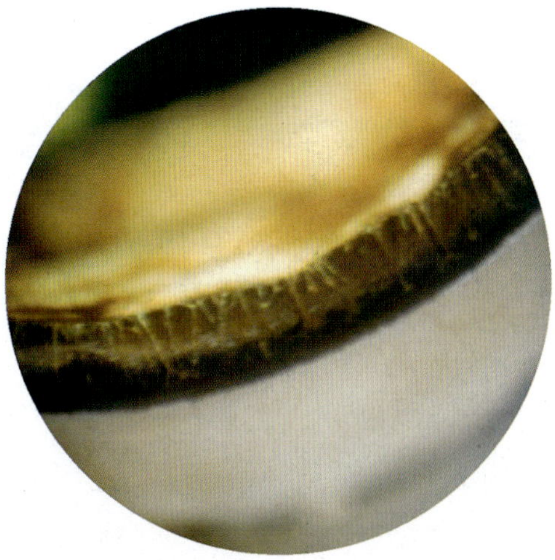

Figure 9-8
Cat with diffuse iris melanoma. A highly pigmented iridocorneal angle is present.

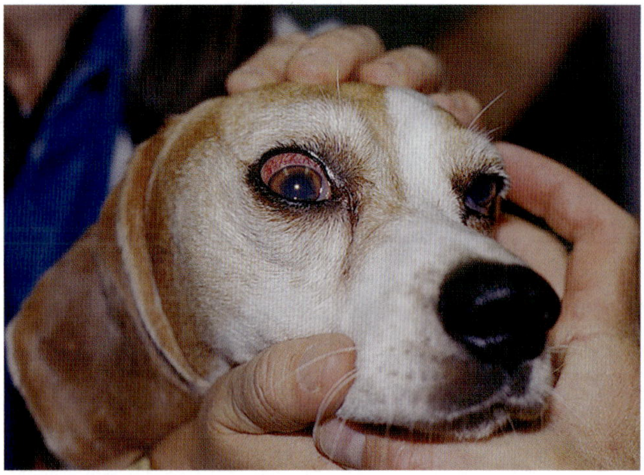

Figure 9-9
Beagle with primary open-angle glaucoma. "Red eye," corneal edema, and dilated pupil are present.

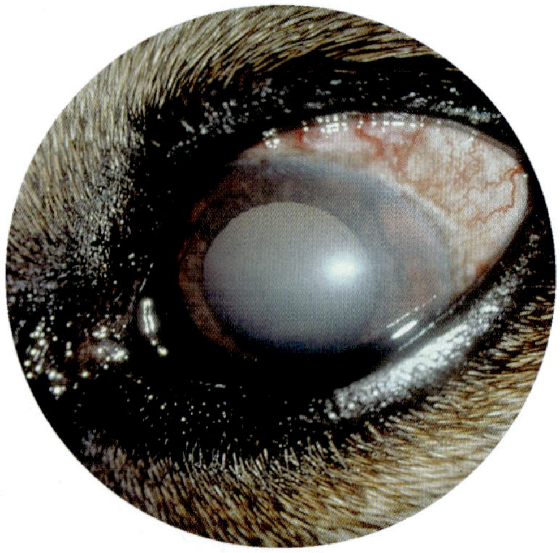

Figure 9-10
Glaucoma in a dog. "Red eye," corneal edema, and dilated pupil are present.

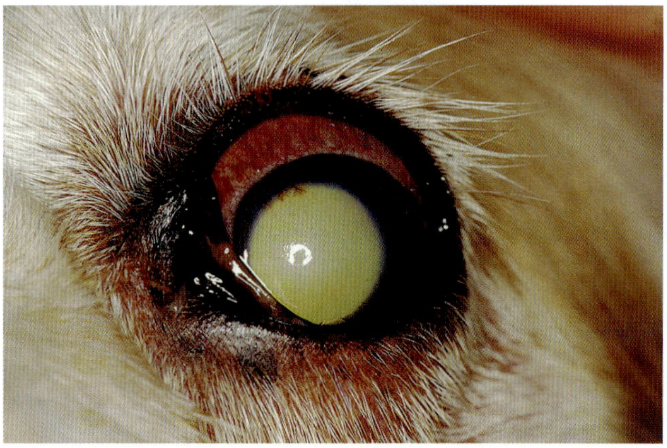

Figure 9-11
American cocker spaniel with fairly acute closed-angle glaucoma. "Red eye," corneal edema, peripheral corneal neovascularization, and dilated pupil are present.

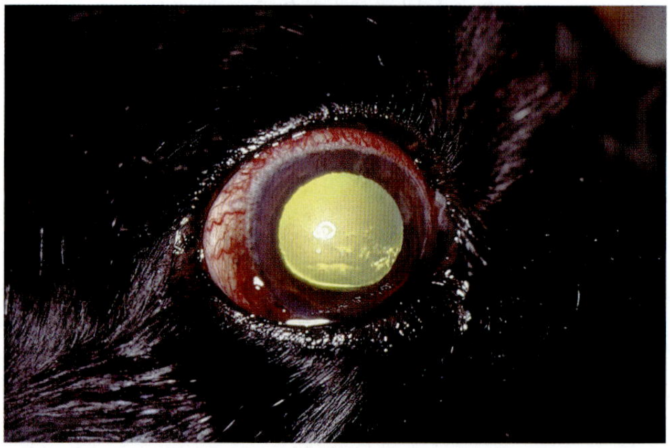

Figure 9-12
Acute glaucoma in a dog. "Red eye," mild corneal edema, and dilated pupil are present.

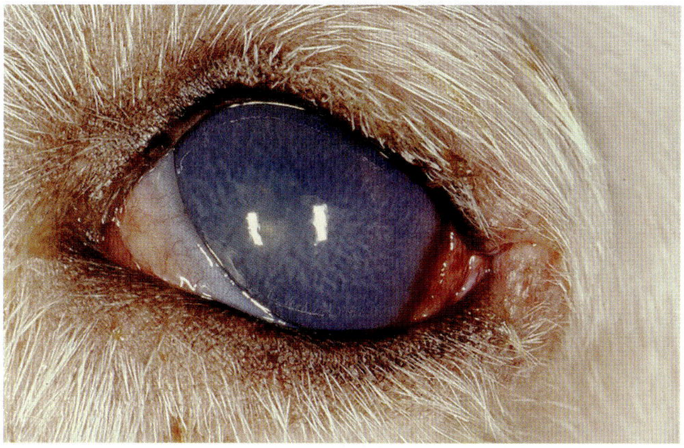

Figure 9-13
Corneal edema resulting from glaucoma in a dog. The intraocular pressure was 60 mm Hg.

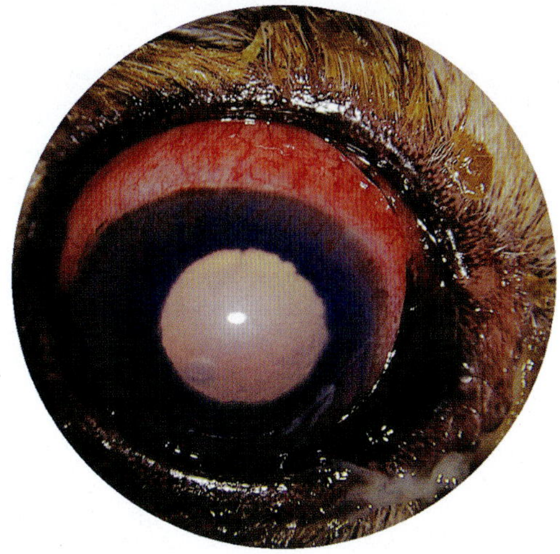

Figure 9-14
"Red eye," corneal neovascularization, and edema in a dog with glaucoma.

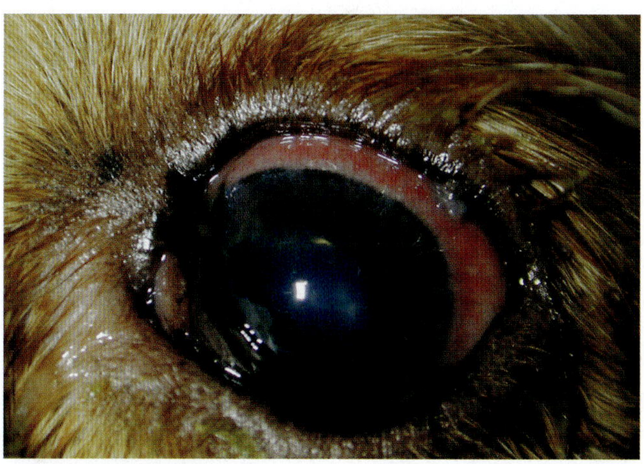

Figure 9-15
Acute glaucoma in an American cocker spaniel. Note the injected conjunctival vessels, corneal edema, and dilated pupil.

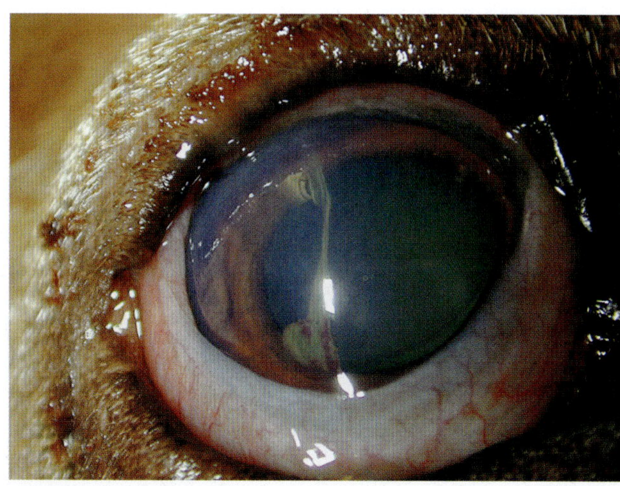

Figure 9-16
Basset hound 48 hours after implantation of an Ahmed valve for glaucoma. Corneal edema and vascularization are present. A strand of fibrin extends to the end of the valve tubing in the anterior chamber.

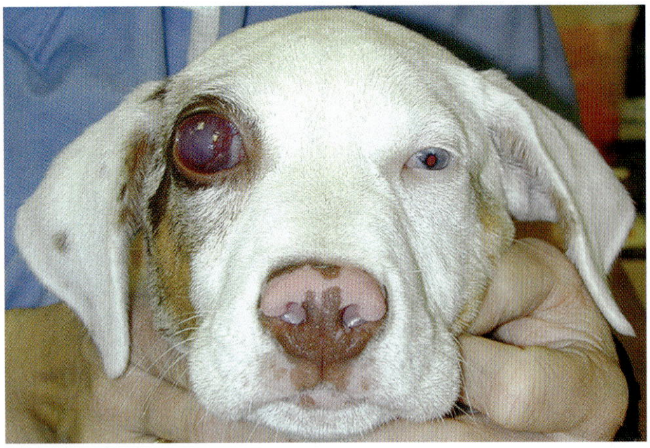

Figure 9-17
Australian shepherd with chronic glaucoma secondary to traumatic uveitis. The right eye is buphthalmic, with corneal edema and vascularization. Buphthalmos in the right eye is accentuated by congenital microphthalmos in the left eye.

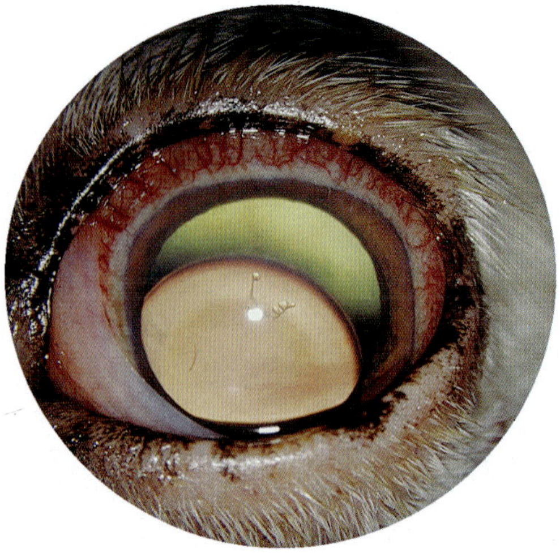

Figure 9-18
Chronic glaucoma in a dog, with buphthalmos, injected conjunctival and scleral vessels, mild corneal edema, dilated pupil, and a posteriorly luxated lens with an aphakic crescent superiorly.

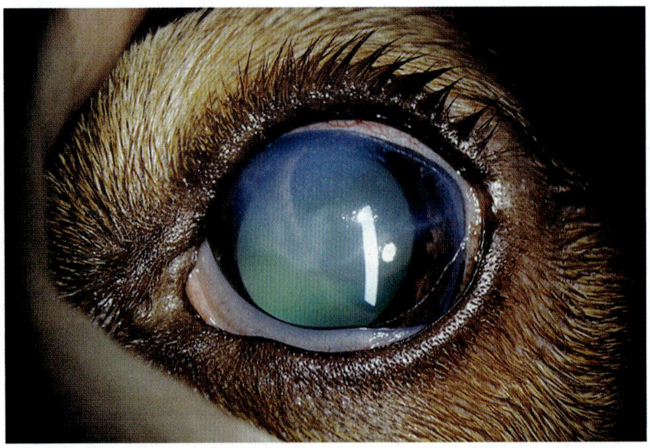

Figure 9-19
Basset hound with chronic glaucoma, buphthalmos, "red eye," corneal edema, dilated pupil, and tears in Descemet's membrane.

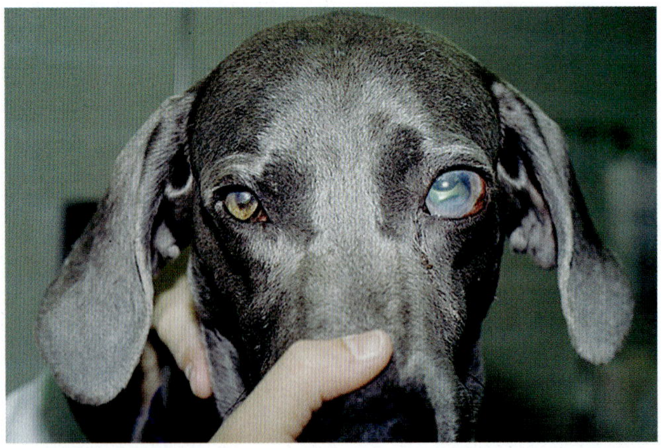

Figure 9-20
Weimaraner with chronic glaucoma in the left eye secondary to bilateral uveitis from *Rickettsia rickettsii* infection. Buphthalmia is present in the left eye, with corneal edema.

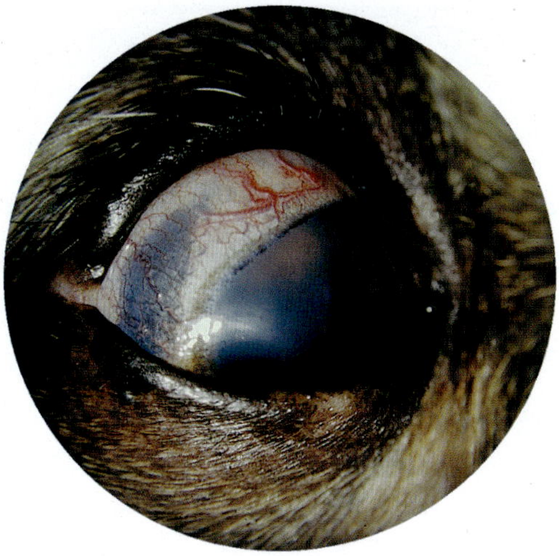

Figure 9-21
Ocular pigment depositions and glaucoma in a Cairn terrier. There is pigment in the sclera and at the limbus, and corneal edema.

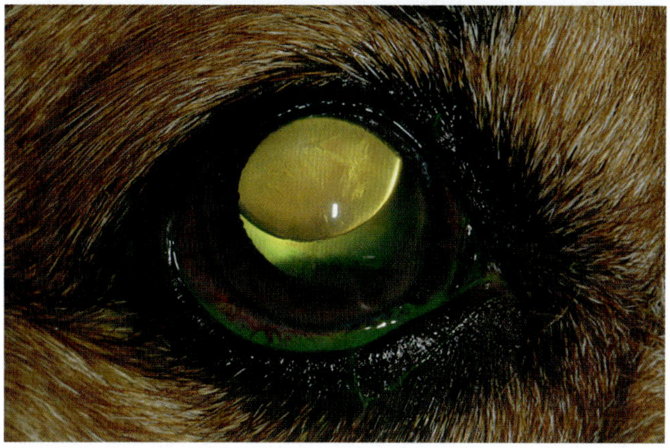

Figure 9-22
Glaucoma with buphthalmos and secondary lens subluxation in a basset hound. A ventral aphakic crescent is seen.

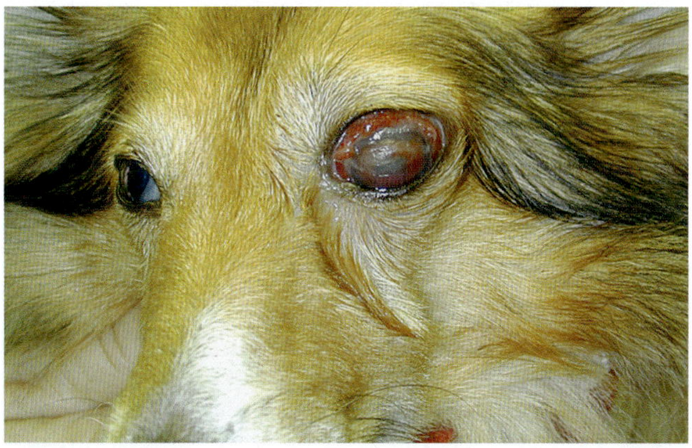

Figure 9-23
Shetland sheepdog with glaucoma, buphthalmos and exposure keratitis secondary to multiple myeloma with ocular involvement.

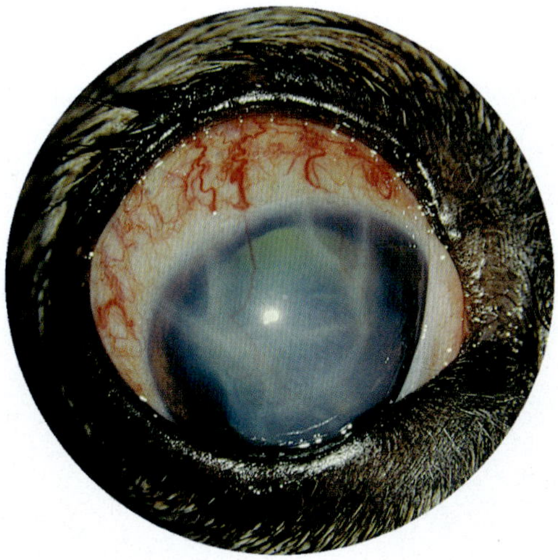

Figure 9-24
Dog with chronic glaucoma, buphthalmos, "red eye," corneal edema, corneal neovascularization, tears in Descemet's membrane, and dilated pupil.

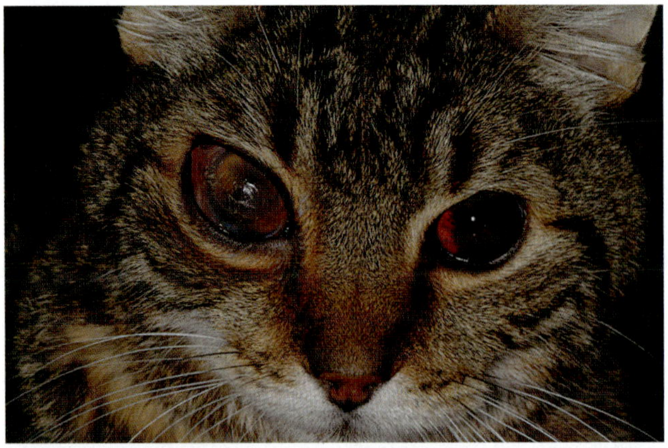

Figure 9-25
Bilateral uveitis with secondary glaucoma in the right eye with buphthalmos and corneal exposure.

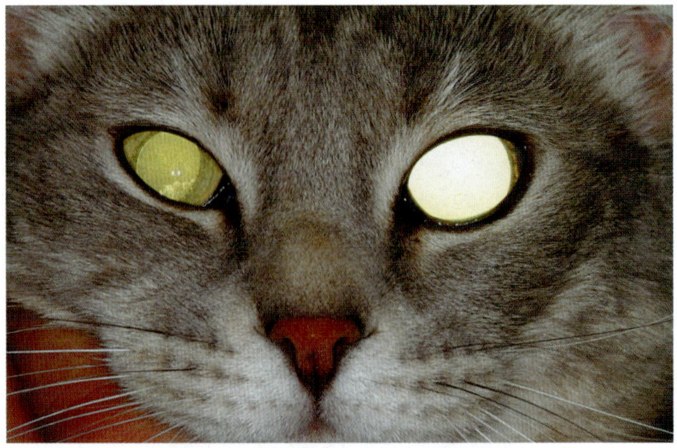

Figure 9-26
Siamese cross-breed with chronic bilateral low-grade uveitis and glaucoma in the left eye. The left pupil is dilated and nonresponsive. Keratic precipitates appear as a faint opacity in the inferonasal portion of the right cornea.

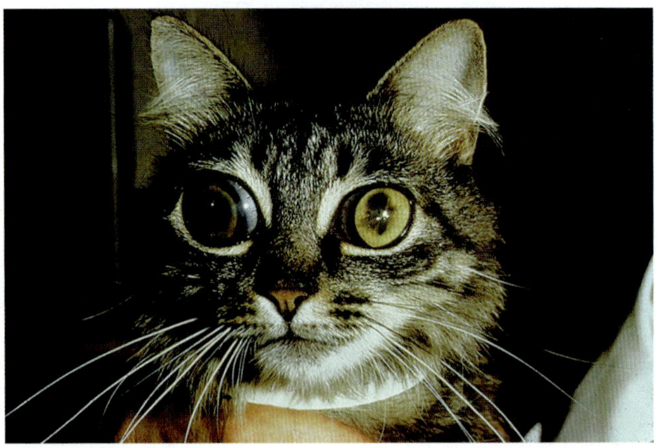

Figure 9-27
Cat with bilateral glaucoma, buphthalmos, and exposure keratitis and drying resulting from the buphthalmos.

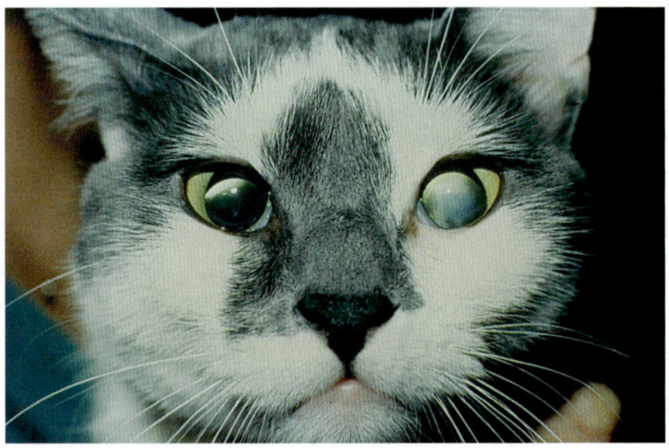

Figure 9-28
Cat with bilateral glaucoma, buphthalmos, dilated pupils, and posteriorly subluxated lenses.

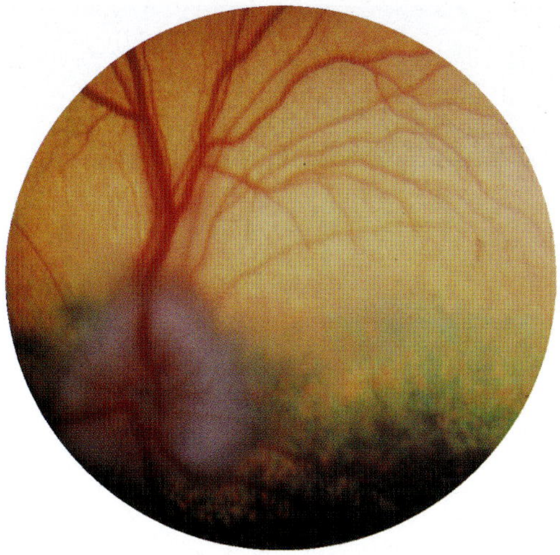

Figure 9-29
Acute optic nerve and peripapillary edema in a dog immediately after emergency treatment for acute glaucoma.

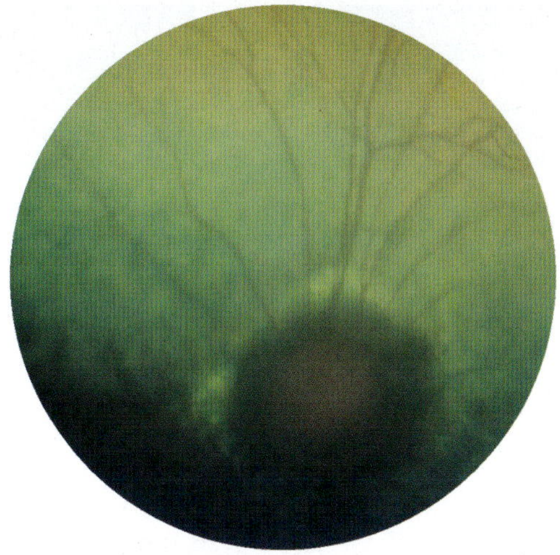

Figure 9-30
Optic nerve and retinal atrophy in a dog with chronic glaucoma.

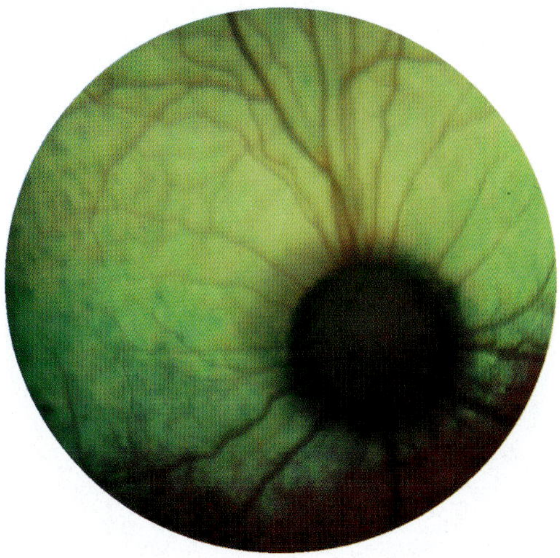

Figure 9-31
Optic nerve cupping and atrophy in a dog with glaucoma. Note the areas of retinal edema in the temporal (left) retina.

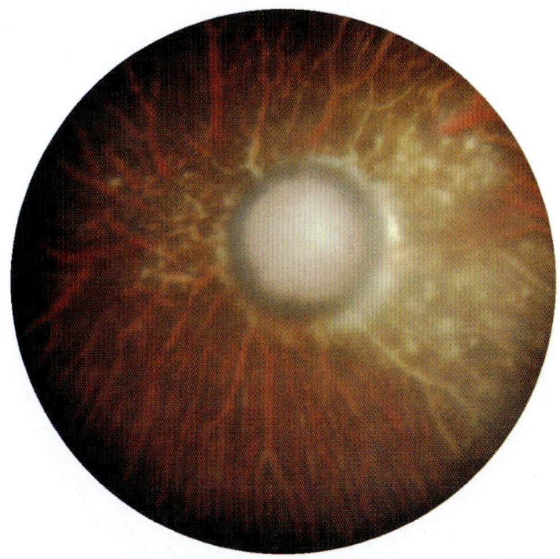

Figure 9-32
Advanced optic nerve cupping and retinal atrophy in a dog with Vogt-Koyanagi-Harada syndrome and secondary glaucoma. Note the loss of all retinal blood vessels.

Chapter 10

Vitreous

INTRODUCTION

The vitreous is a gel composed of collagen fibrils, mucopolysaccharides, and water (98%). It is normally optically transparent. It maintains the shape of the eye and aids in keeping the retina opposed to the underlying layers. Pathologically it may be affected by changes associated with aging (asteroid hyalosis); liquefaction (syneresis), which often accompanies inflammation of the uvea and retina; degeneration; and the deposition of various chemical and cellular infiltrates (inflammatory and neoplastic cells), blood, or cholesterol (synchysis scintillans).

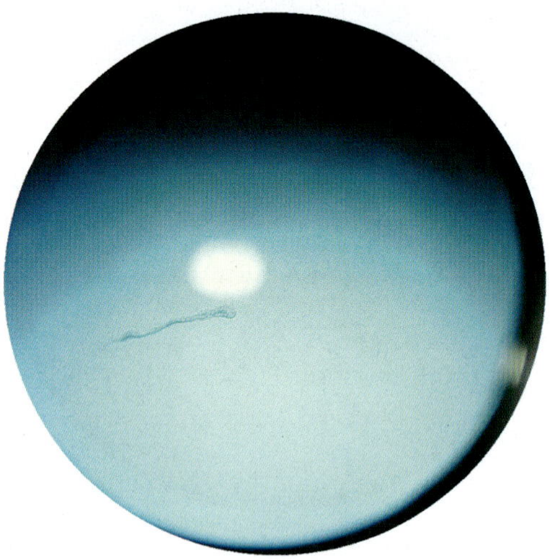

Figure 10-1
Persistent hyaloid remnant in an Old English sheepdog. The hyaloid artery supplies blood to the developing eye in utero. Around the time of birth, it normally atrophies and disappears. The hyaloid remnant in this figure remains attached axially to the posterior lens capsule. It is not patent.
(Courtesy Dr. E. Dan Wolf.)

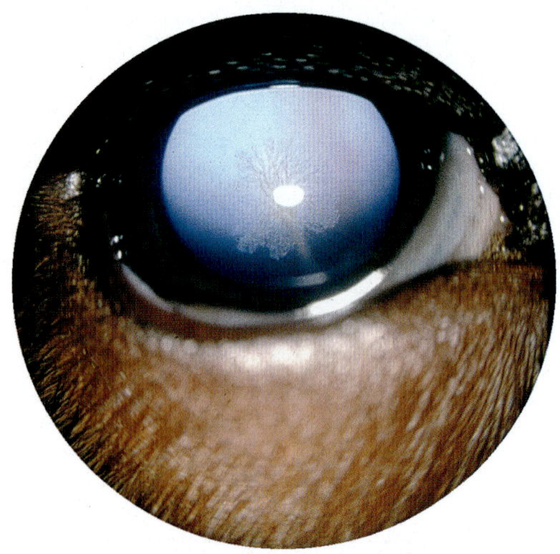

Figure 10-2
Persistent hyperplastic tunica vasculosa lentis (PHTVL) and persistent hyperplastic primary vitreous (PHPV) in a young Doberman pinscher. This is a hereditary, congenital lesion, shown in this figure as vessels on the posterior lens capsule. More severe lesions can cause blindness.

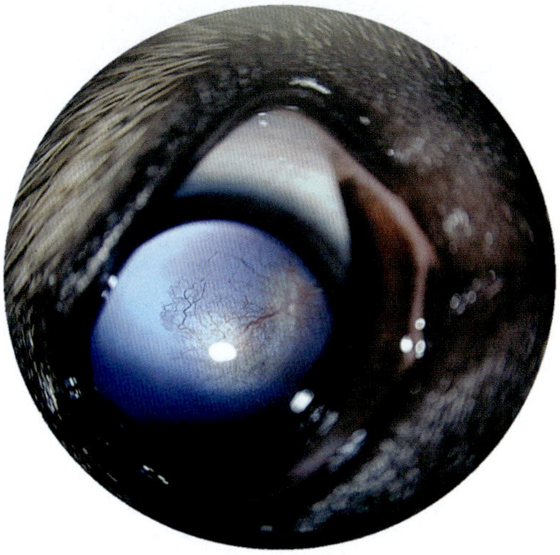

Figure 10-3
PHTVL and PHPV in a dog with blood vessels over the posterior lens capsule. A posterior capsular opacity is seen above the flash reflection.

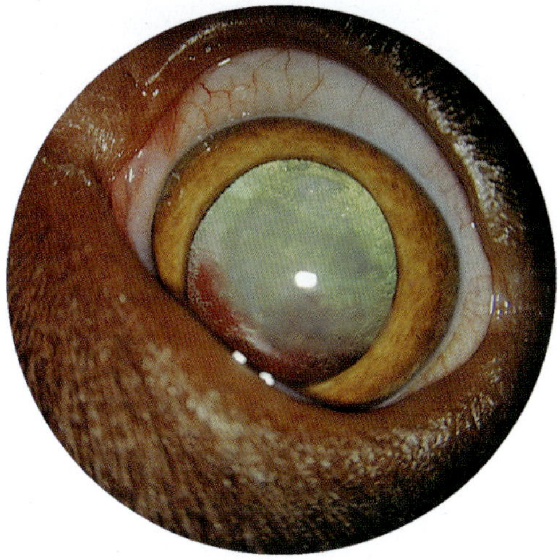

Figure 10-4
Cataract, PHTVL, and PHPV in a pointer. Intralenticular hemorrhage is seen inferiorly.

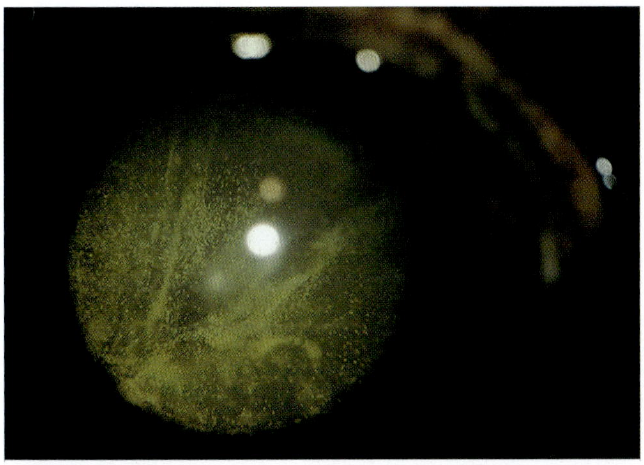

Figure 10-5
Asteroid hyalosis in a golden retriever.

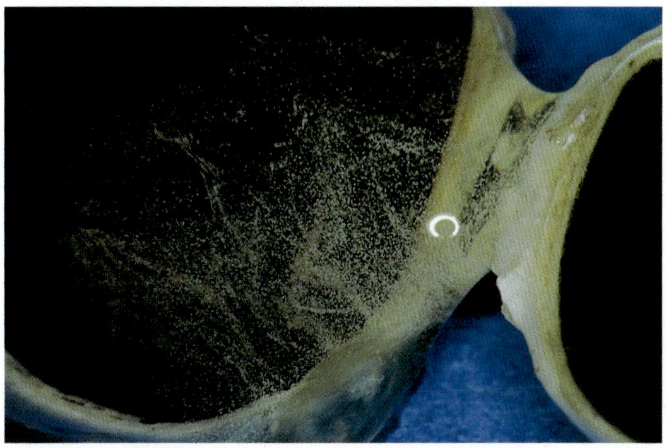

Figure 10-6
Asteroid hyalosis in the opened eye of an aged dog. Asteroid hyalosis is characterized by small refractile opacities in the vitreous. These lipid-laden opacities are usually seen in older dogs, can be unilateral or bilateral, and rarely cause visual problems.

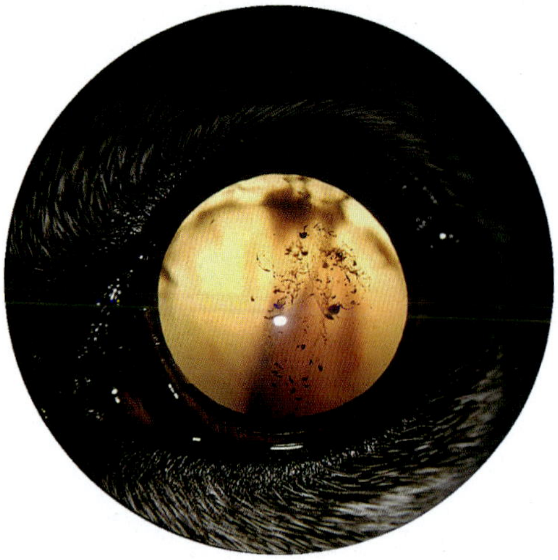

Figure 10-7
Hyphema and vitreal hemorrhage. Causes of bleeding in the eye include systemic clotting disorders, vasculitis, intraocular tumor, and retinal detachment.

Chapter 11

Retina, Choroid, Sclera

INTRODUCTION

The retina is a multicellular layer 100 to 250 μm thick that lines the posterior segment of the eye. It is sandwiched between the vitreous and retinal pigment epithelium (RPE) and choroid, from which its outer layers receive nutrition. The normal retina is almost transparent; the cellular arrangement is such that light can pass through the retina with limited impediment to reach the photoreceptors (rods and cones) that absorb light and convert it into electrochemical energy. The photoreceptors are adjacent to the RPE. Some light is absorbed by the retinal layers, however, which becomes evident when the retina undergoes degeneration and becomes thinner. In dogs and cats some of the light incident on the retina is absorbed as it passes through the photoreceptor layer. The light then hits the tapetum cellulosum in the choroid, which acts as a mirror and reflects the light back via the retina, where more is absorbed to maximize the light-gathering power of the eye. For this to be possible, little light must be absorbed in the intervening RPE cell layer, and it is for this reason that the RPE is largely nonpigmented over the area of the tapetal fundus. The tapetal fundus occupies the upper hemisphere of the fundus. The nontapetal fundus occupies the lower hemisphere of the posterior segment and also surrounds the periphery of the tapetal fundus superiorly, nasally, and temporally.

The layered structure of the retina, RPE, choroid, and sclera can be reduced to a schematic to illustrate how in various areas of the normal fundus the ophthalmoscopic view appears as it does. The appearance of and variations in the fundus owe much to the pigmentation in the eye as a whole, which can vary considerably among species and individual animals or even between the two eyes of an animal.

NORMAL FUNDUS IN DOGS

Normal Tapetum in Dogs

When a dog's tapetal fundus is viewed ophthalmoscopically, retinal vessels are superimposed on the highly colored tapetum. The only visible components of the retina are the blood vessels. The RPE in this region is nonpigmented to allow light to reach and be reflected by the tapetum. Therefore, the RPE layer is not visible either. The tapetum is visible as the aggregate of numerous tapetal cells that overlap one another to make a layer of variable thickness, depending on the location in the posterior segment, and varies between eyes according to the amount of pigment in the eye because the tapetum consists of modified pigment cells. The tapetum may be gray, violet, blue, green, yellow, or reddish orange. The surface area of the posterior segment covered by the tapetum also may vary, tending to occupy a larger area in larger dog breeds (and including the optic nerve in the tapetal area) and a smaller area (usually more on the temporal area of the fundus) in small breeds. Some dogs have no tapetum at all. The border of the tapetal and nontapetal fundus may be sharply defined (usually more likely in short-coated breeds) or irregular with interlocking of tapetal and nontapetal regions (in longer-coated animals). Dogs of same breeds often have the same tapetal appearance and often color.

Because the tapetum acts as a mirror to reflect light for a second pass through the retina, the underlying choroid and sclera in the tapetal area of the fundus are not usually visible (at least if the tapetum is well developed).

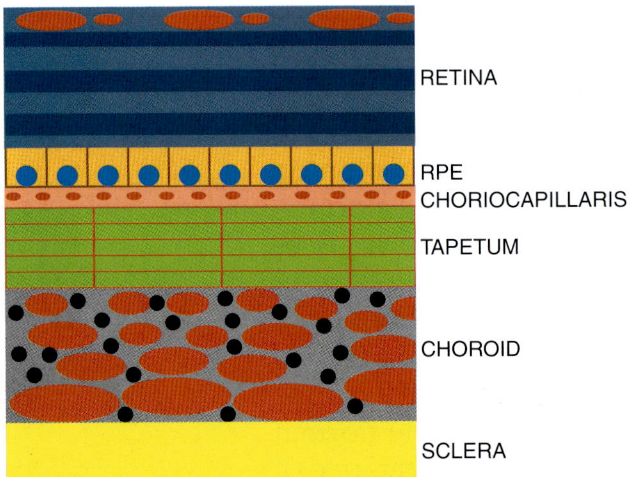

Figure 11-1
This schematic shows a cross-section through a normally pigmented tapetal area of the fundus. The vitreous is not shown but would be above the retina in this figure. RPE overlying the tapetum is not pigmented. Black dots in the choroid represent melanin, because the choroid in these animals is pigmented, although this cannot be seen ophthalmoscopically. The viewer looks down on these layers from above.

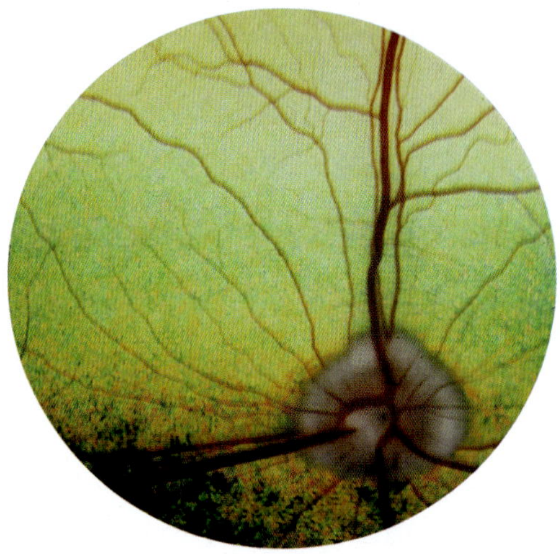

Figure 11-2
Normal retina. Some myelination of the optic disc is visible.

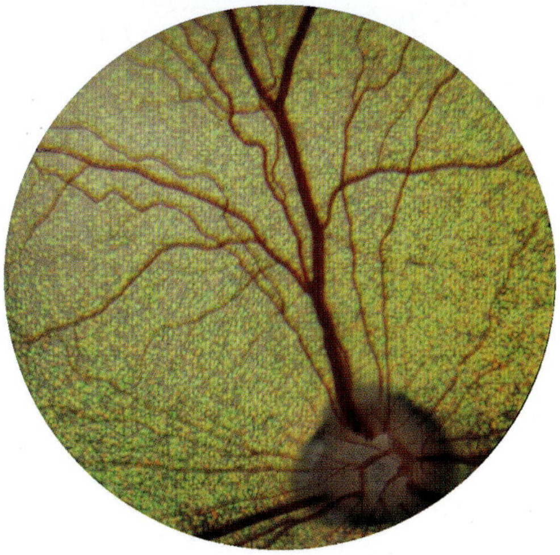

Figure 11-3
Normal retina with a speckled tapetum, the result of variable thickness of the tapetal cell layer.

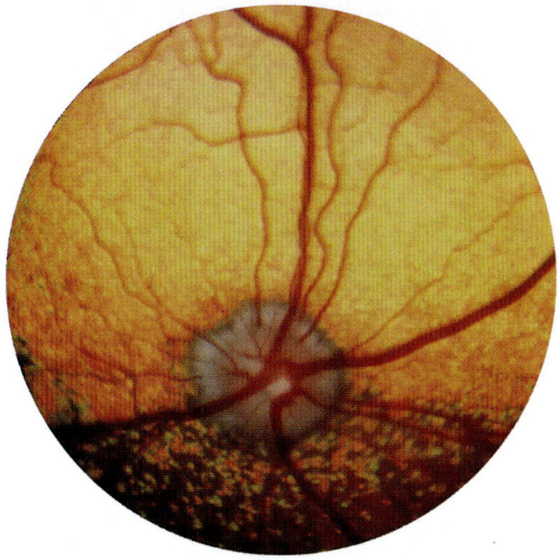

Figure 11-4
Normal retina in a springer spaniel. The tapetum is orange.

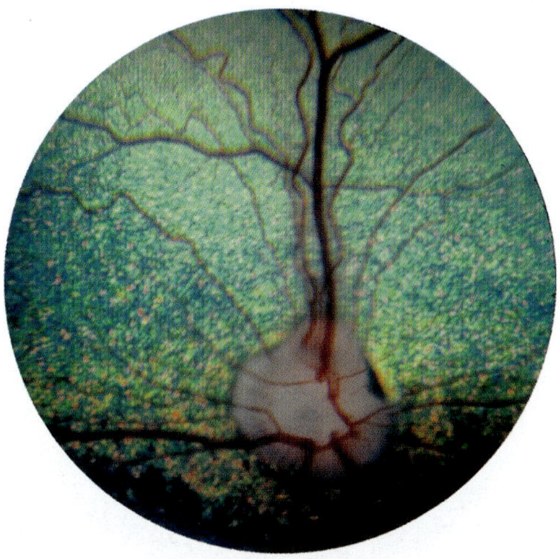

Figure 11-5
Normal retina. The tapetum is speckled.

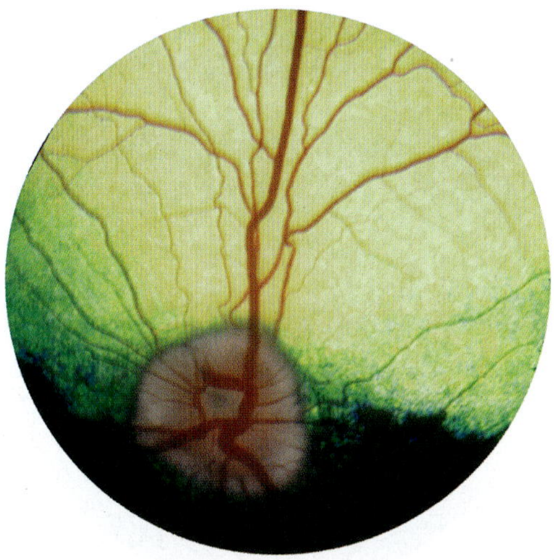

Figure 11-6
Normal retina in a black Labrador retriever. Typical tapetum in many canine breeds.

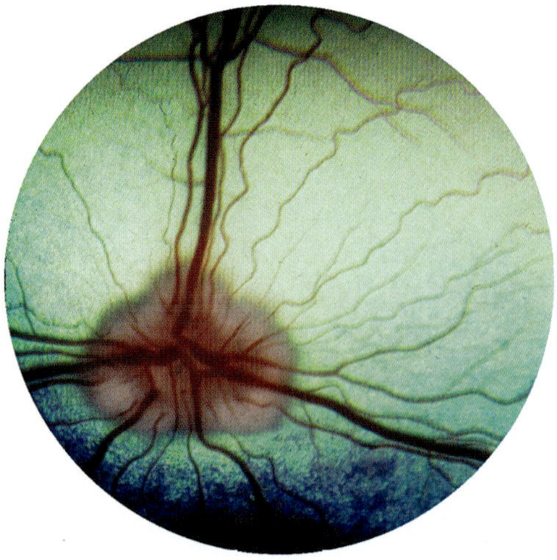

Figure 11-7
Normal fundus in a German shorthaired pointer with a large amount of optic nerve myelination.

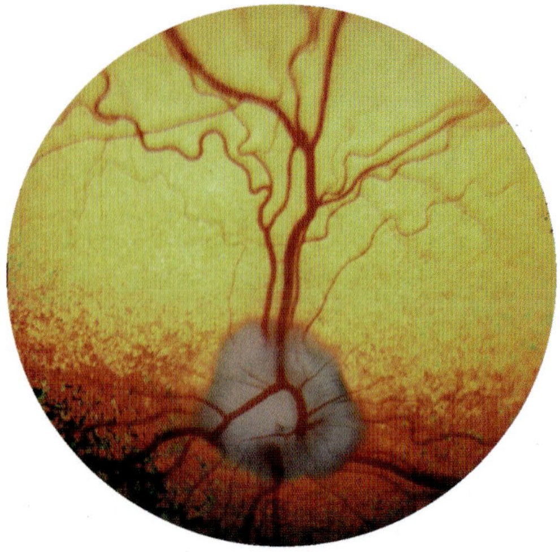

Figure 11-8
Normal retina with a yellow-orange tapetum in a golden retriever.

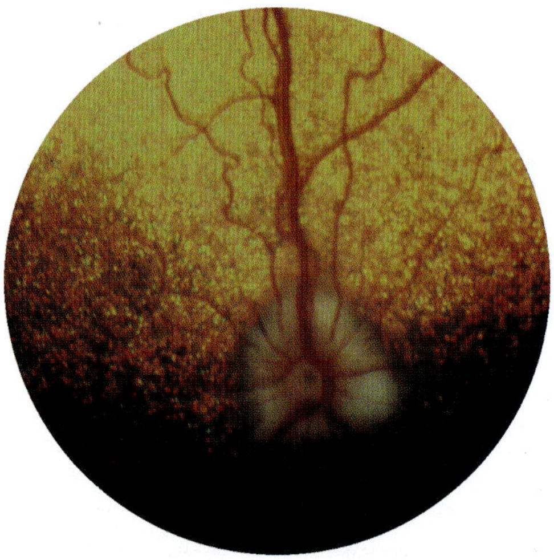

Figure 11-9
Normal retina with a yellow-red tapetum and a well-myelinated disc.

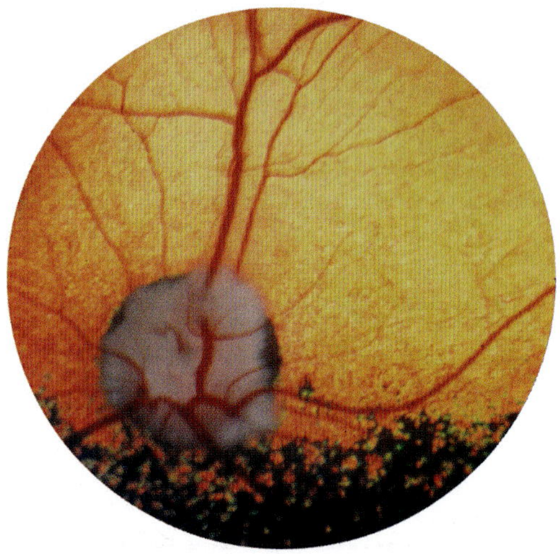

Figure 11-10
Normal retina. The dark areas around the disc are areas where the tapetum ends before the optic disc begins; choroidal pigment is visible here (sometimes called *conus*).

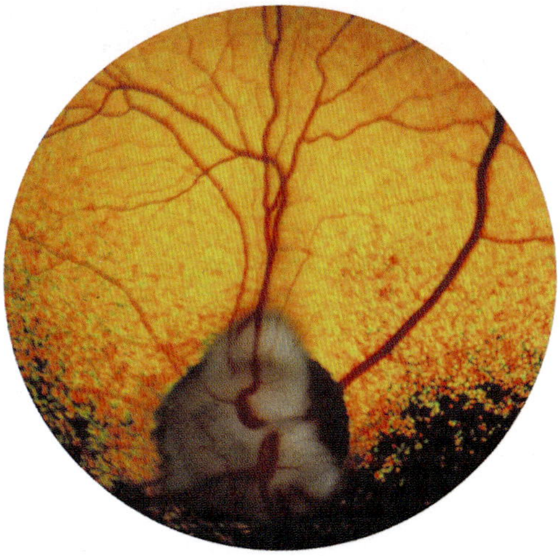

Figure 11-11
Normal retina with odd myelination of the optic disc. The dark areas around the disc are areas where the tapetum ends before the optic disc begins; choroidal pigment (conus) is visible here.

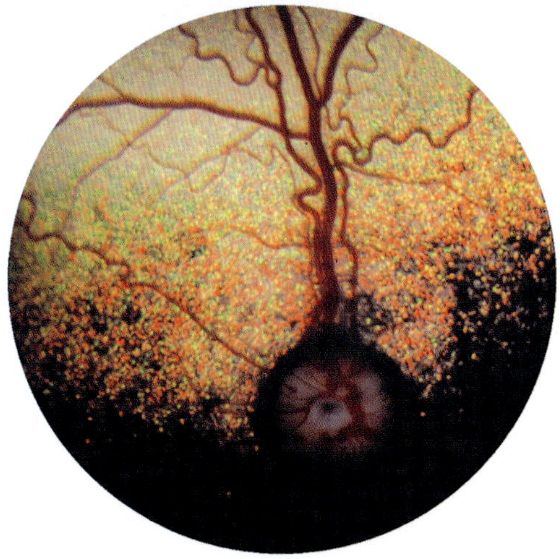

Figure 11-12
Normal retina. Tapetal and nontapetal junction is feathered (scalloped); the disc is circular, because little extension of myelination is present along the axons in the retina around the disc.

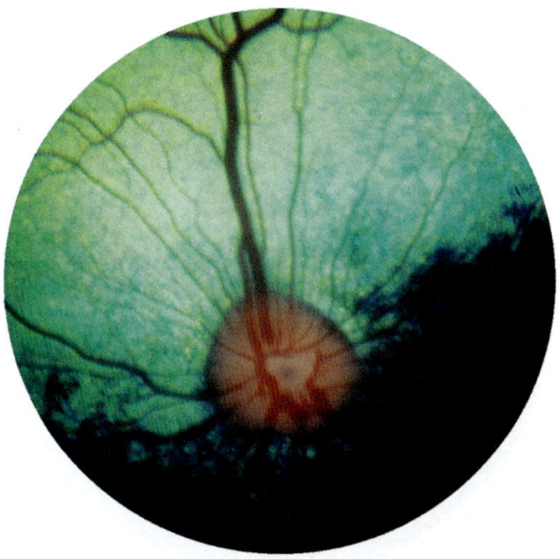

Figure 11-13
Normal retina. Extension of myelin out from the disc is limited, and a small pigmented conus surrounds the disc.

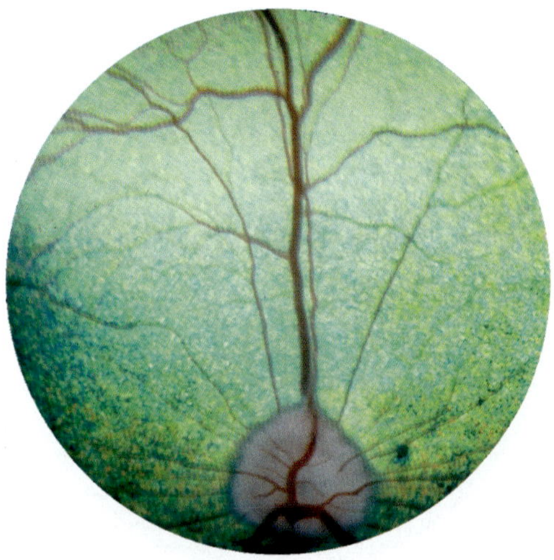

Figure 11-14
Normal retina. A physiologic cup is visible in the center of the optic nerve. The circular outline of the optic nerve can be seen inside the myelinated area of the nerve head. The neurons at the edge of the nerve are losing myelin (hence the gray tint to the nerve).

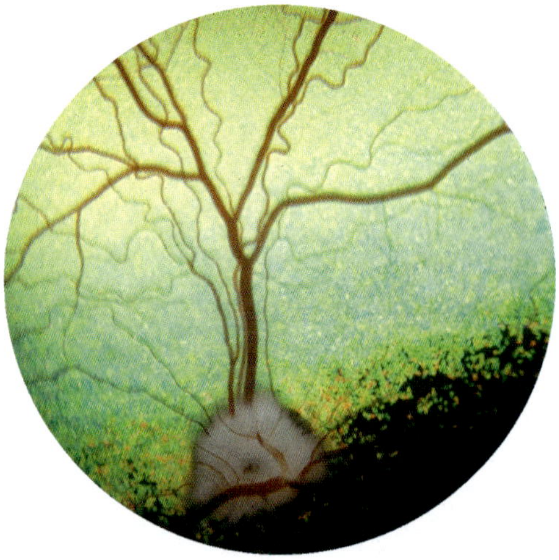

Figure 11-15
Normal retina. Variable color is present in the tapetum. Note the variable filling of the vessels on the disc. Arterioles tend to be more tortuous than the retinal veins.

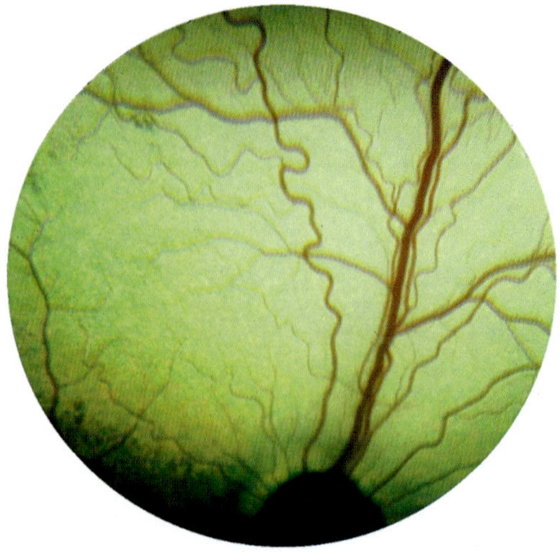

Figure 11-16
Normal retina. The arterioles are tortuous but still within normal limits.

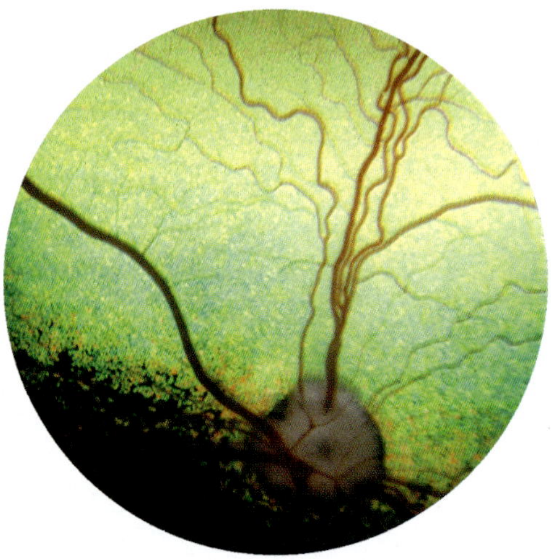

Figure 11-17
Normal retina. End-on capillaries (regularly spaced dark spots) can be seen in parts of the tapetum (similar to stars of Winslow in the horse).

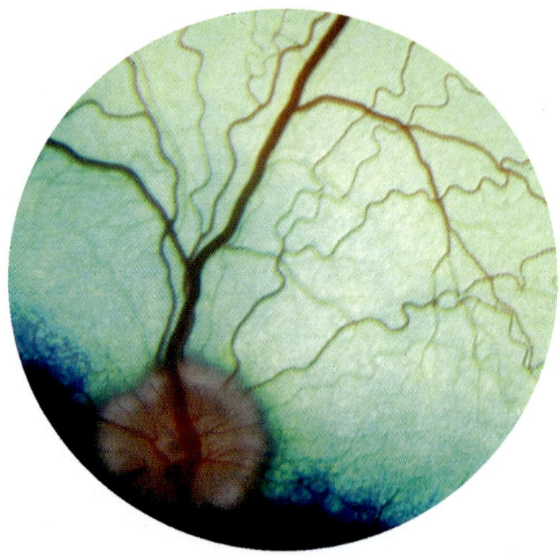

Figure 11-18
Normal retina. The vessels over the optic nerve are prominent; the arterioles are tortuous but normal.

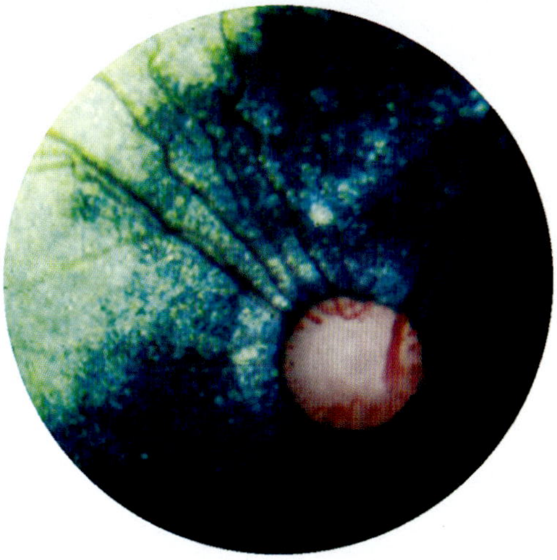

Figure 11-19
Normal canine retina with poor myelination in the optic nerve. A pigmented conus is present around the nerve. The arrangement of both arterioles and veins arising toward the edge of the nerve is more typical of the feline fundus. In dogs the veins usually arise more centrally on the optic nerve.

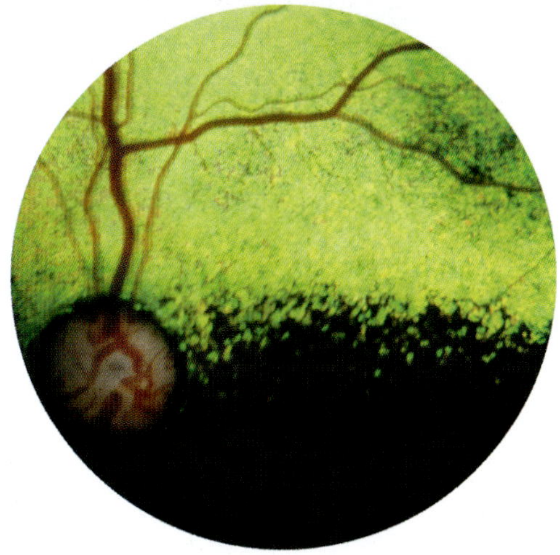

Figure 11-20
Normal retina. Pigment varies at the tapetal-nontapetal junction; pigment is present in the tapetum.

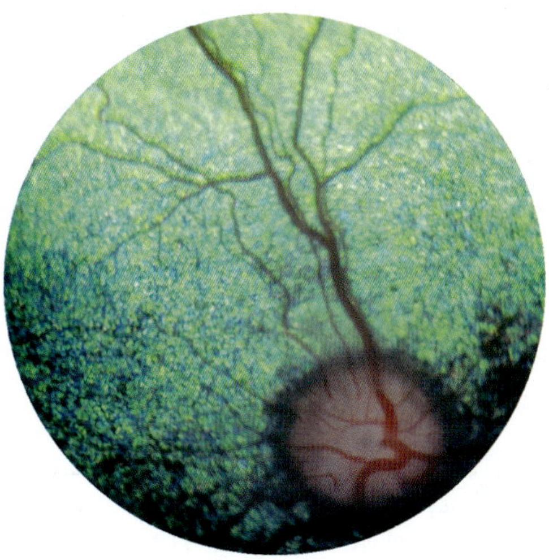

Figure 11-21
Normal retina. A pigmented conus is present around the optic disc; the blue-green speckling throughout the tapetum is the result of variable thickness of the tapetal cell layer.

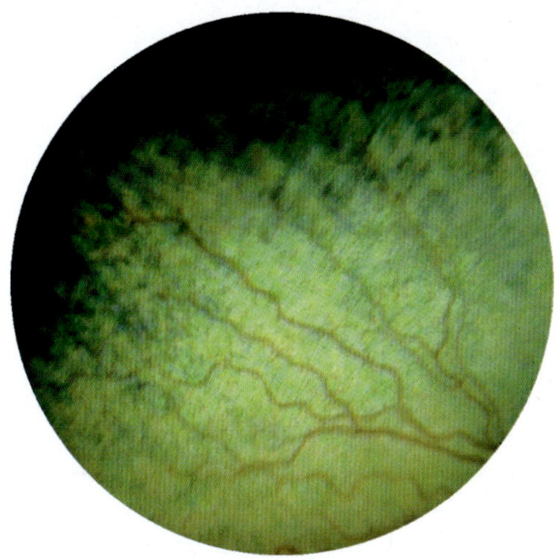

Figure 11-22
Peripheral tapetum in a normal dog. The radiating dark lines appear to correspond to underlying choroidal blood vessels. This should be differentiated from thinning of the peripheral retina in dogs with degenerative retinopathies (e.g., progressive retinal atrophy [PRA]).

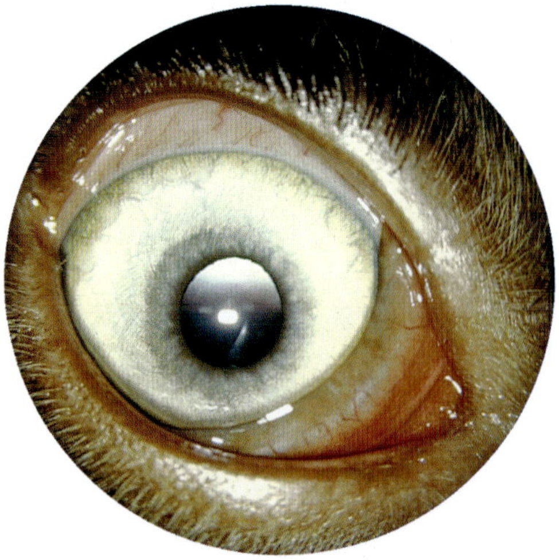

Figure 11-23
Normal weimaraner. The tapetal reflex through the pupil is white.

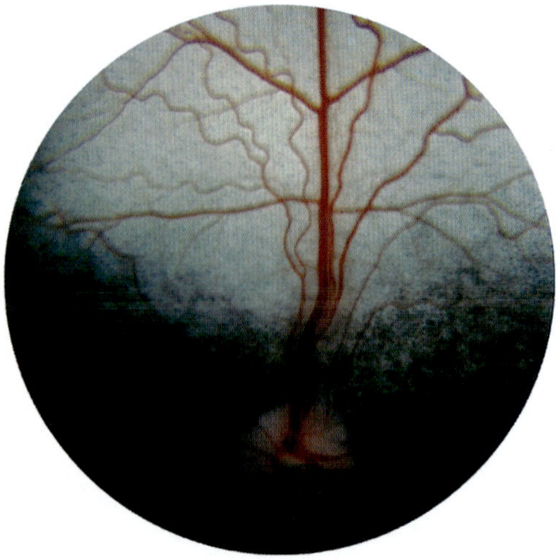

Figure 11-24
Normal retina in an Australian shepherd with a light-colored tapetum.

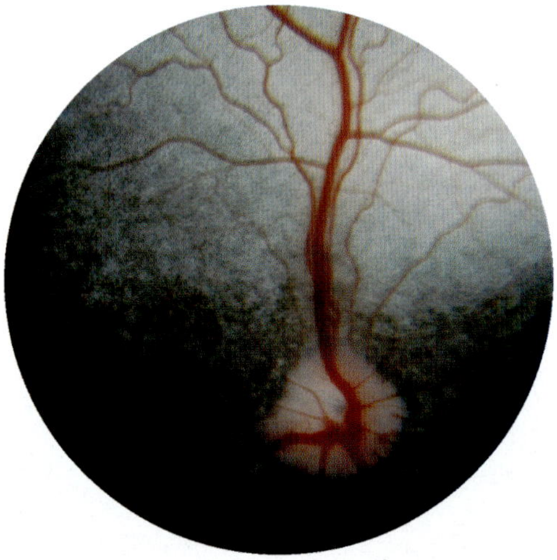

Figure 11-25
Normal retina with a gray tapetal color.

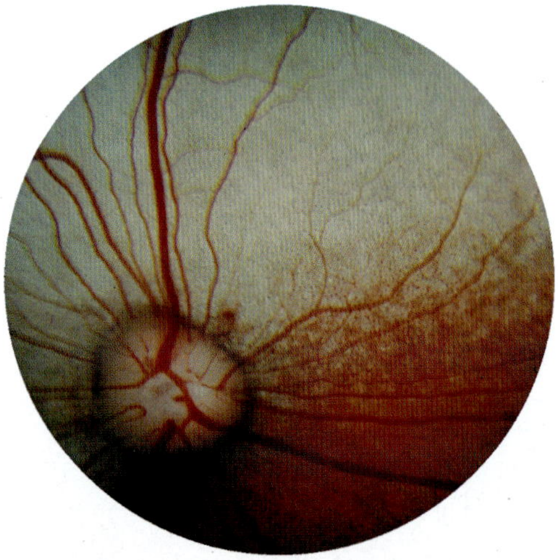

Figure 11-26
Normal retina. The tapetum is white with dark spots, which are the end-on view of capillaries passing through the tapetum from the deeper choroidal vessels to reach the choriocapillaris layer beneath the RPE. The nontapetum is subalbinotic.

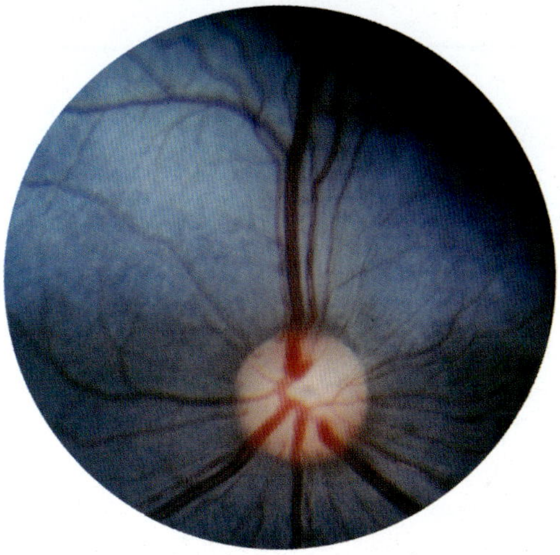

Figure 11-27
Juvenile fundus. In a very young dog the tapetum is a gray to lilac color, which changes to mature tapetal color during the first 3 months of life.

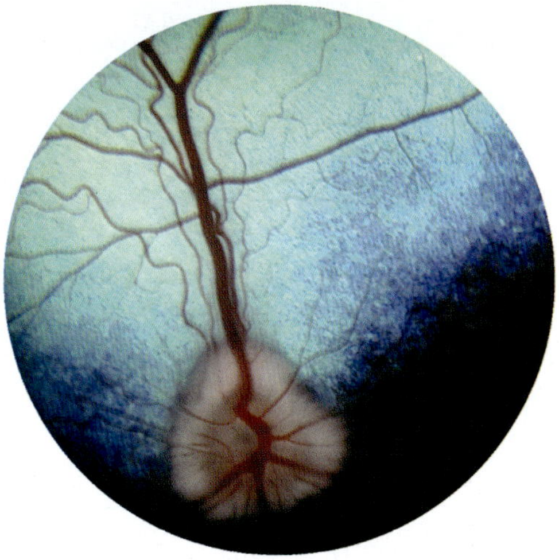

Figure 11-28
Normal retina in a young dog; the tapetum is starting to take on its adult color.

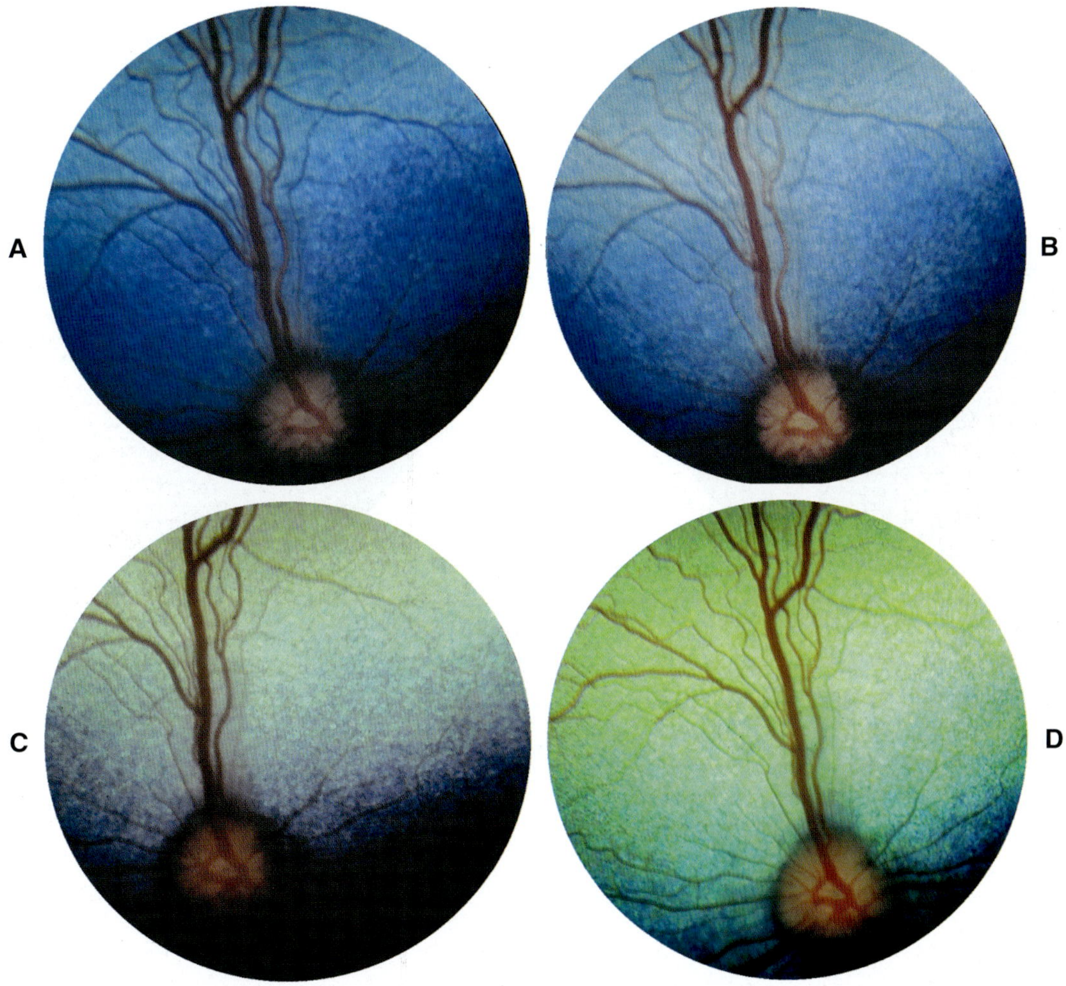

Figure 11-29 A-D
Normal basset hound puppy at ages **A,** 4, **B,** 8, **C,** 13, and **D,** 18 weeks. A change in tapetal color occurs with the change in age.

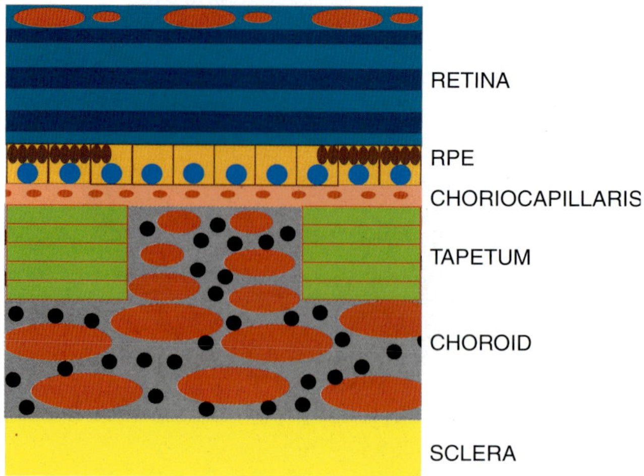

Figure 11-30
Tapetal hypoplasia. If the pigment is absent in the RPE, as it is in the diagram, an area of thin or absent tapetum reveals choroidal vessels and pigment as islands within the tapetal fundus. Areas of absent tapetum may also be present with pigment in the RPE, which is visible as pigmented spots in the superior fundus or as a greatly enlarged nontapetum and reduced-to-absent tapetum (this is not illustrated).

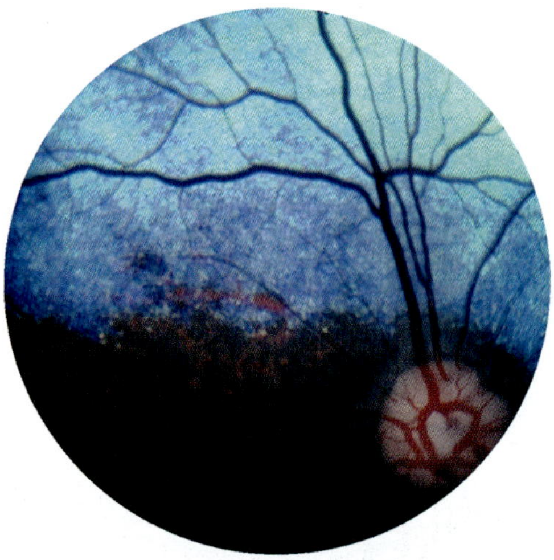

Figure 11-31
Normal retina in a young dog. Small focal absences of tapetum are present, and RPE pigment at the tapetal-nontapetal junction and choroidal vessels is visible.

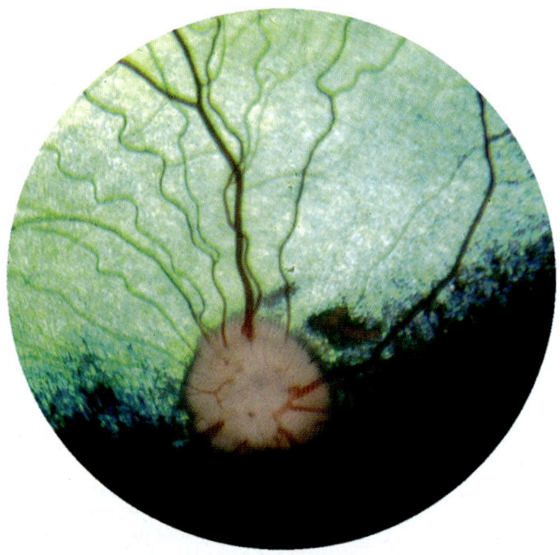

Figure 11-32
Normal retina. The tapetum has thinned areas through which choroidal vessels are showing.

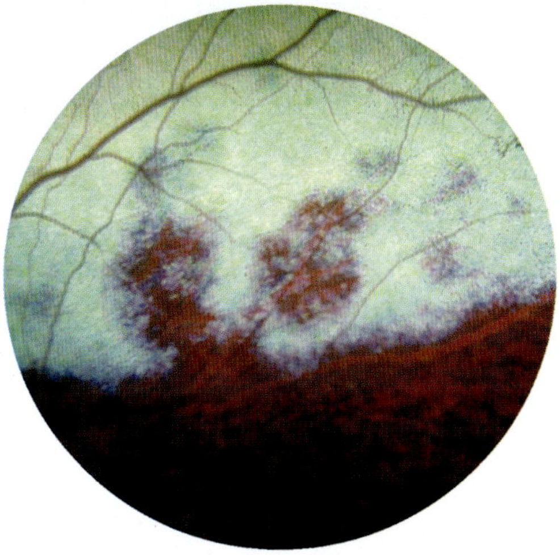

Figure 11-33
Normal tapetal-nontapetal junction in a dalmatian. Choroidal vessels are showing through in patches where the tapetum is missing and the RPE is nonpigmented.

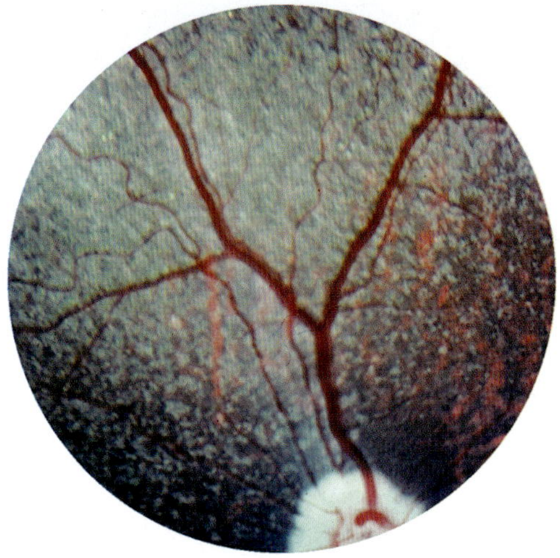

Figure 11-34
Normal retina in a collie. The tapetum consists of sparse, white islets of tapetal cells. The RPE is sparsely pigmented, resulting in the showing of choroidal vessels through the retina.
(Courtesy Dr. E. Dan Wolf.)

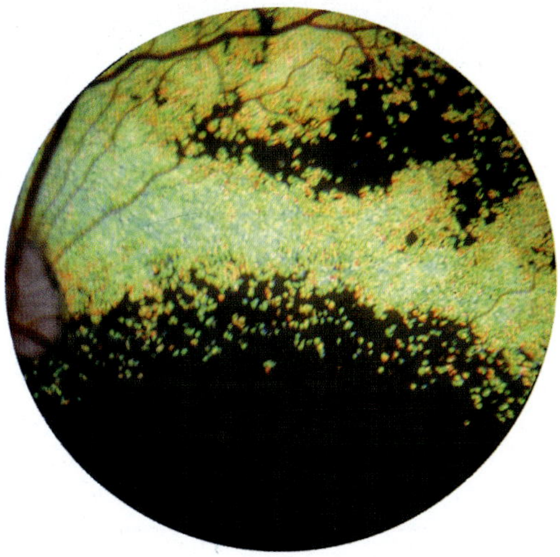

Figure 11-35
Normal retina. The tapetal-nontapetal junction is scalloped, the tapetum is missing in large areas, and the RPE is heavily pigmented.

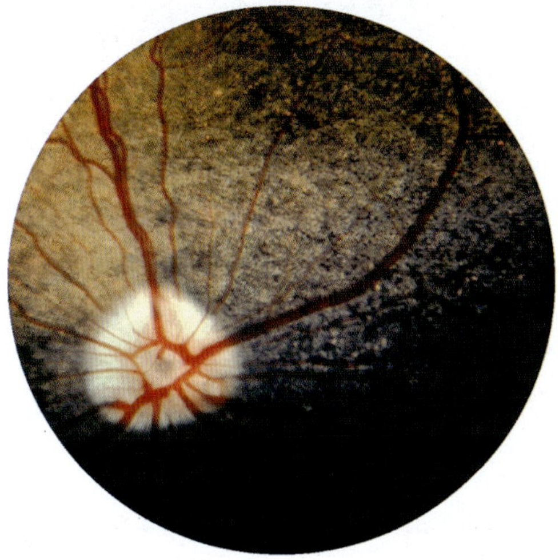

Figure 11-36
Normal retina in an Australian shepherd. Few tapetal cells are present, and RPE is pigmented in the superior fundus. End-on vessels can be seen in the tapetum.

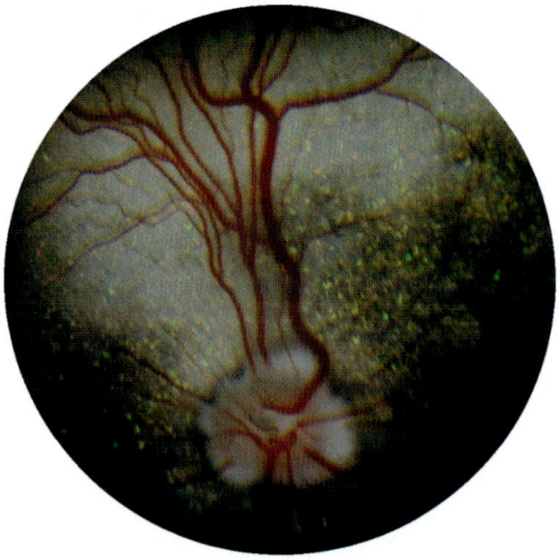

Figure 11-37
Normal retina. The tapetum is poorly developed; speckled tapetal cells of green and yellow predominate. Superiorly the tapetal color is somewhat diluted and is highlighted by reflection from the inner limiting membrane of the retina.

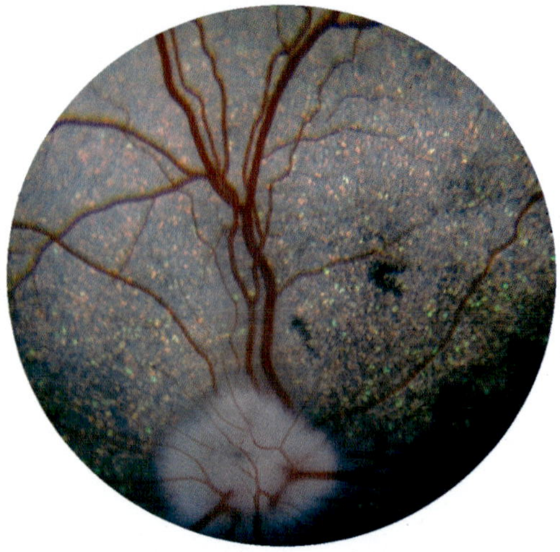

Figure 11-38
Normal Australian shepherd. The thin tapetum shows speckles of color throughout the superior fundus. The grayish reflex is a reflection from the inner limiting membrane of the retina.

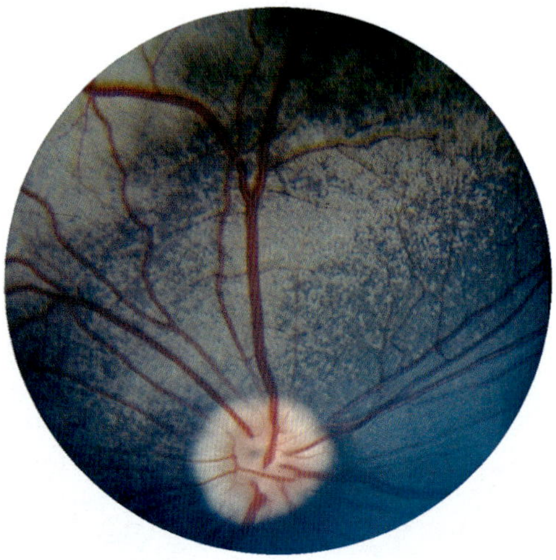

Figure 11-39
Normal retina with a sparse, white tapetum.

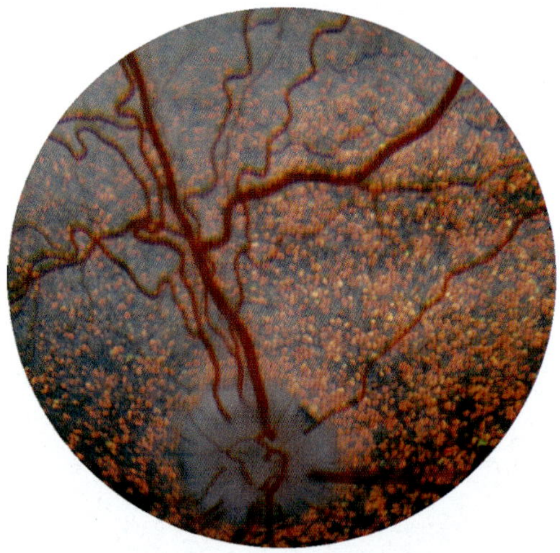

Figure 11-40
Normal tapetum in a Border collie. Sparse tapetum is visible as red tapetal islets. The superior gray color is a flash artifact from the inner limiting membrane.

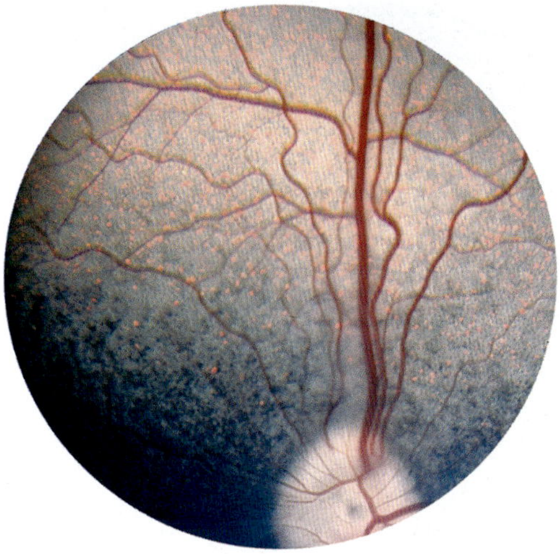

Figure 11-41
Normal retina. Small areas of tapetum are visible. Superiorly choroidal vessels can be seen through a sparsely pigmented RPE.

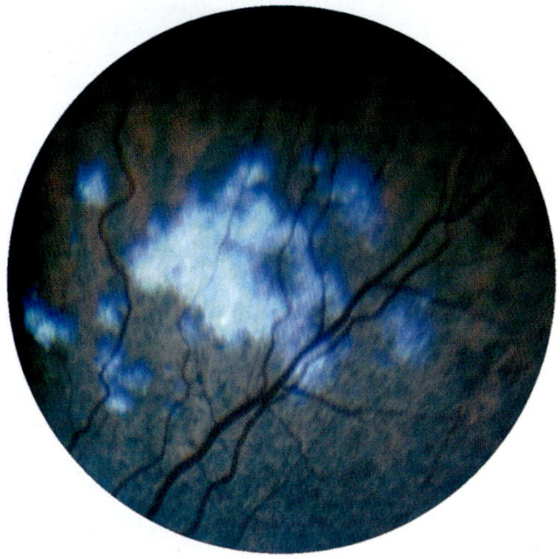

Figure 11-42
Normal retina. Small islets of tapetum are present in the superior fundus.

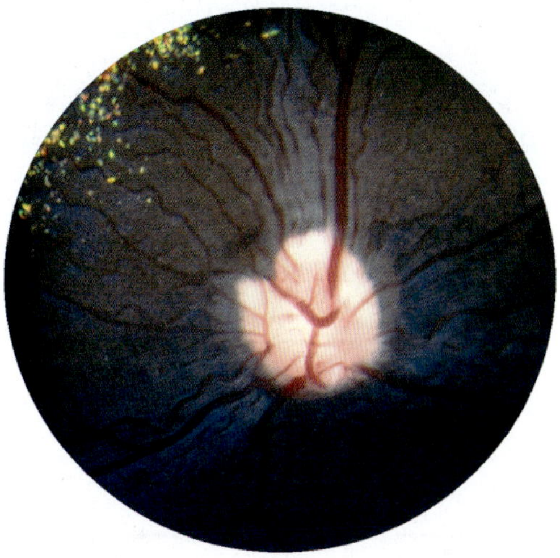

Figure 11-43
Normal retina. A few islets of tapetal cells are present superiorly. When such islets are present they are often in the temporal area of the fundus.

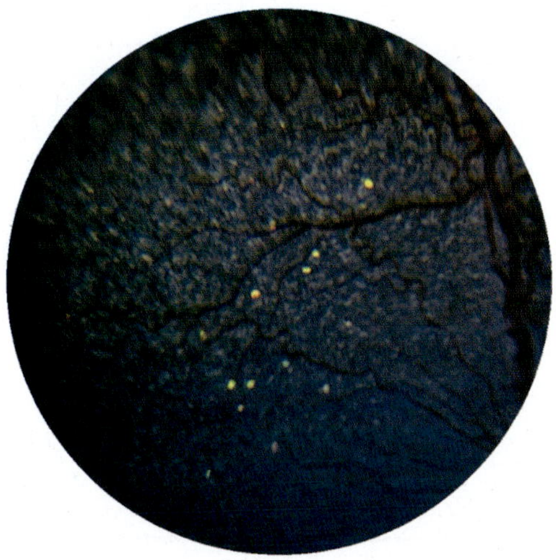

Figure 11-44
Normal retina. Several tapetal islets are shown.

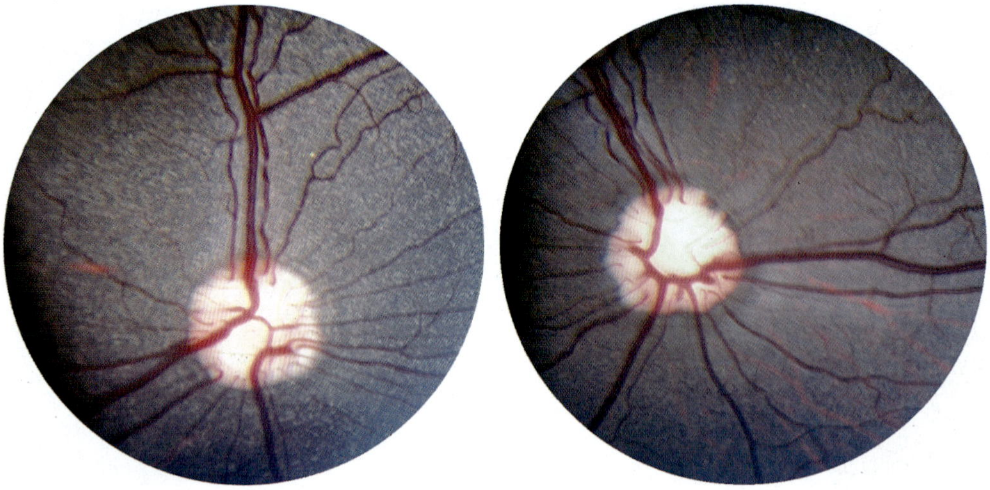

Figure 11-45
Normal retinas in a miniature longhaired dachshund. The tapetum is very poorly developed; choroidal vessels can be seen through sparsely pigmented RPE.

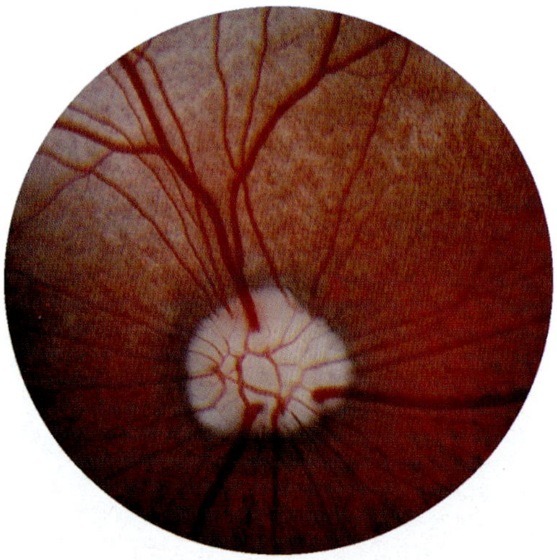

Figure 11-46
Normal retina in an Australian shepherd. The tapetum is sparse and white; choroidal vessels can be seen through a minimally pigmented RPE.

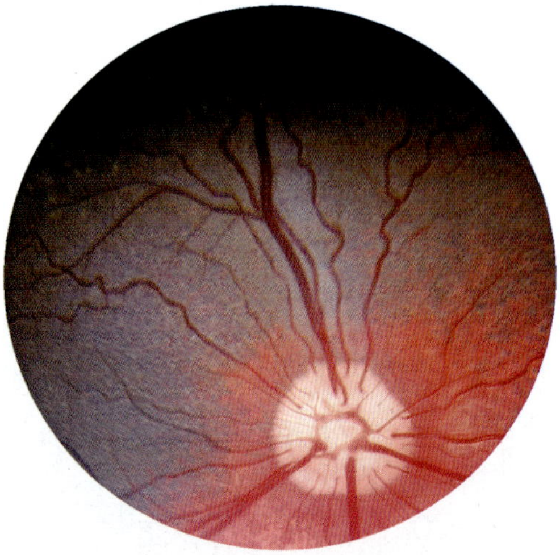

Figure 11-47
Normal retina. No tapetum is present. The RPE is pigmented superiorly, so this part of the fundus looks dark brown. The RPE is sparsely pigmented inferiorly where the red glow from the choroidal vessels is visible.

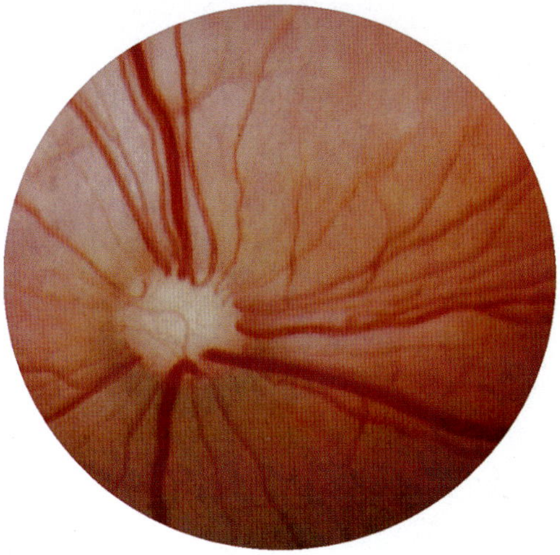

Figure 11-48
Normal, juvenile fundus. Disc is not well myelinated. The tapetum is poorly developed at this age.

Normal Nontapetum in Dogs

In the nontapetum of a normally pigmented dog the RPE is pigmented. The ophthalmoscopic appearance of the nontapetum is brown to black, with retinal vessels overlying the RPE.

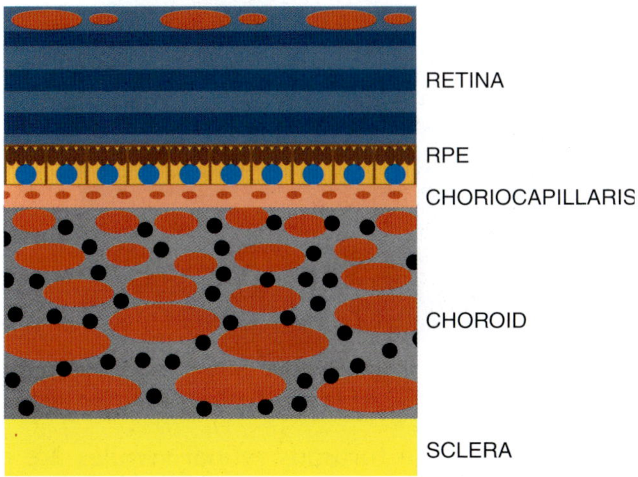

Figure 11-49
Schematic diagram of the nontapetum of a dog. The RPE is pigmented (brown ovals in the cells represent pigment granules). When the fundus is viewed, the choroid and sclera cannot be seen because of the overlying RPE pigment.

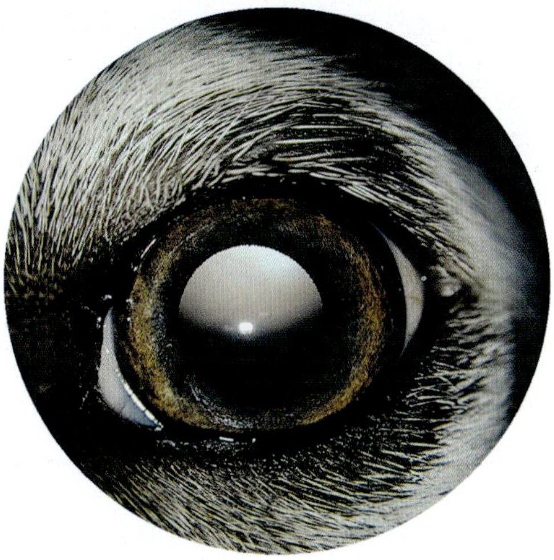

Figure 11-50
Normal dark-colored canine iris, which would be associated with a well-pigmented fundus. (Courtesy Dr. Robert Playter.)

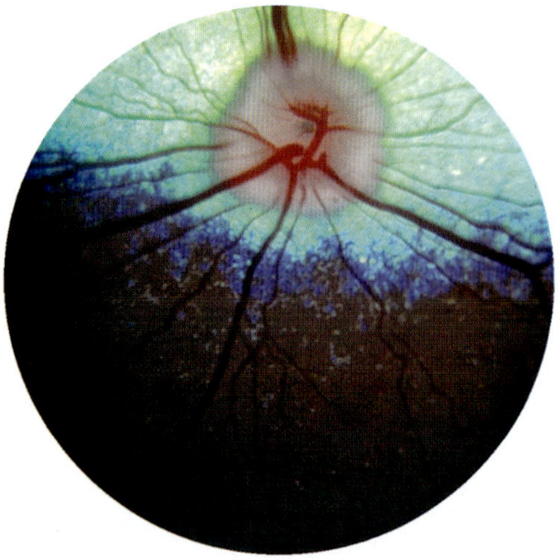

Figure 11-51
Normal dog. The nontapetal color is dark brown.

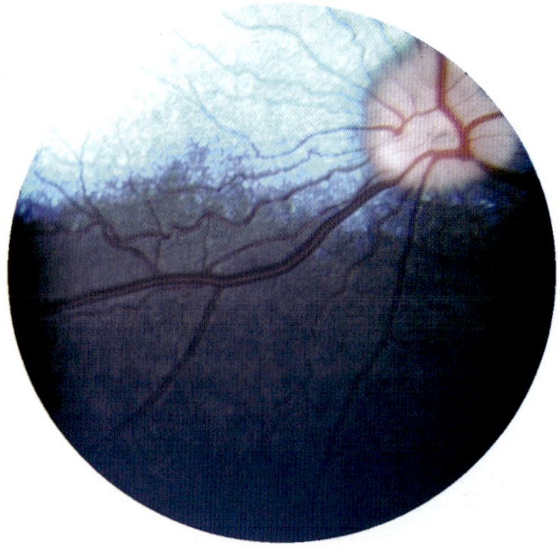

Figure 11-52
Normal dog. This is a typical dark-brown nontapetum.

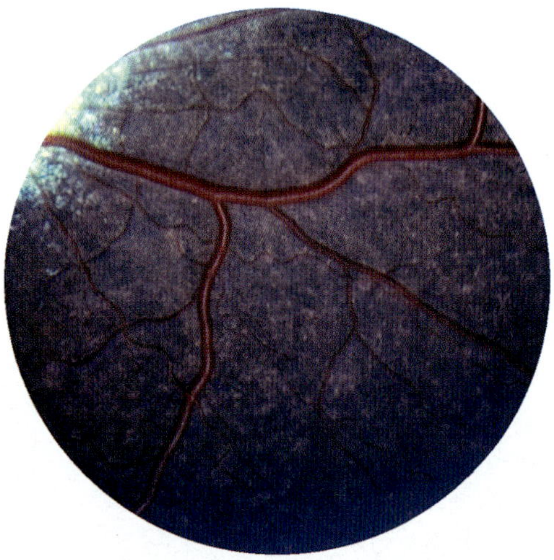

Figure 11-53
Normal dog. The diffuse mottling of the superior nontapetum is common.

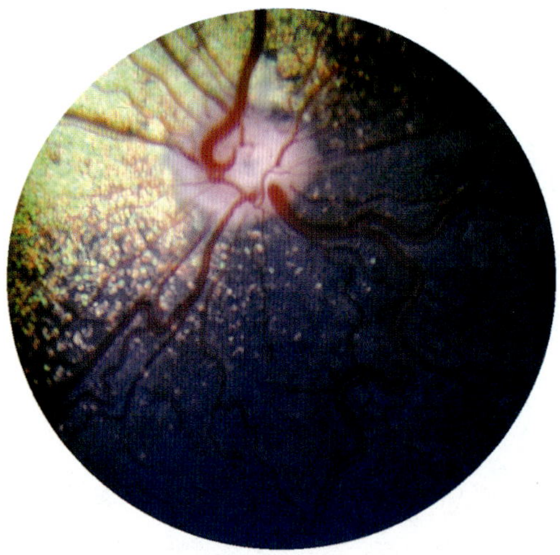

Figure 11-54
Normal dog. The tortuous retinal venules are a normal variation.

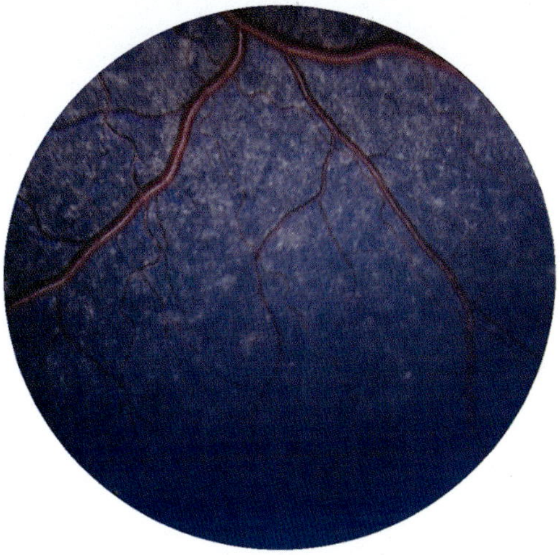

Figure 11-55
Normal dog nontapetum; the blue color is the effect of the camera flash distributed across the retina. This view is of a more peripheral area of the nontapetum seen in Figure 11-53.

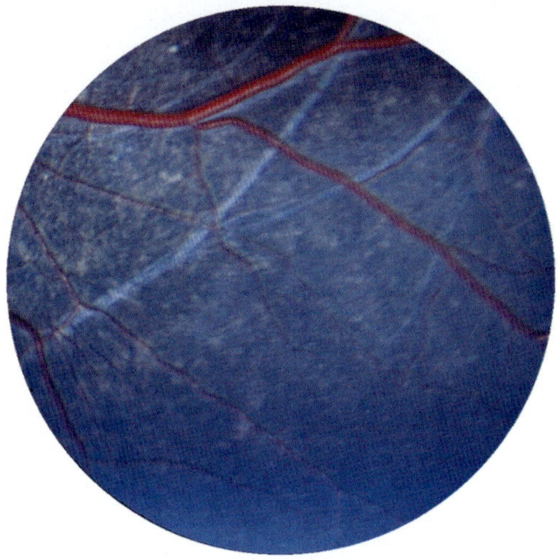

Figure 11-56
Normal dog. Myelinated nerve fibers are visible as arcing white lines in an American cocker spaniel (blue color is camera flash artifact).

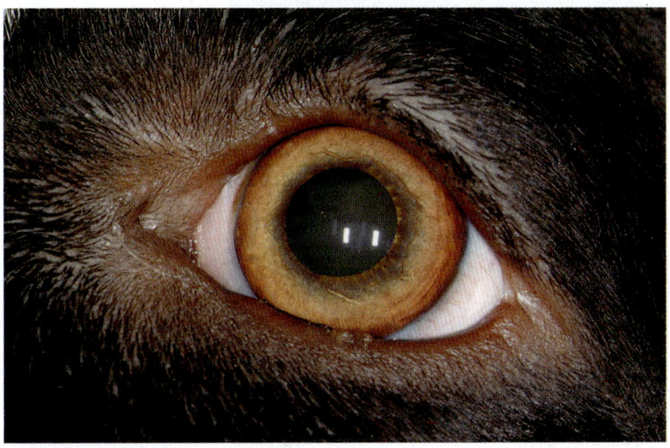

Figure 11-57
In dogs with a light (color dilute) coat color (e.g., chocolate Labrador retriever) the iris is a light brown, as in this German short-haired pointer, and fundus pigmentation can be expected to be correspondingly reduced.

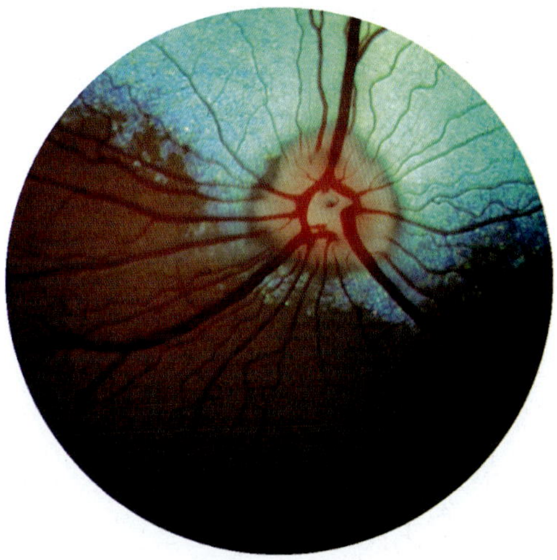

Figure 11-58
Normal dog. The chocolate-brown color of the nontapetum is usually associated with a color dilute coat (e.g., a chocolate Labrador retriever).

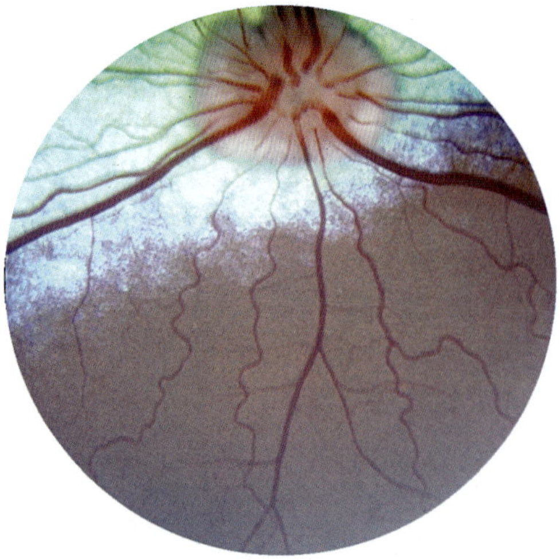

Figure 11-59
Normal fundus in a liver-colored German short-haired pointer. The RPE in the nontapetum is less pigmented than that of non–color-dilute dogs and looks reddish brown because of the underlying choroidal vessels and the bright reflection from the flash.

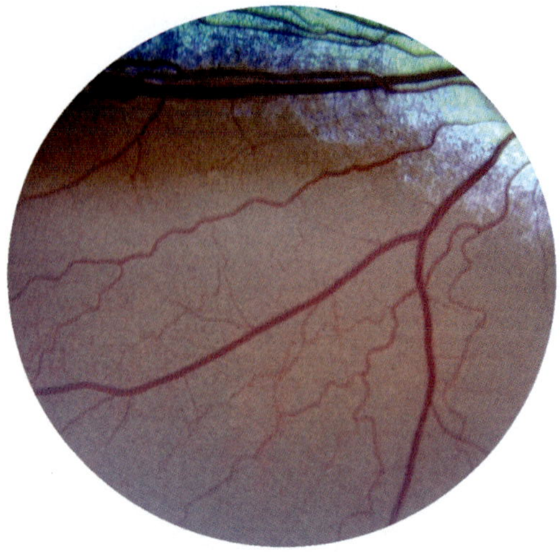

Figure 11-60
Normal dog with a color-dilute coat and reddish-brown nontapetum.

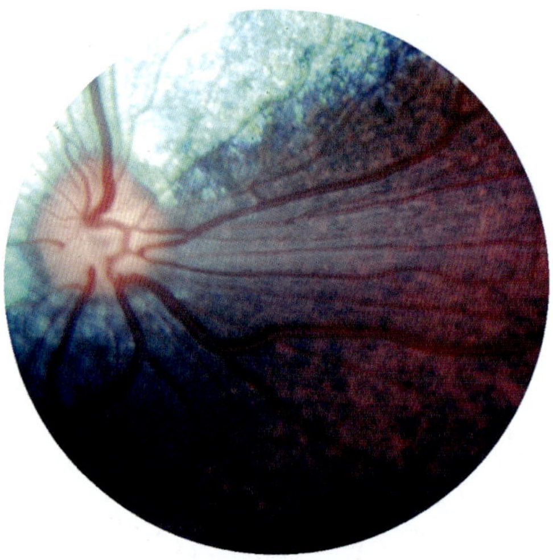

Figure 11-61
Normal greyhound; choroidal vessels can be seen in the periphery of the nontapetum because of absence of pigment in the RPE.

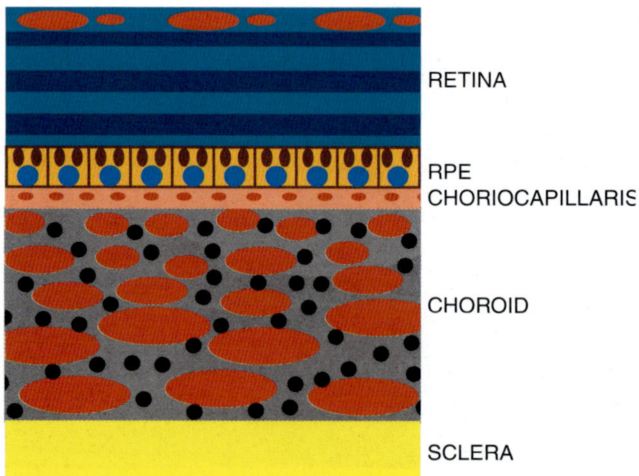

Figure 11-62
Red fundus. This phenomenon appears in some breeds with a poorly developed or absent tapetum but with some pigment in the RPE. The red appearance is assumed to be an optical effect of viewing red blood in the choroidal vessels through a thin layer of pigment.

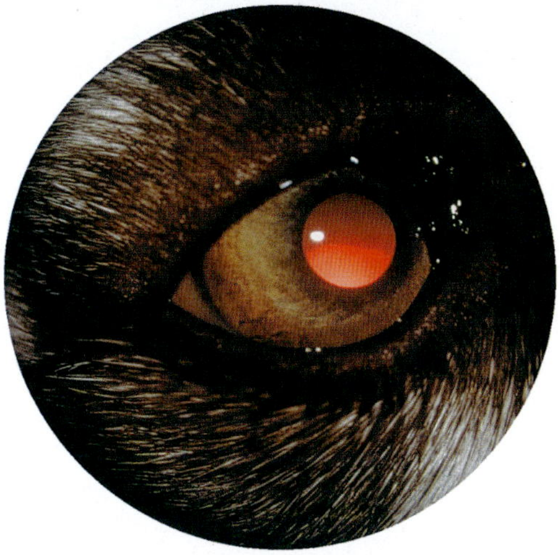

Figure 11-63
Normal Siberian husky. A light-colored iris with reduced pigment in the fundus gives a reddish glow to the fundic reflex visible through the pupil.

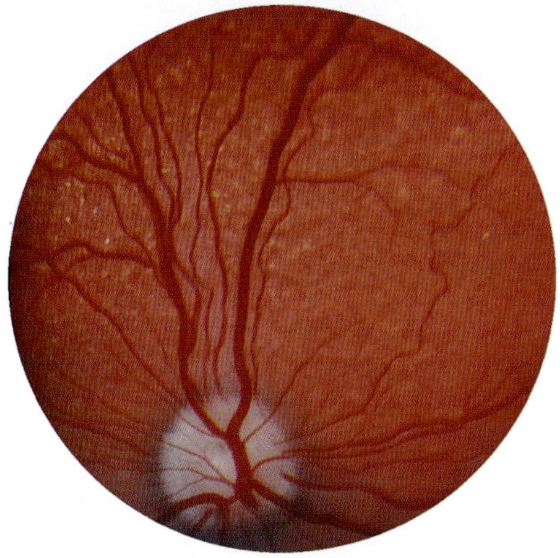

Figure 11-64
Normal Australian shepherd. Development of the tapetum is very limited, most evident in the temporal fundus.

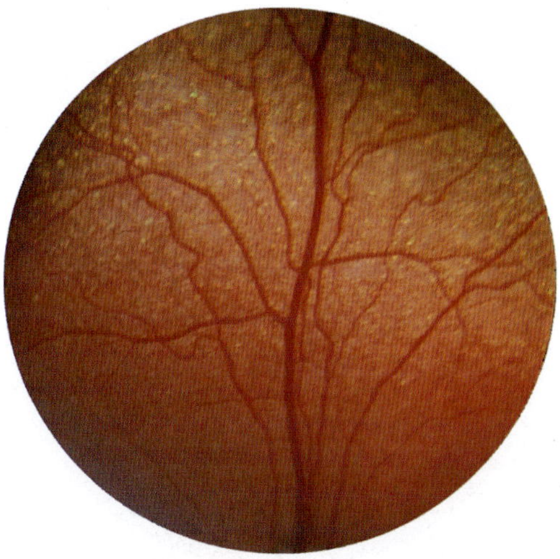

Figure 11-65
Normal tapetal fundus. Note scattered tapetal islets.

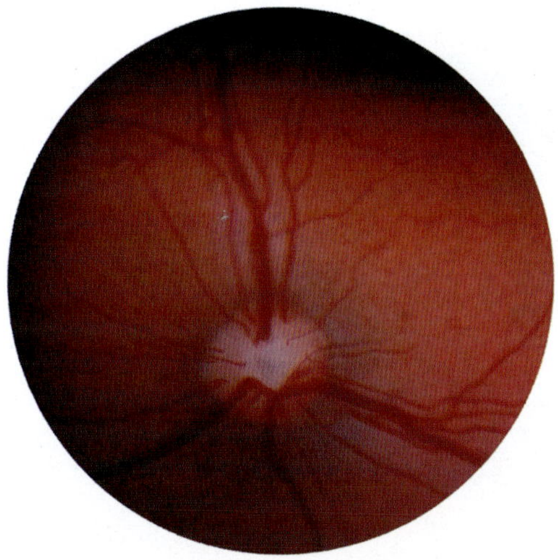

Figure 11-66
Normal juvenile fundus.

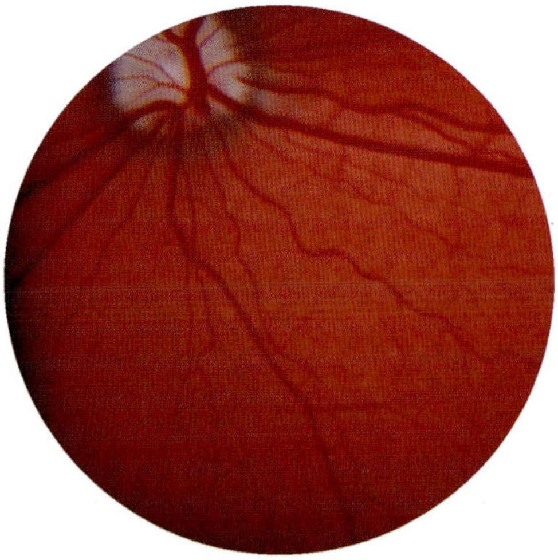

Figure 11-67
Nontapetum in a normal Australian shepherd.

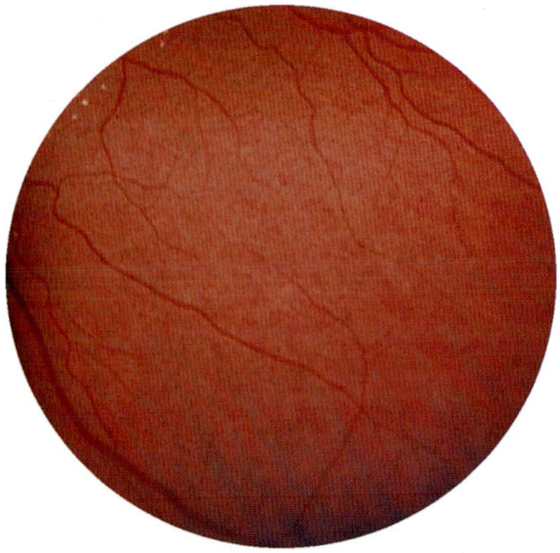

Figure 11-68
Nontapetum in a normal Australian shepherd. Distinct choroidal vessels can be seen inferiorly in the far periphery.

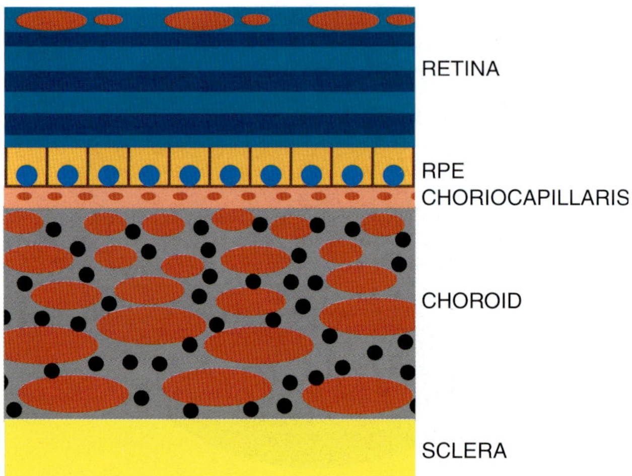

Figure 11-69
Tigroid nontapetal fundus, so called because of the tiger-striped appearance of the choroidal vessels and choroidal pigment. The pigment is reduced or absent in the RPE, which allows the viewer to see retinal vessels superimposed on a background of choroidal vessels and pigment. The sclera is not visible because the choroidal pigment absorbs any light incident on it.

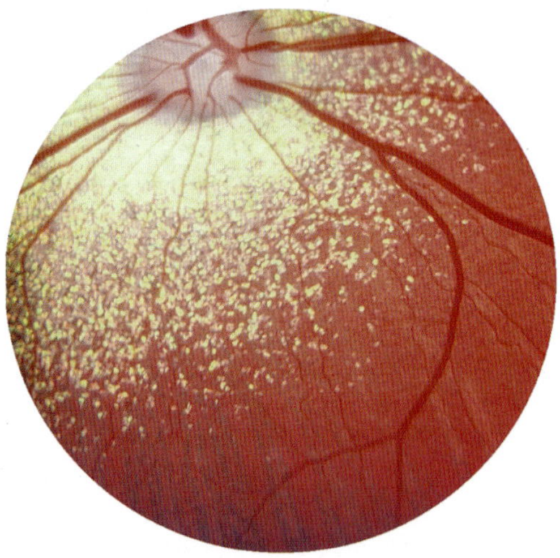

Figure 11-70
Normal dog. Tigroid fundus.

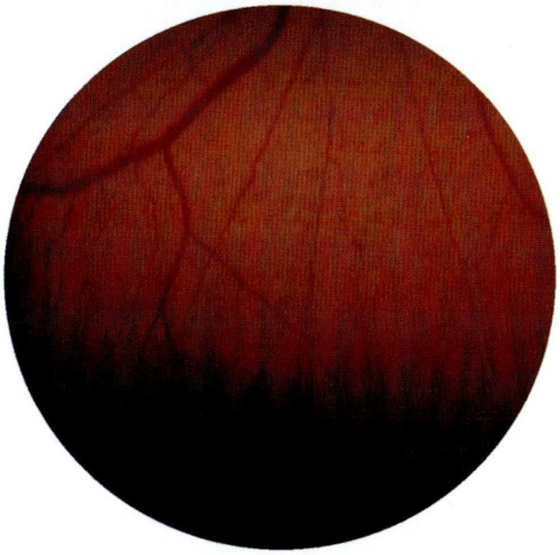

Figure 11-71
Normal Australian shepherd. Tigroid fundus.

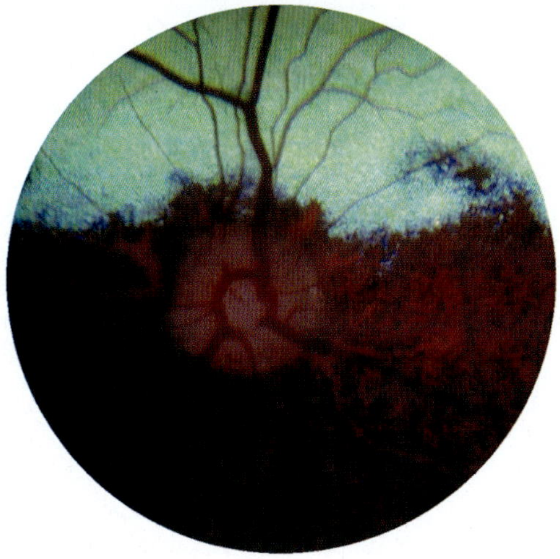

Figure 11-72
Normal retina with choroidal vessels visible in nontapetum.

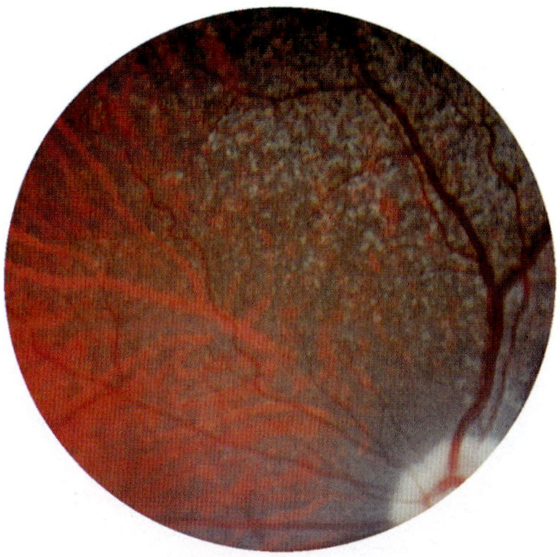

Figure 11-73
Normal merle collie. Choroidal vessels are visible on left side of photograph.
(Courtesy Dr. E. Dan Wolf.)

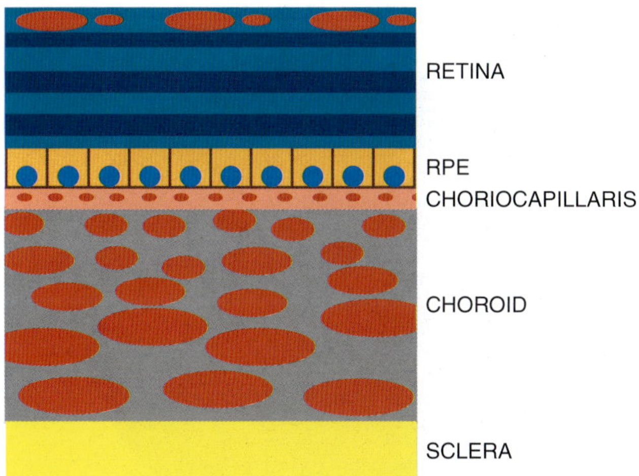

Figure 11-74
Subalbinotic fundus. Pigment is reduced or absent in the RPE and choroid. The resulting funduscopic appearance is of retinal vessels superimposed on choroidal vessels, all superimposed on the white background of the sclera.

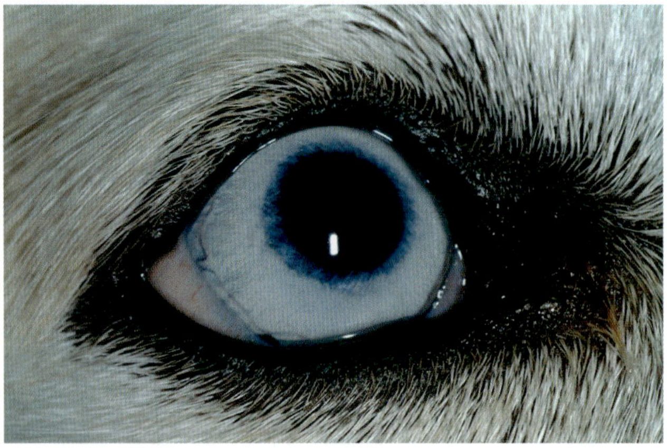

Figure 11-75
Subalbinotic iris in a Siberian husky.

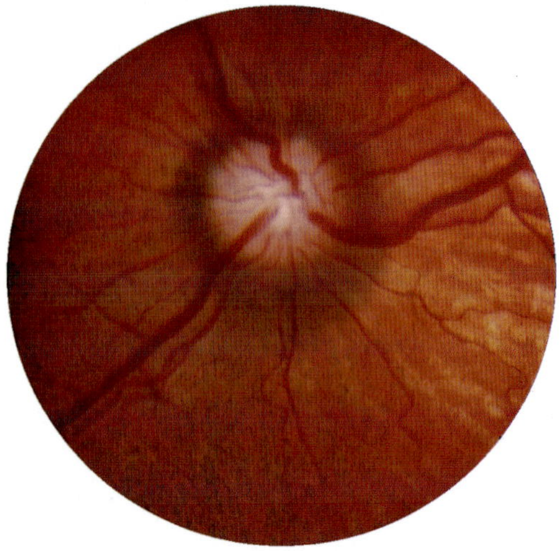

Figure 11-76
Normal Australian shepherd. No tapetum is visible in this photograph, and the tiger stripes of the choroidal vessels are visible on the right.

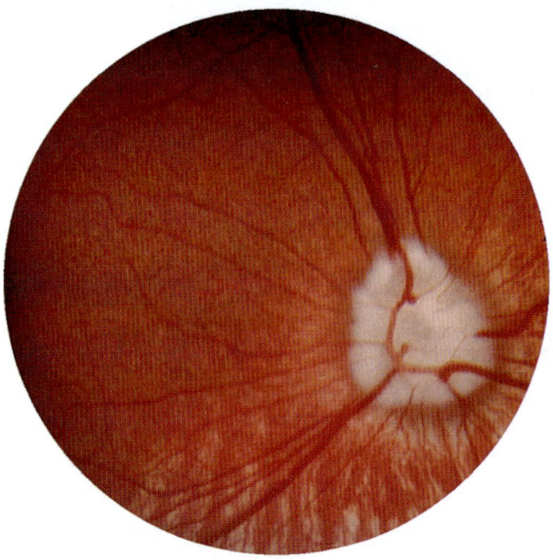

Figure 11-77
Normal dog. No tapetum is visible in this photograph, and the tiger stripes of the choroidal vessels are visible in the nontapetum.

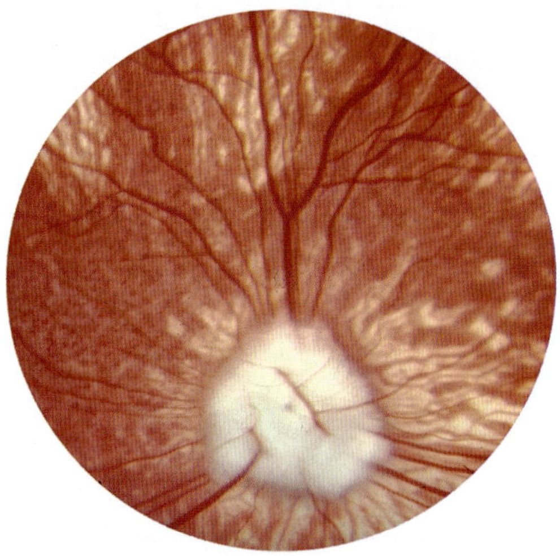

Figure 11-78
Normal dog. Choroidal vessels are visible throughout the fundus.

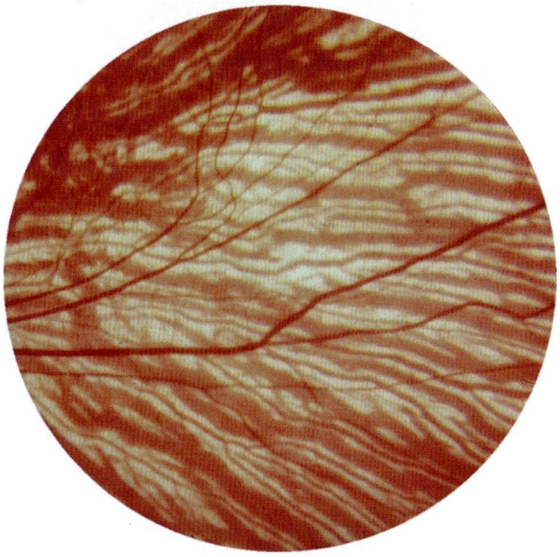

Figure 11-79
Normal dog. Choroidal vessels are visible throughout the fundus. More peripheral area of the same fundus as shown in Figure 11-78.

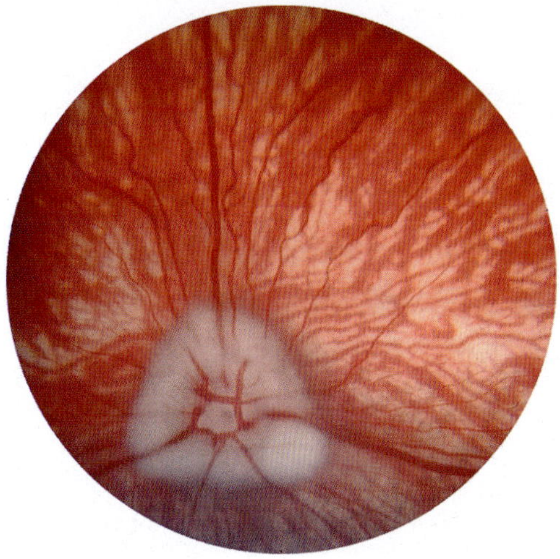

Figure 11-80
Normal Siberian husky. Choroidal vessels are visible throughout the fundus.

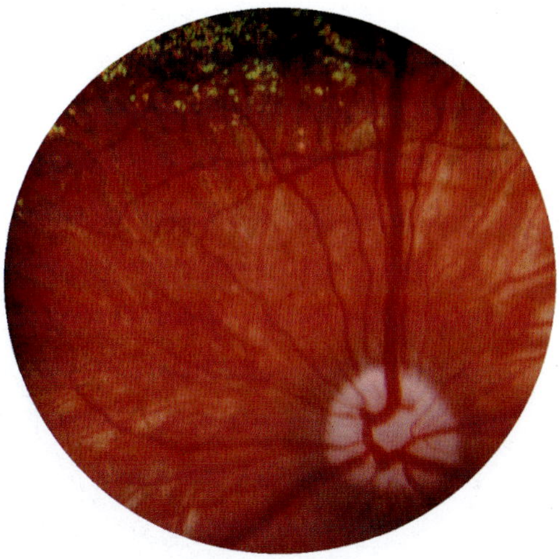

Figure 11-81
Normal dog. Islets of tapetal cells are visible superiorly; choroidal vessels are visible throughout the rest of the fundus.

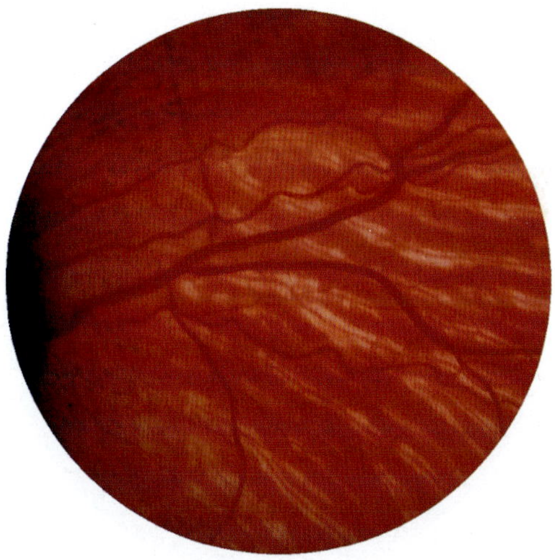

Figure 11-82
Normal Australian shepherd. Choroidal vessels are visible throughout the fundus.

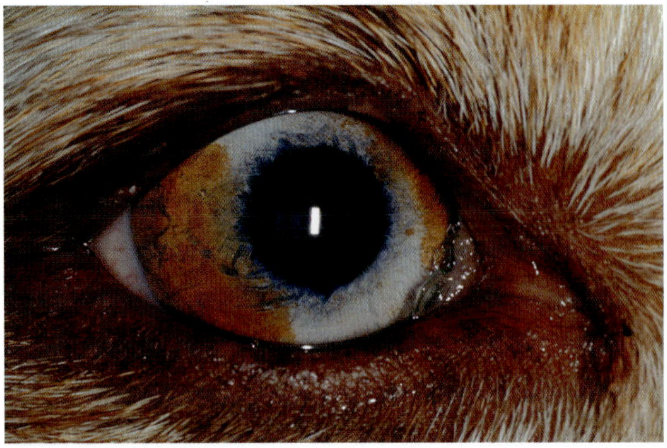

Figure 11-83
Heterochromia in an Australian shepherd.

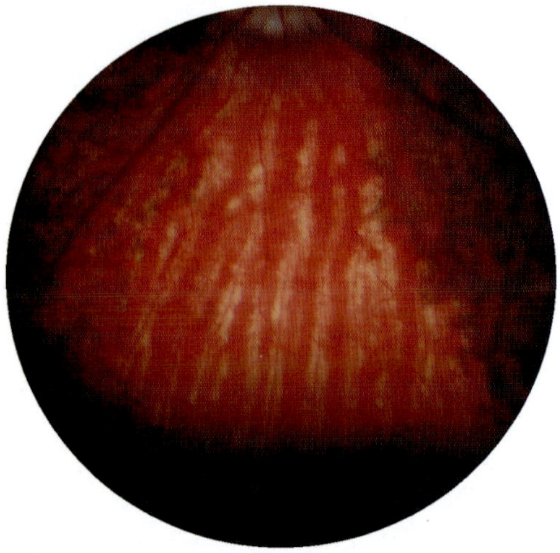

Figure 11-84
Australian shepherd from Figure 11-83. Some areas of RPE are normally pigmented; other areas are nonpigmented, and choroidal vessels can be seen.

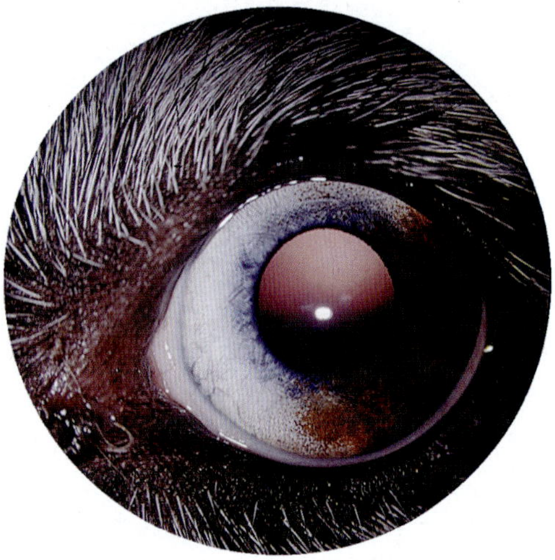

Figure 11-85
Normal dog. Heterochromia with a fundus similar to Figure 11-86.

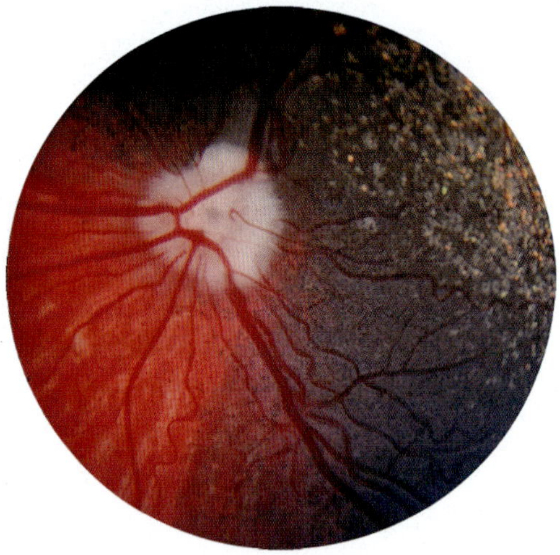

Figure 11-86
Normal dog. Tapetum is sparse superiorly. Some areas of RPE are normally pigmented; other areas are unpigmented, and choroidal vessels can be seen.

NORMAL FUNDUS IN CATS

As in the dog, the ophthalmoscopic view of the tapetal fundus of the cat shows retinal vessels superimposed on the highly colored tapetum. The only visible components of the retina are the blood vessels. The RPE in this region is nonpigmented to allow light to reach and be reflected by the tapetum. Therefore the RPE layer is not visible either. Compared with dogs, cats have fewer variations in the tapetum. Usually the tapetal color is yellowish, and the optic nerve is usually in the tapetum. The nontapetum in cats is usually dark brown, with retinal vessels superimposed. Blue-eyed white cats usually have no tapetum and have a subalbinotic fundus, similar to blue-eyed dogs. Blue-eyed cats with Siamese point coloring (e.g., Siamese, Himalayan) usually have a normal tapetum, but the nontapetum is subalbinotic.

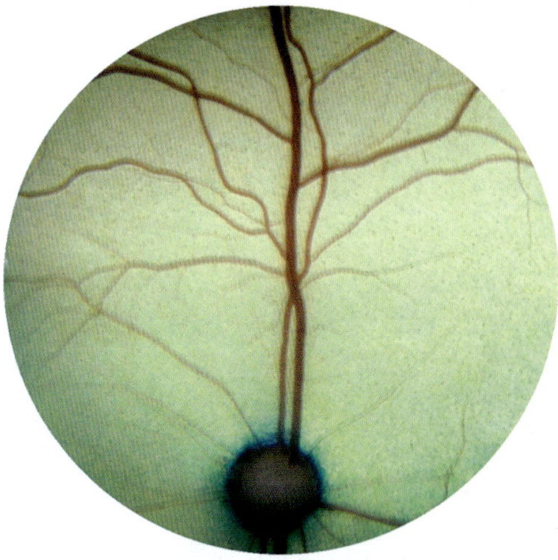

Figure 11-87
Normal cat. The tapetal color is typical, and the optic nerve is surrounded by tapetum.

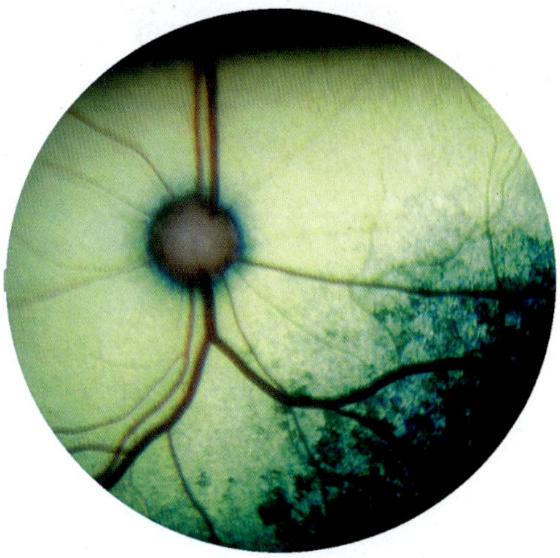

Figure 11-88
Normal cat.

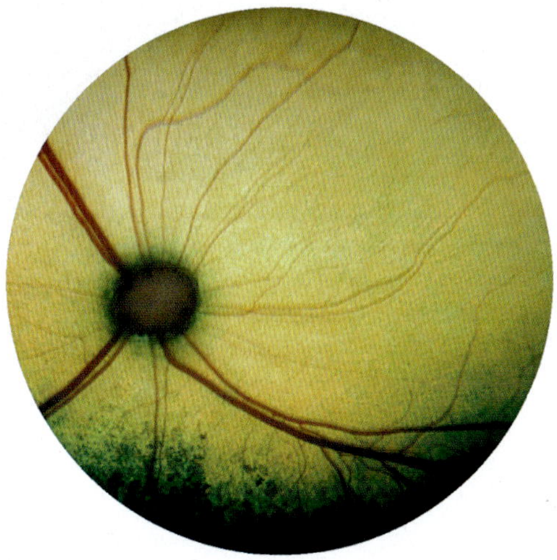

Figure 11-89
Normal cat.

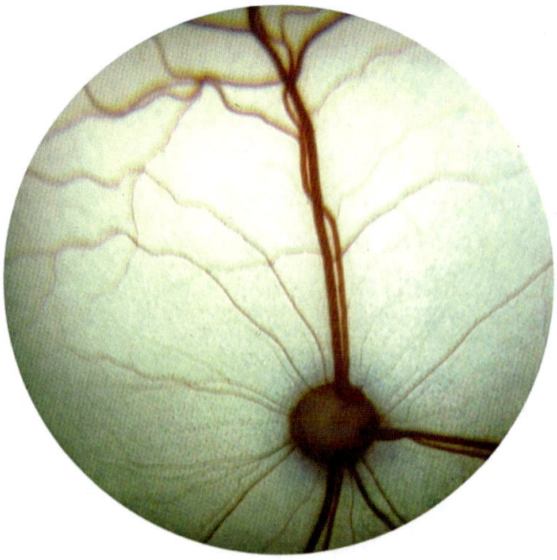

Figure 11-90
Normal cat with an odd variation on tapetal color.

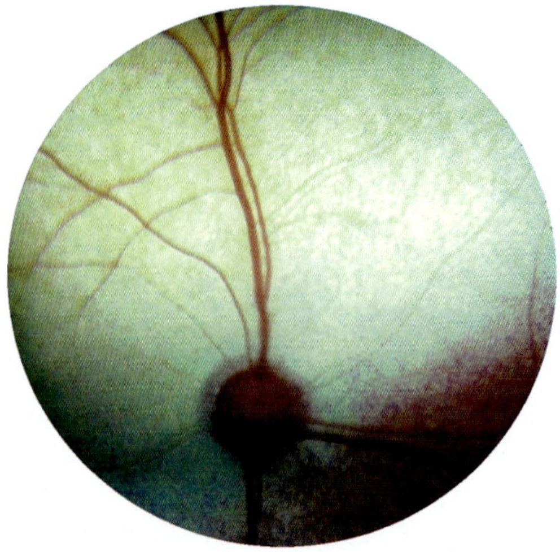

Figure 11-91
Normal cat.

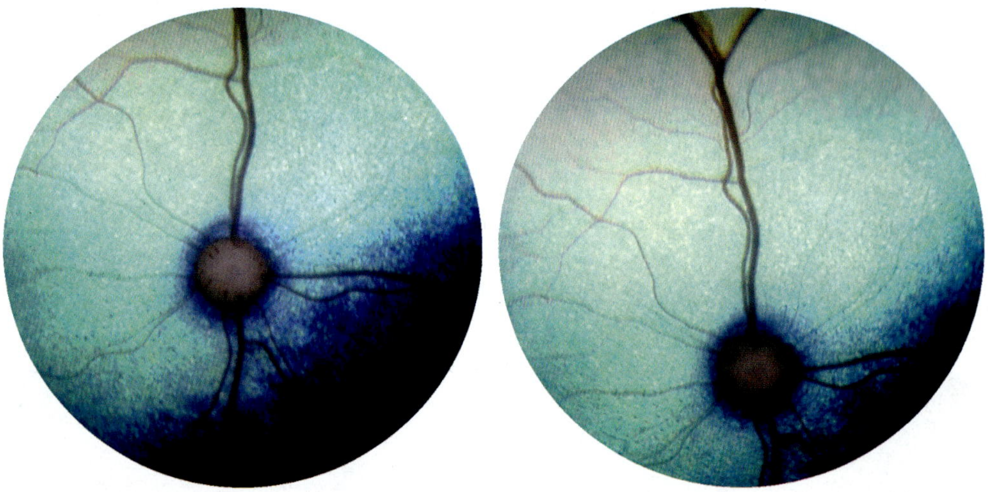

Figure 11-92
Two views of a normal fundus in a cat.

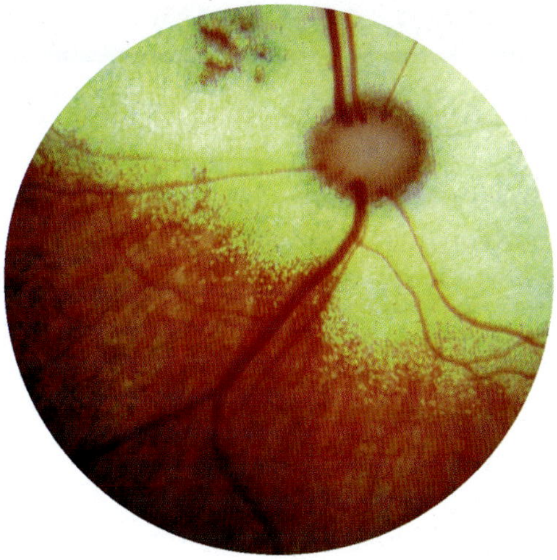

Figure 11-93
Normal Siamese-type fundus. Note the area of missing tapetal cells at the 11 o'clock position, with choroid showing through. The nontapetum is subalbinotic with choroidal vessels seen.

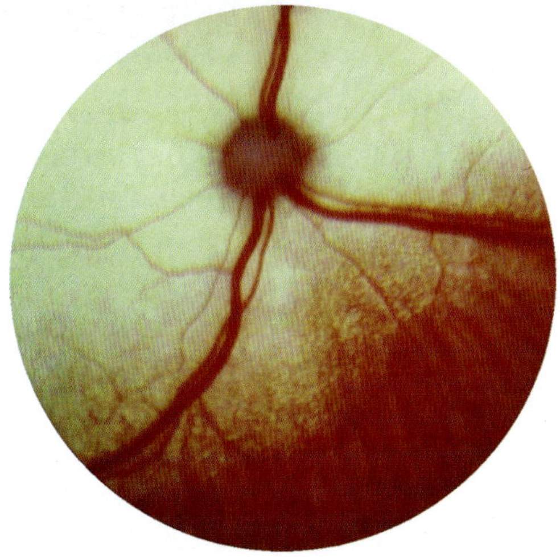

Figure 11-94
Normal Siamese-type fundus.

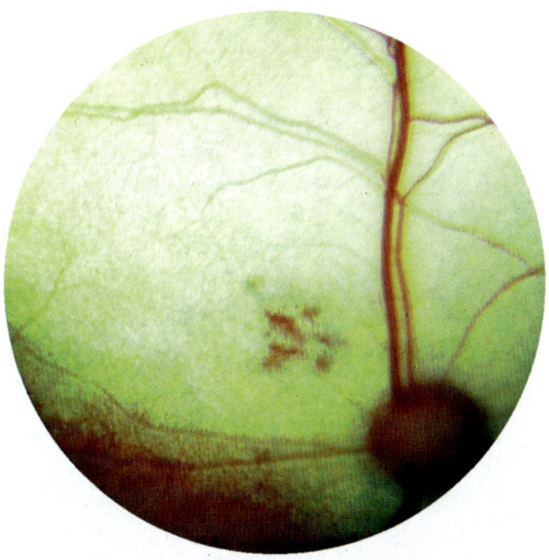

Figure 11-95
Normal cat. Choroidal vessels are showing through the tapetum of a Siamese cat.

CANINE PROGRESSIVE RETINAL ATROPHY

Progressive retinal atrophy (PRA) is a catch-all term used to describe retinal degenerations that are bilateral, progressive, inherited (and therefore breed associated), and eventually blinding. Because PRA usually begins as a rod abnormality, the first clinical sign noticed is night blindness. Because cones are also involved in the disease, day blindness follows. Ophthalmoscopically the first signs of PRA are altered tapetal reflectivity in the peripheral tapetum and mild retinal vessel attenuation. With progression the tapetum becomes diffusely hyperreflective, retinal vessels are markedly attenuated, pigment alteration occurs in the nontapetum, and the optic nerve becomes atrophic. Cataracts are often present secondary to PRA. Age of onset can vary considerably depending on the particular breed involved.

Photoreceptor dysplasias are inherited forms of PRA characterized by an early onset of clinical signs. Histologically, affected dogs never develop normal photoreceptors. In photoreceptor degenerations, rods and cones develop normally but undergo degeneration later in life. Clinical signs depend on whether rods, cones, or both are affected.

Progressive Retinal Atrophy and the Tapetum

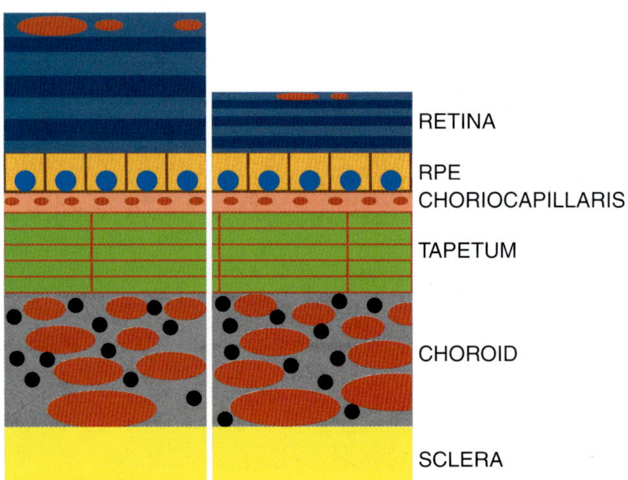

Figure 11-96
The schematic drawing on the left illustrates a normal retina; the one on the right illustrates a retina affected by PRA. The thinning of the retina in the tapetal fundus allows more reflection of light from the tapetum, visible as hyperreflectivity.

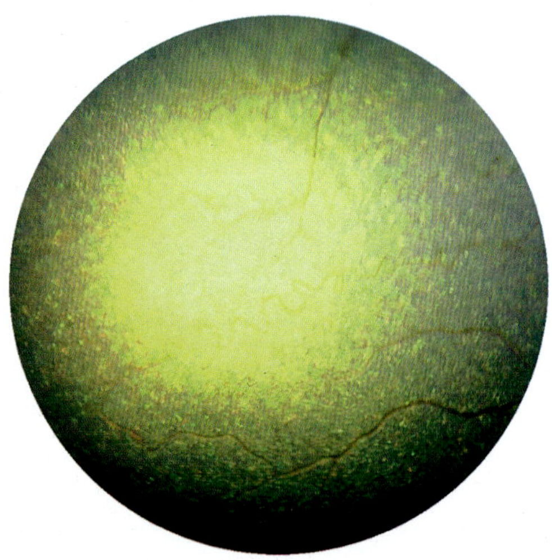

Figure 11-97
Rod-cone dysplasia type 1 in a 14-month-old Irish setter—the same dog as shown in Figures 11-98 and 11-99. This photograph shows the peripheral tapetum and marked tapetal hyperreflectivity and vessel attenuation.

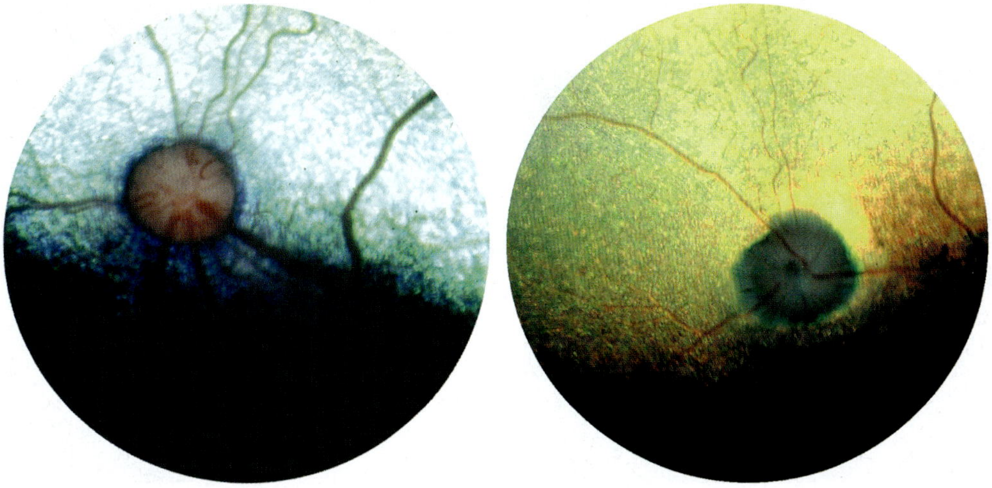

Figure 11-98 A-B
A, Rod-cone dysplasia type 1 in an Irish setter at 4 months of age. Note the juvenile fundus, which ophthalmoscopically appears normal. **B**, Rod-cone dysplasia type 1 in the same dog at 10 months of age. This photograph is of the same dog as shown in Figures 11-97 and 11-99. Tapetal hyperreflectivity, vessel thinning, and optic atrophy can be seen.

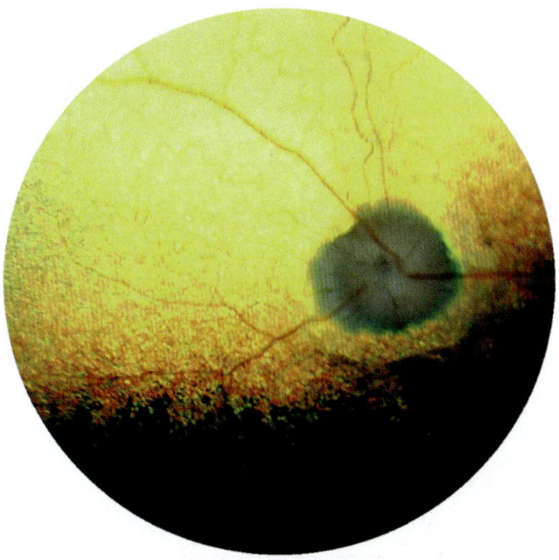

Figure 11-99
Rod-cone dysplasia type 1 in a 14-month-old Irish setter—the same dog as shown in Figures 11-97 and 11-98. Tapetal hyperreflectivity, vessel thinning, optic atrophy, and glial proliferations at edge of the nerve (gliosis) can be seen.

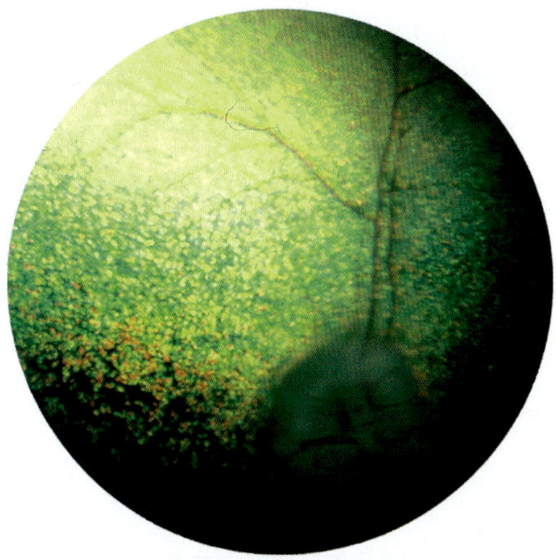

Figure 11-100
Progressive retinal atrophy in a Gordon setter. Retinal blood vessels are attenuated, and tapetal hyperreflectivity is present.

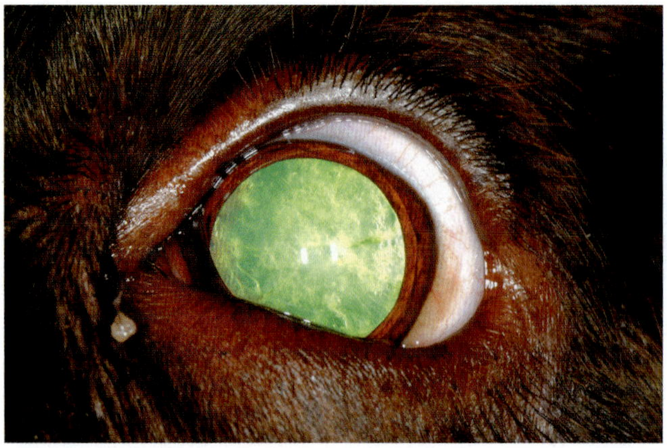

Figure 11-101
PRA in a 5-year-old Labrador retriever. Note the relatively bright tapetal reflection and the associated cataract.

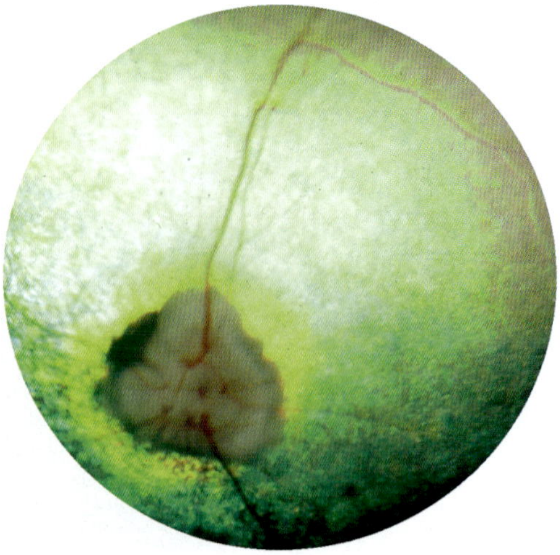

Figure 11-102
PRA in a 3-year-old Labrador retriever with hyperreflective tapetum, decreased blood vessels, and optic atrophy.

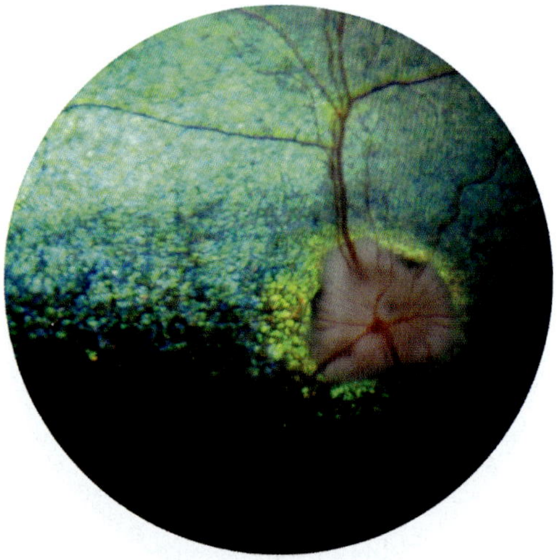

Figure 11-103
PRA in a 4-year-old Labrador retriever. Tapetal hyperreflectivity, notable color change around the optic nerve, and vessel attenuation are present.

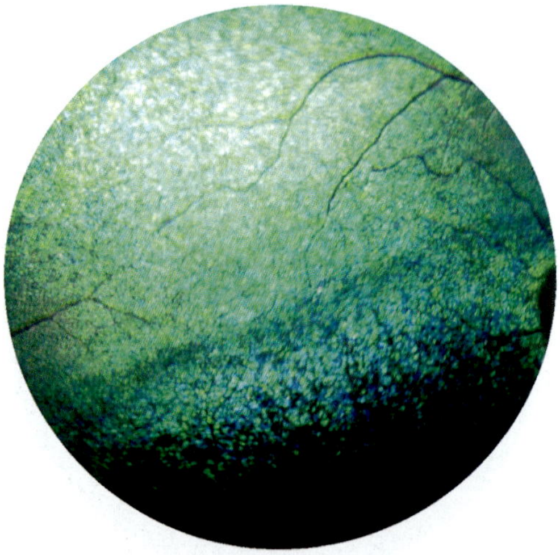

Figure 11-104
PRA in a 4-year-old Labrador retriever (same dog as shown in Figure 11-103). Peripheral tapetum with hyperreflectivity is shown, with altered reflectivity and vessel attenuation.

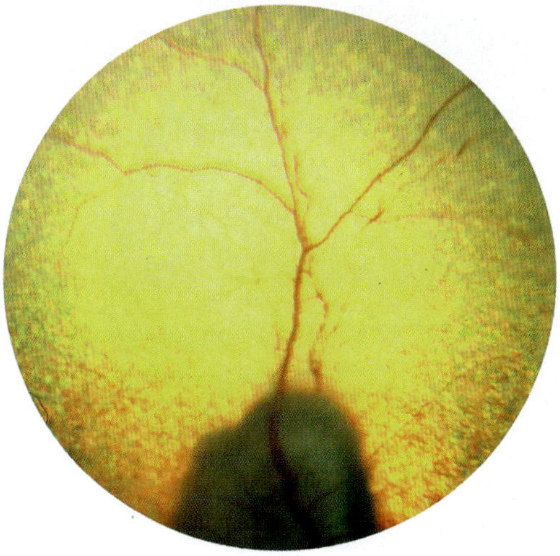

Figure 11-105
PRA in a 7-year-old golden retriever. Vessel attenuation, "boxcarring" of retinal vessels, and tapetal hyperreflectivity are visible.

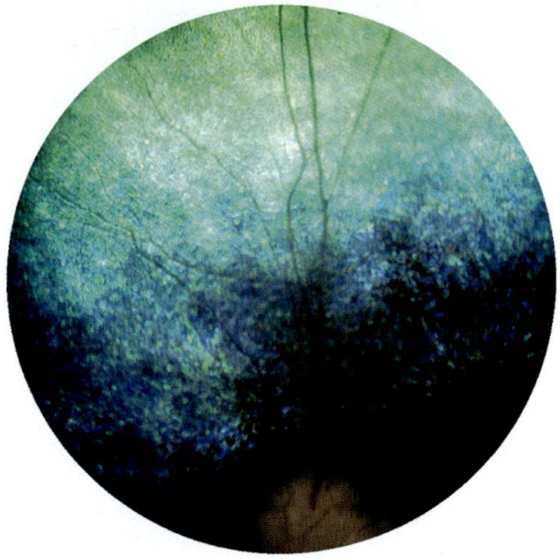

Figure 11-106
PRA in a pug. Tapetal hyperreflectivity and attenuated retinal vessels are visible.

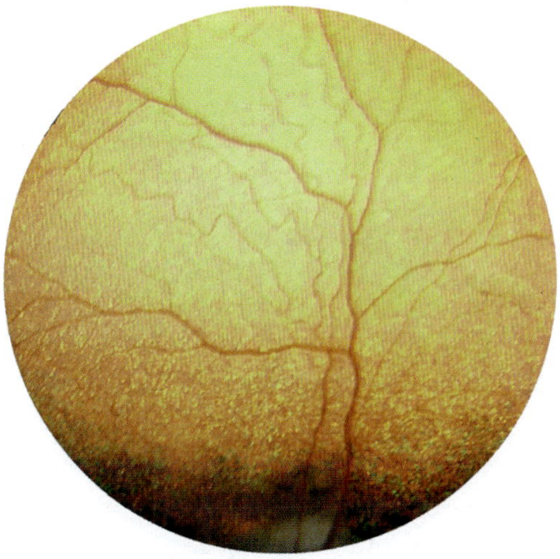

Figure 11-107
Early PRA in a cocker spaniel. Mild vascular attenuation and the beginning of peripheral tapetal hyperreflectivity are present.

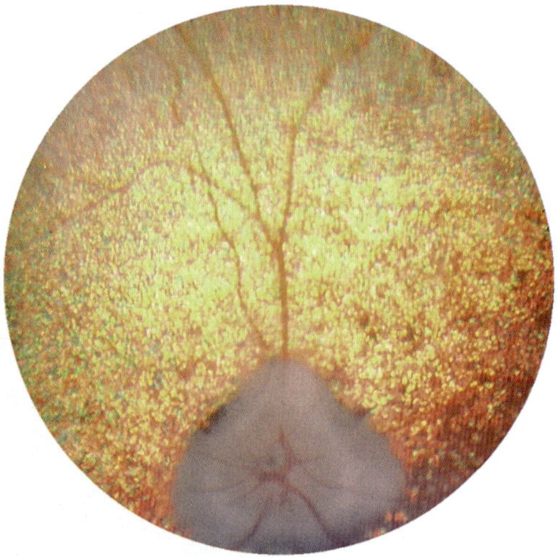

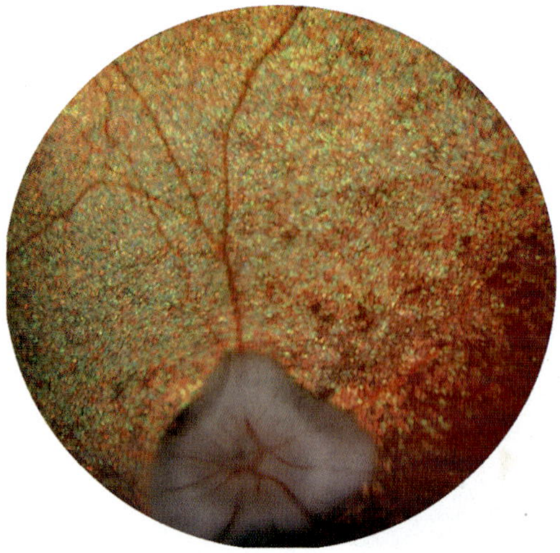

Figure 11-108
Advanced PRA in a springer spaniel. The photograph on the right was taken with less light exposure than the photograph on the left. Marked vessel attenuation, tapetal hyperreflectivity, and optic atrophy are present. Note how the appearance of the tapetum changes with the changes in the light intensity.

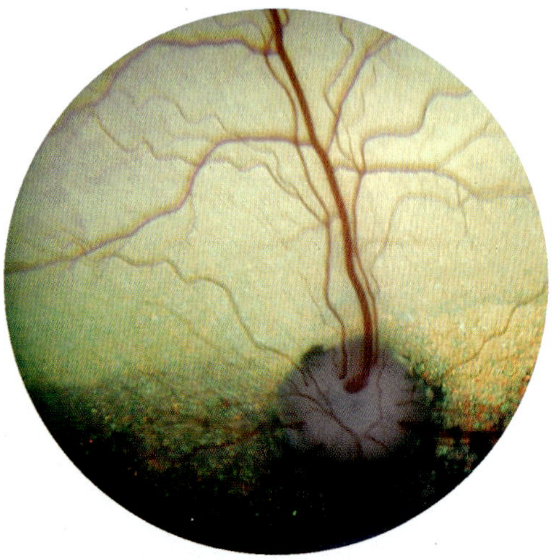

Figure 11-109
PRA in an American water spaniel. Note the tapetal hyperreflectivity superiorly and the color change in the band above the disc.

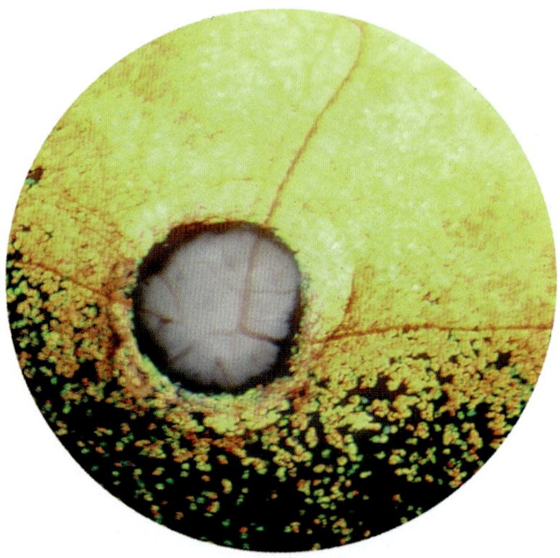

Figure 11-110
Advanced PRA in a 2-year-old miniature long-haired dachshund. Loss of myelin around disc, vessel attenuation, and tapetal hyperreflectivity are present.

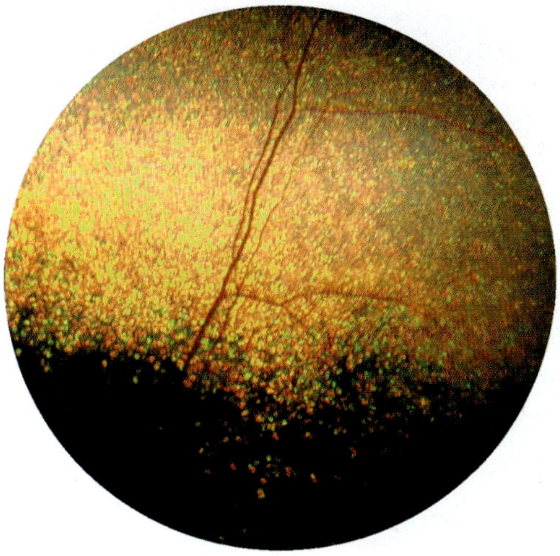

Figure 11-111
PRA in an 18-month-old miniature longhaired dachshund. Retinal vascular attenuation and hyperreflectivity in the periphery of the tapetum are present. This area actually looks darker in this photograph because of the angle of incident lighting. This effect is also visible with the indirect ophthalmoscope, depending on the angle of viewing.

A

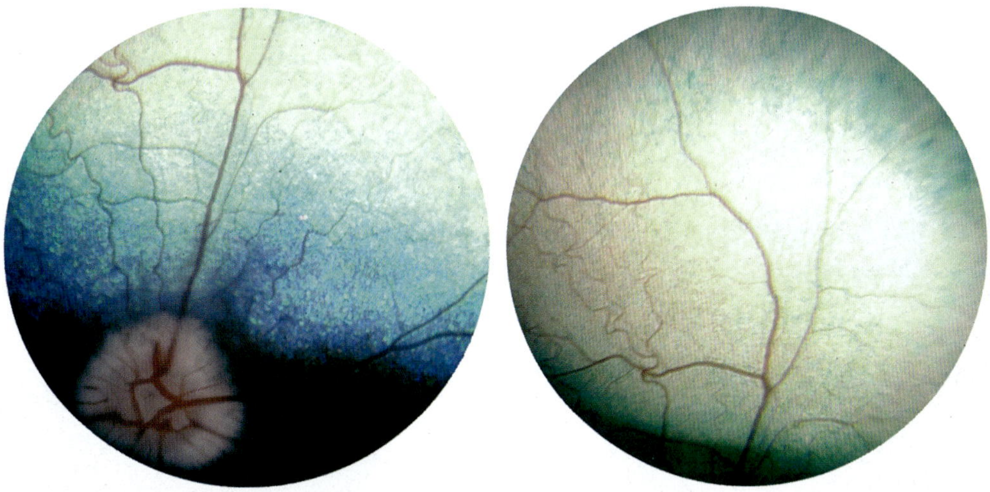

B

Figure 11-112 A-B
A, PRA in a miniature schnauzer. Vascular attenuation is visible. **B**, PRA in the equatorial fundus of the same dog, but with more hyperreflectivity than at the posterior pole.

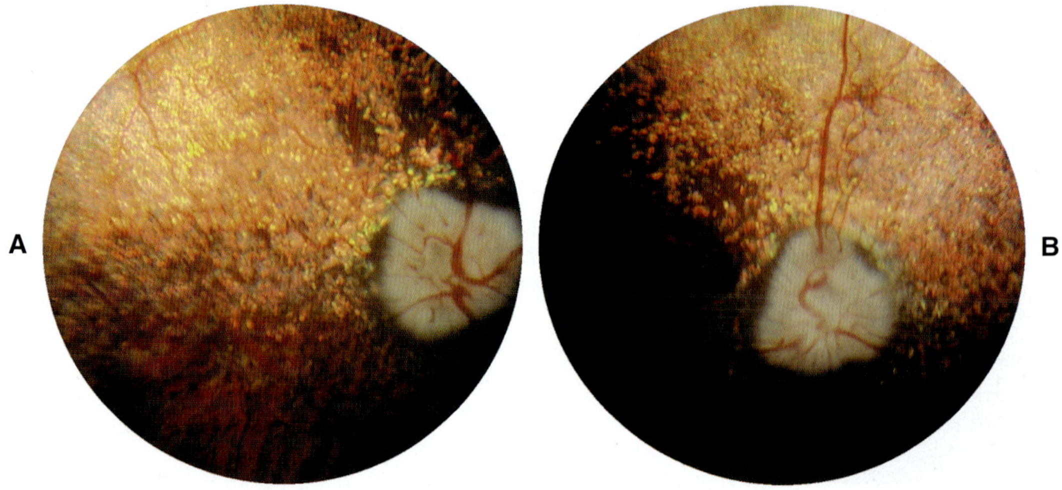

Figure 11-113 A-B
PRA in a poodle. **A**, Right eye. Central and peripapillary hyperreflectivity are present in the tapetal fundus. **B**, Left eye. Note the hyperreflective tapetum, loss of retinal arterioles, and attenuation of retinal veins.

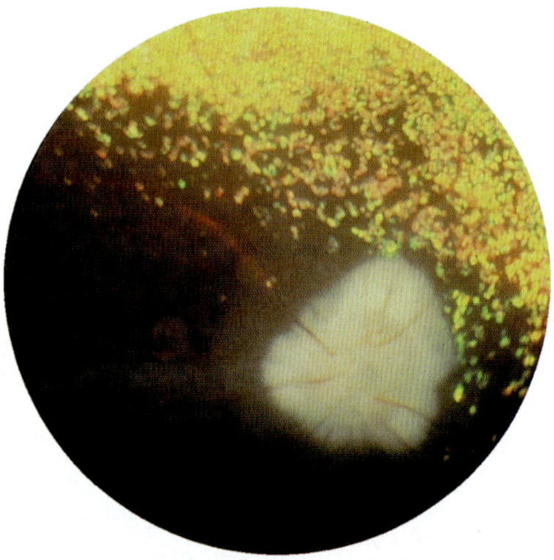

Figure 11-114
PRA in a poodle. Note the depigmentation and hyperpigmentation near the optic nerve. Vascular attenuation is present. The optic nerve is atrophic; myelin loss reveals the circular outline of the optic nerve head.

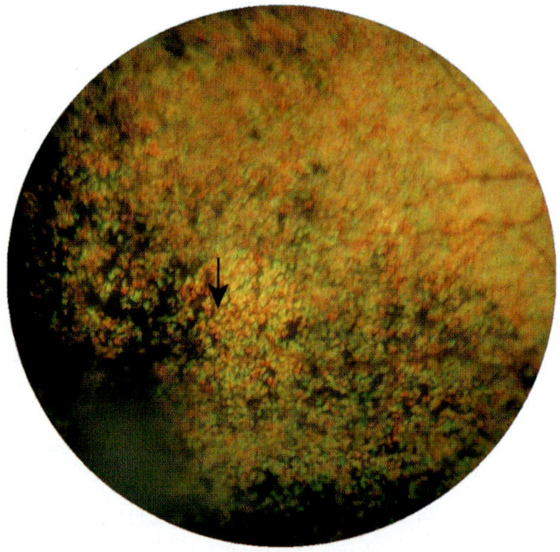

Figure 11-115
Early PRA in a 5-year-old poodle. Focal tapetal hyperreflectivity is visible in the periphery. This is the earliest ophthalmoscopic sign of progressive rod-cone degeneration–1 (PRCD-1) in a poodle.

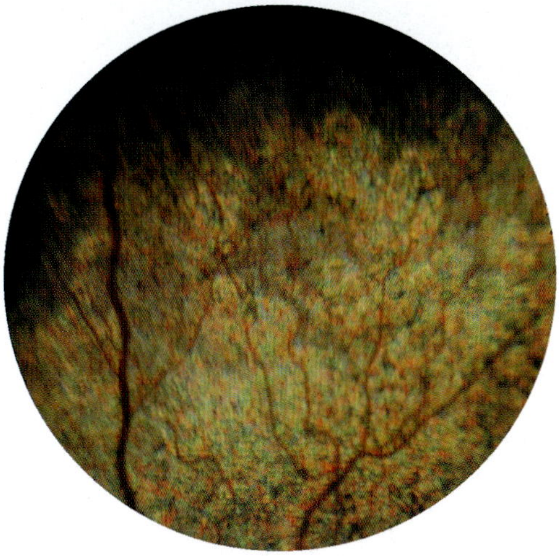

Figure 11-116
PRA in a poodle. Note the segmental hyperreflectivity in the peripheral tapetum.

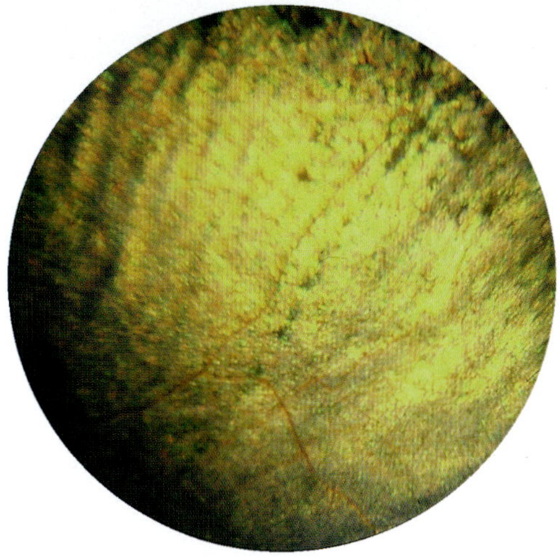

Figure 11-117
PRA in a poodle. The photograph is underexposed; despite this, note the marked tapetal reflectivity. The ridged (striped) effect represents the appearance of choroidal vessels through thinned retina. Vascular attenuation is also present.

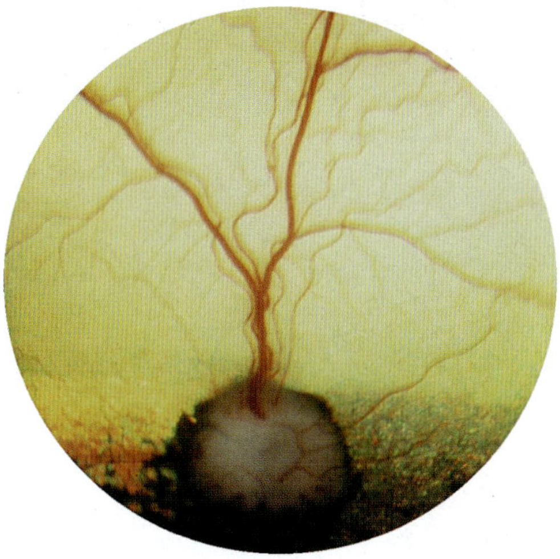

Figure 11-118
PRA in a Portuguese water spaniel. A hyperreflective horizontal band is present adjacent to the disc; diffuse hyperreflectivity is present in the rest of the tapetum.

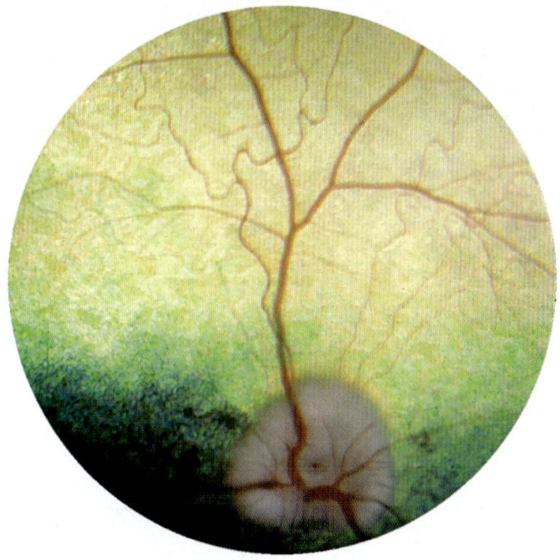

Figure 11-119
Retinal degeneration in a 5-year-old mixed-breed dog. Note the patchy variability in the yellow color of the tapetum and caliber variations in the retinal arterioles.

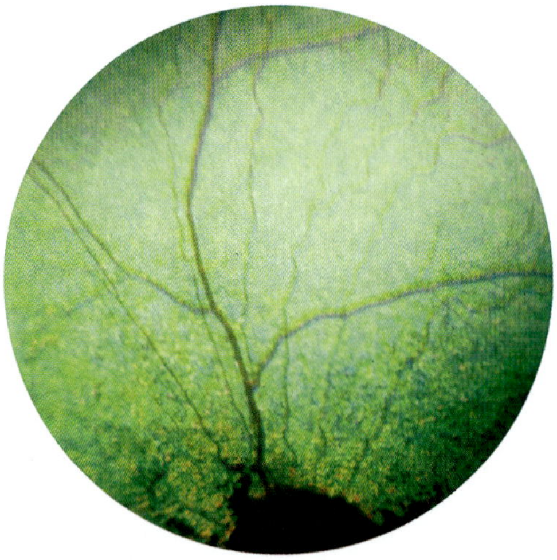

Figure 11-120
PRA in a Tibetan terrier. Tapetal hyperreflectivity and vascular attenuation are present.

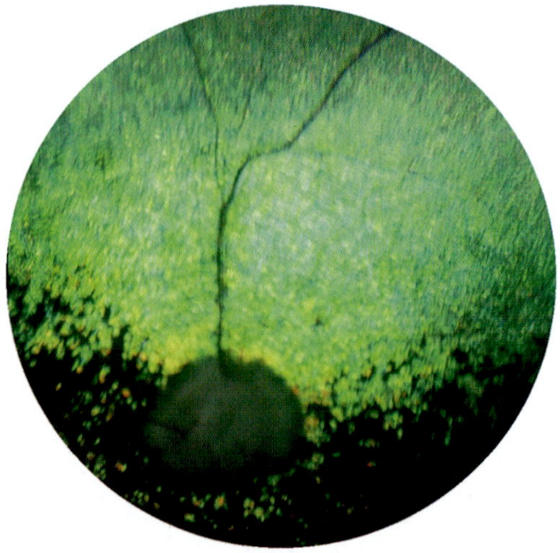

Figure 11-121
Advanced PRA in a Tibetan terrier. Vessel attenuation, tapetal hyperreflectivity, and optic atrophy are present.

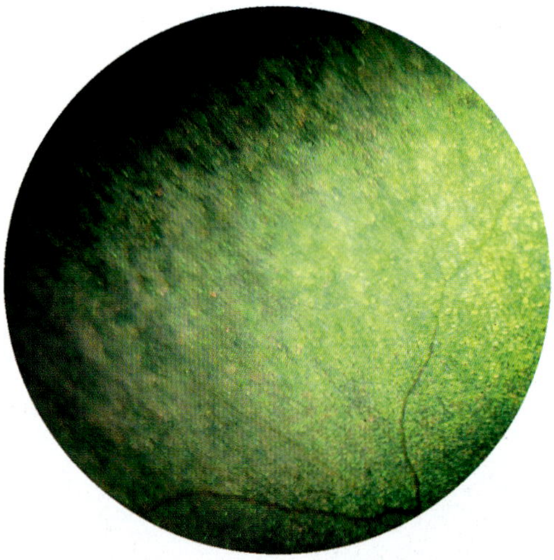

Figure 11-122
Advanced PRA in a Tibetan terrier. Note the tapetal hyperreflectivity and ridging (striping) caused by choroidal vessels showing through a thinned retina.

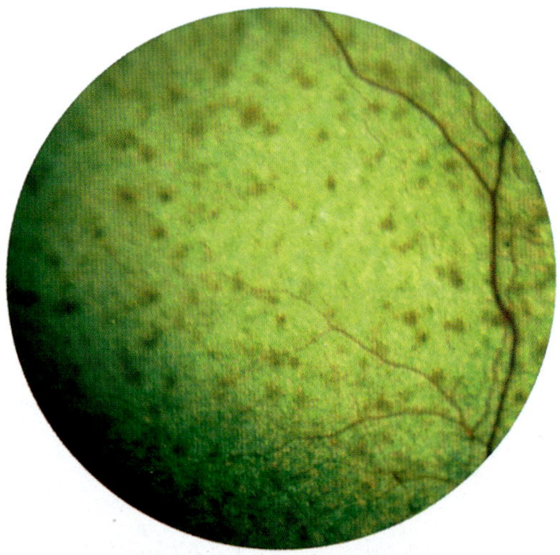

Figure 11-123
Central PRA (CPRA) in a briard. CPRA is an RPE dystrophy, and foci of lipofuscin can be seen in the RPE as golden brown spots. This disease is similar to retinopathies caused by vitamin E deficiency.

Progressive Retinal Atrophy and the Nontapetum

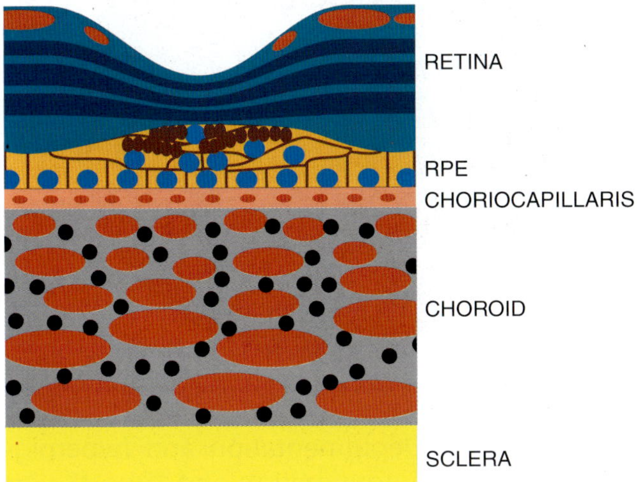

Figure 11-124
Schematic diagram of retinal degeneration (here shown as a focal lesion) in the nontapetal fundus. The RPE responds to overlying retinal degeneration by undergoing variable degrees of depigmentation and RPE cell hypertrophy and hyperplasia with nests of cells with increased pigmentation.

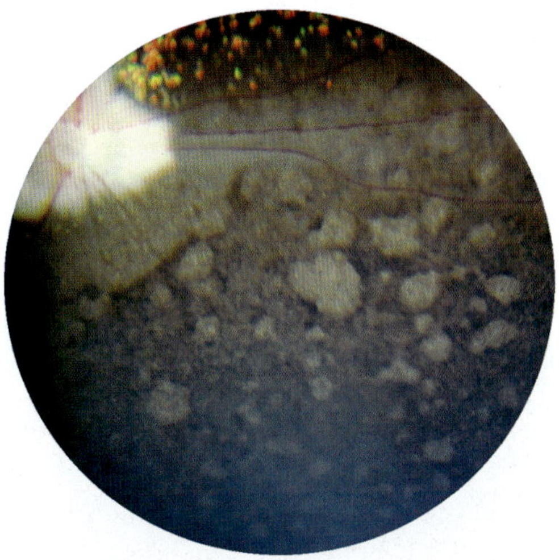

Figure 11-125
PRA in a cocker spaniel. RPE depigmentation and focal areas of pigment proliferation are present within the level of the RPE.

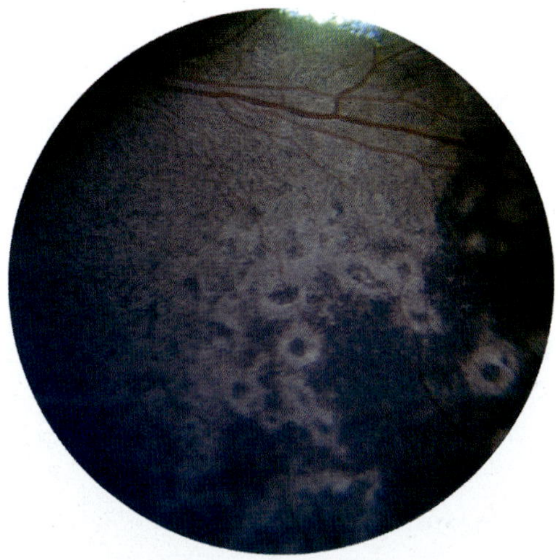

Figure 11-126
PRA in a Labrador retriever. Note the depigmentation and hyperpigmentation in the nontapetum.

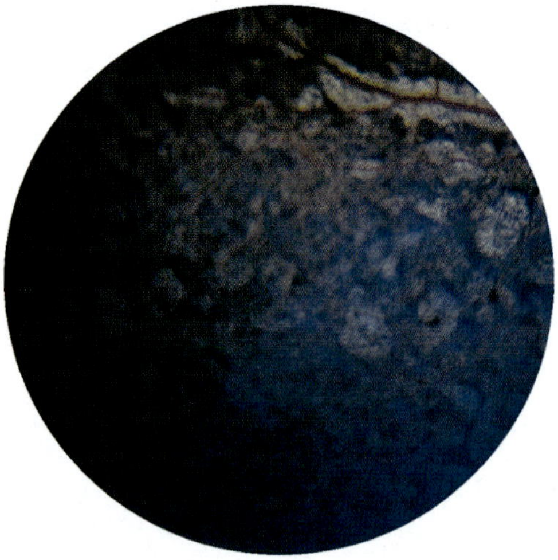

Figure 11-127
PRA in a 4-year-old Labrador retriever. Note the depigmentation and hyperpigmentation in nontapetum.

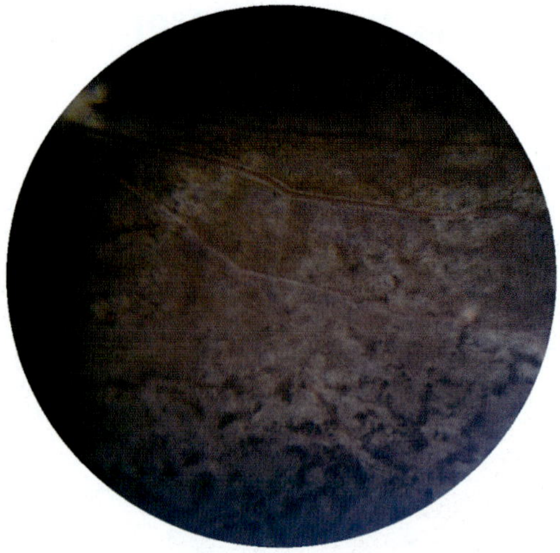

Figure 11-128
PRA in a pug. Depigmentation and hyperpigmentation in the nontapetum and "ghost" vessels (vessels through which blood no longer flows) are present.

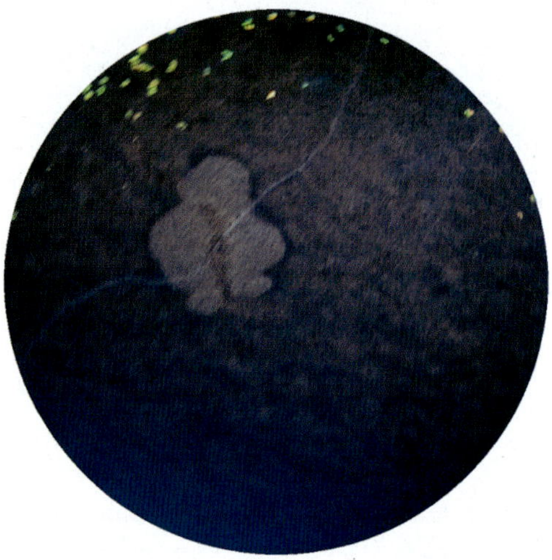

Figure 11-129
Advanced PRA in a miniature longhaired dachshund. A ghost vessel, RPE depigmentation, and pigment clumping are visible.

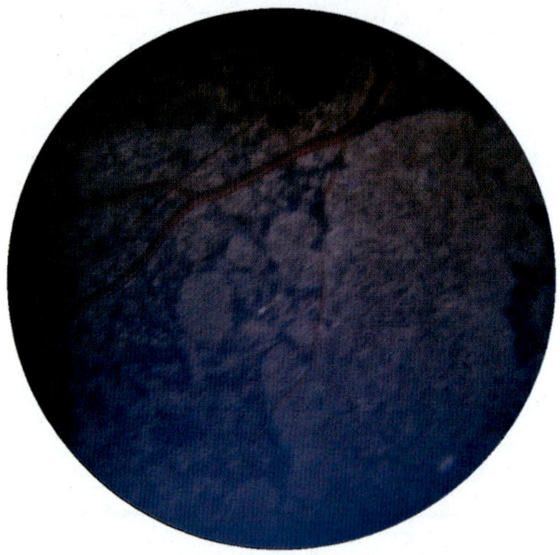

Figure 11-130
PRA in a 6-year-old rottweiler. Diffuse patches of RPE depigmentation (reduced pigment) and areas of increased pigmentation in the nontapetum are present.

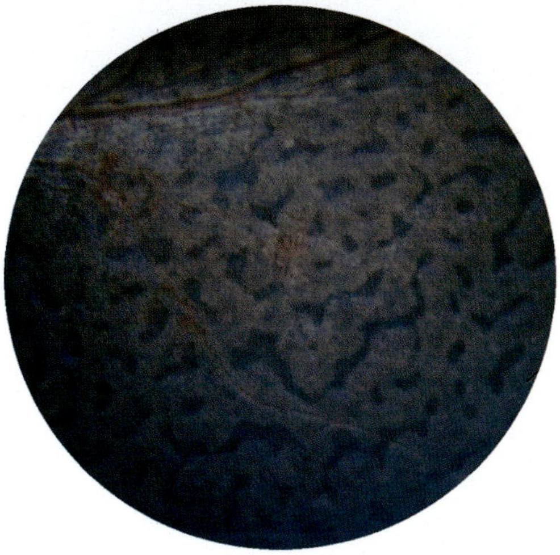

Figure 11-131
PRA in a poodle. Splotchy depigmentation and hyperpigmentation are present, with ghost vessels in the nontapetum; also present is multifocal retinal hemorrhage of unknown cause.

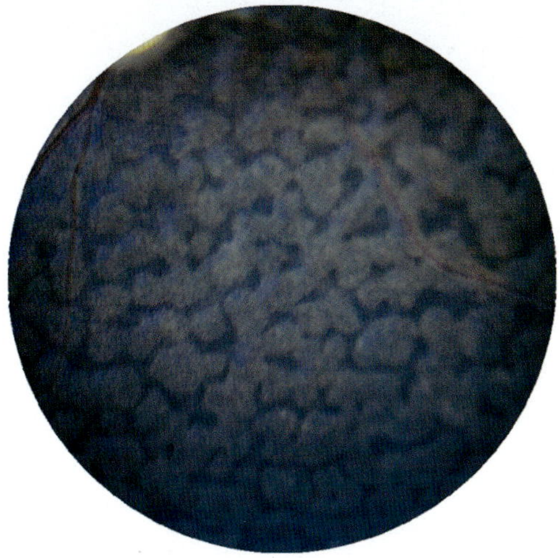

Figure 11-132
PRA in a mixed-breed dog. Depigmentation and hyperpigmentation are present in the nontapetum.

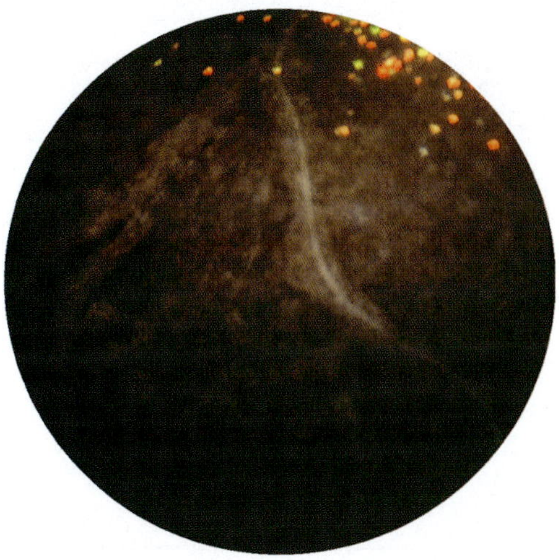

Figure 11-133
PRA in a poodle. Vascular loss and foci of depigmentation accentuated around the vessels are present.

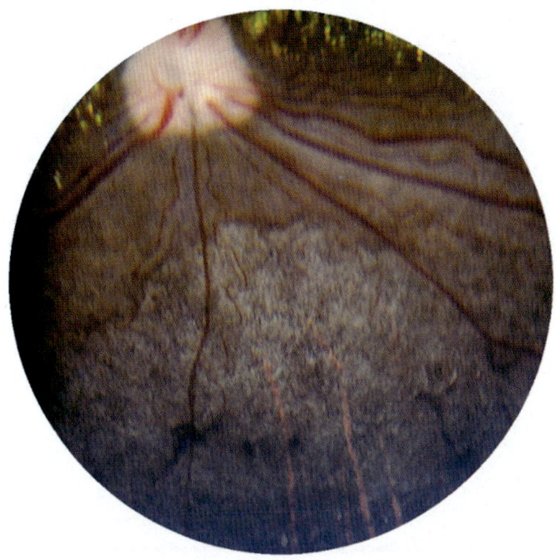

Figure 11-134
PRA in a poodle. Depigmentation of the RPE in the nontapetum reveals choroidal vessels.

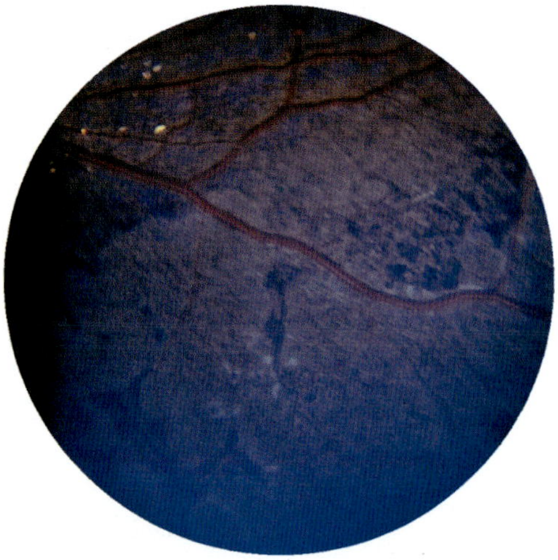

Figure 11-135
PRA in a poodle. Note the patchy depigmentation and white foci with focal hyperpigmentation.

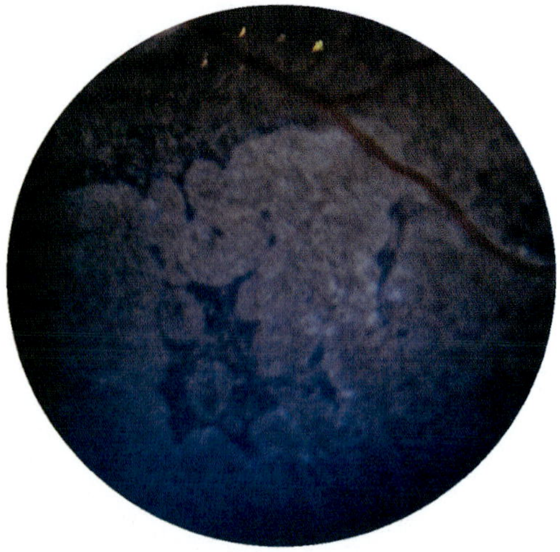

Figure 11-136
PRA in the same poodle as shown in Figure 11-135. Focal depigmentation, hyperpigmentation, and white foci are present.

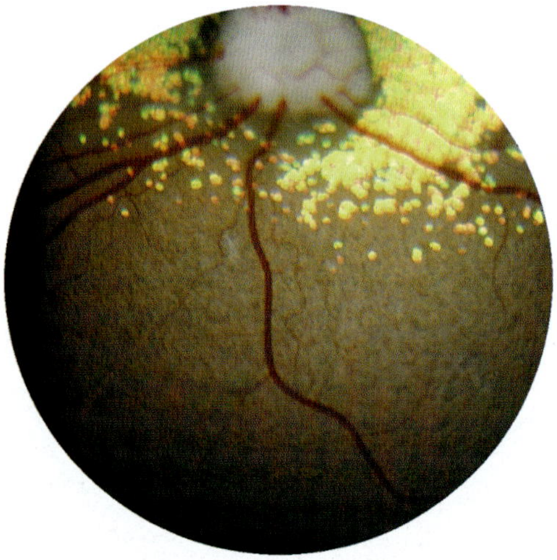

Figure 11-137
PRA in a Portuguese water spaniel. Depigmentation reveals choroidal vessels and small foci of hyperpigmentation.

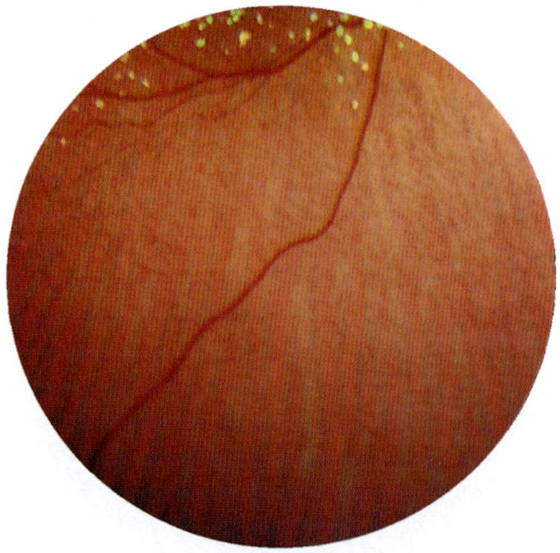

Figure 11-138
PRA in a Tibetan terrier. Arteriolar attenuation and depigmentation of the choroid are present.

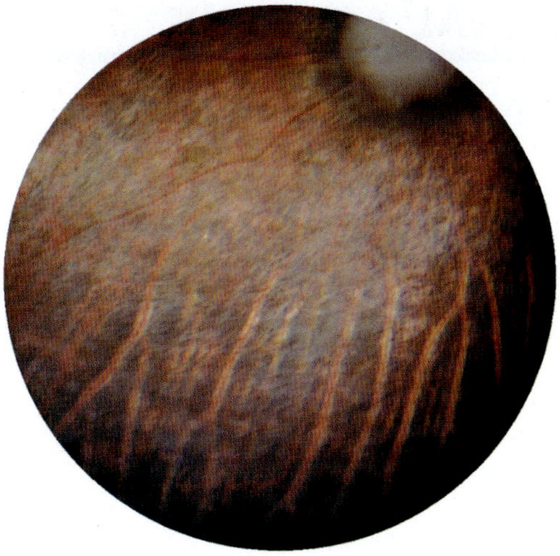

Figure 11-139
PRA in an English pointer. An atrophic disc and attenuated retinal vessels in a subalbinotic fundus are present.

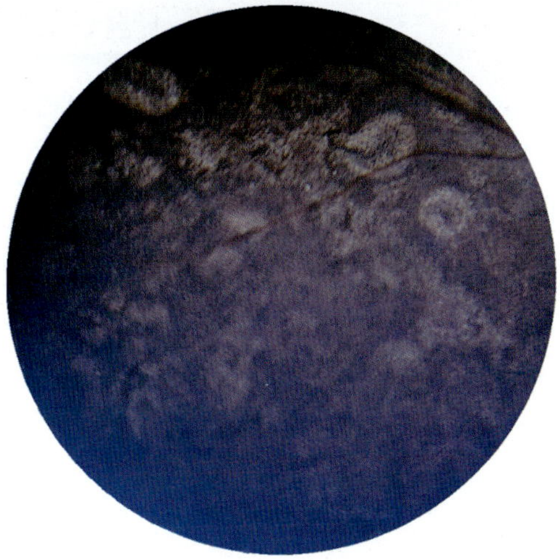

Figure 11-140
PRA in a 5-year-old mixed-breed dog. Note depigmentation in the nontapetum.

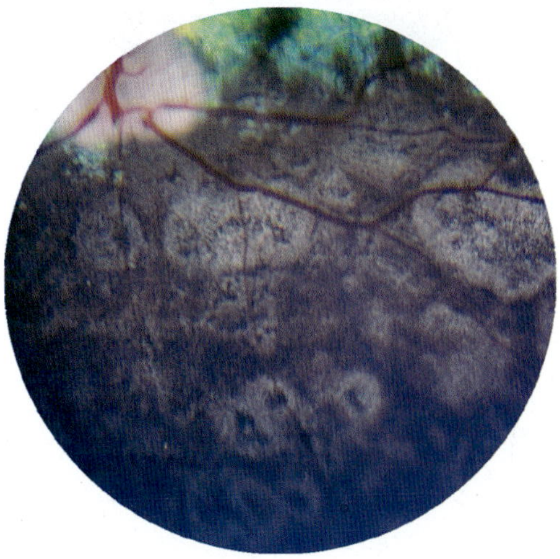

Figure 11-141
PRA in a mixed-breed dog. Note the depigmentation and hyperpigmentation in the nontapetum.

FELINE PROGRESSIVE RETINAL ATROPHY

In dogs diffuse retinal degeneration is usually diagnosed as PRA, implying a hereditary basis. PRA has been described in several breeds of cats, but ophthalmoscopically, end-stage taurine deficiency mimics end-stage PRA. If these two diseases cannot be separated, the catch-all term *retinal degeneration* is used. Another important cause of retinal degeneration in cats is associated toxicity from systemically administered enrofloxacin (and possibly other quinolones).

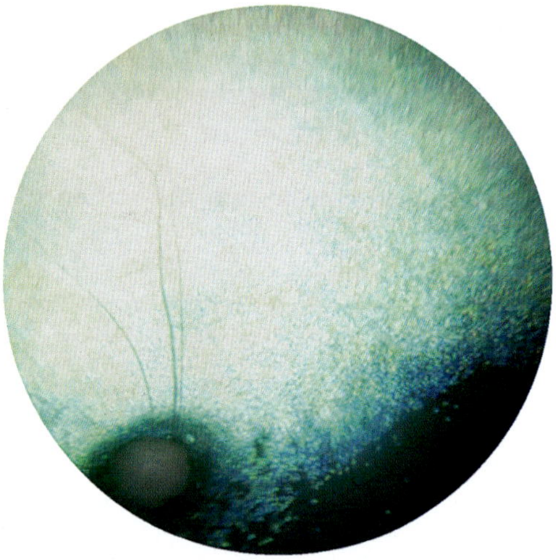

Figure 11-142
PRA in a cat. Attenuated retinal vessels and a hyperreflective tapetum are present.

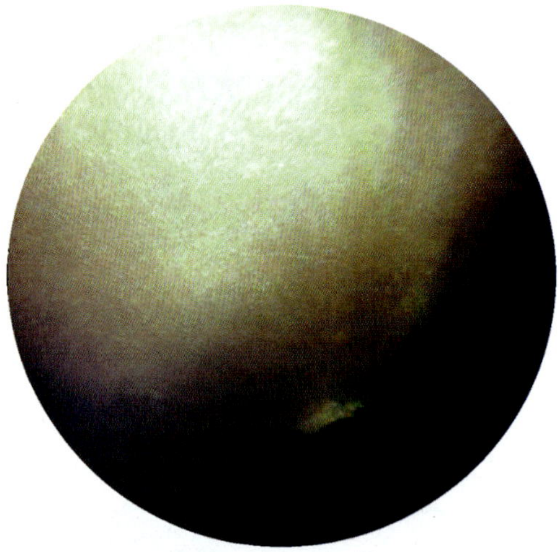

Figure 11-143
Retinal degeneration in a cat. Tapetal hyperreflectivity is present, and the blood vessels have all but disappeared.

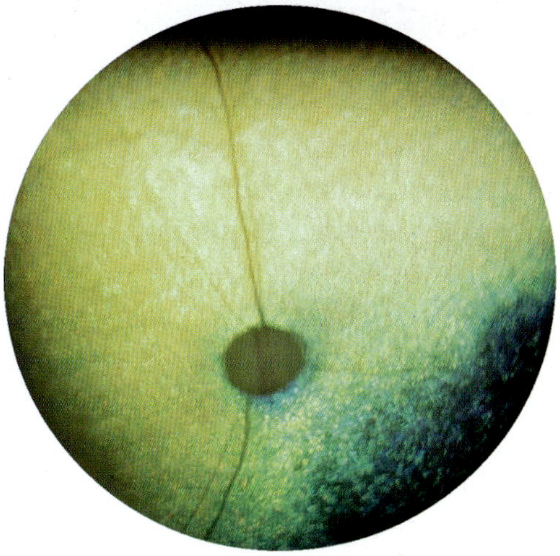

Figure 11-144
Retinal degeneration in a cat. Blood vessel diameter is decreased, and tapetal hyperreflectivity is present. An incidental finding is the presence of blood vessels running through the optic disc.

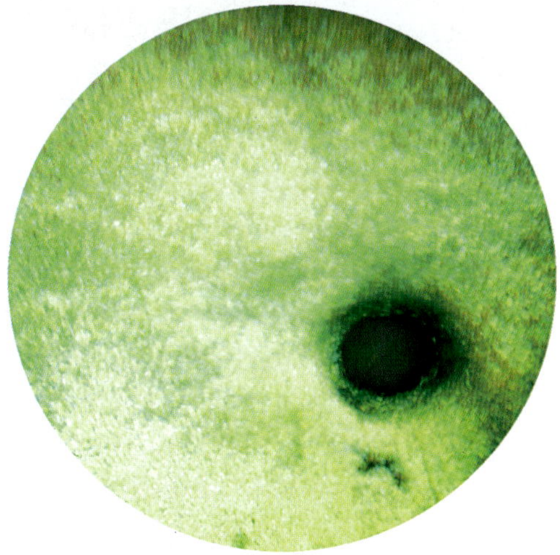

Figure 11-145
Retinal degeneration in a cat. Tapetal hyperreflectivity, almost complete disappearance of blood vessels, and optic atrophy are present.

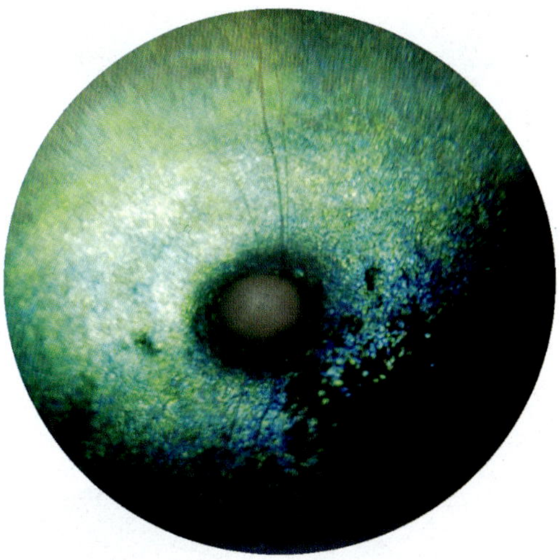

Figure 11-146
Retinal degeneration in a cat, with tapetal hyperreflectivity, vascular attenuation, and optic atrophy.

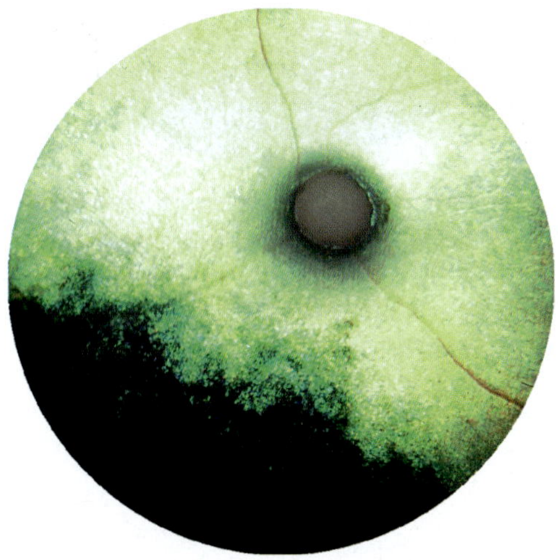

Figure 11-147
Abyssinian with late PRA, with advanced tapetal hyperreflectivity, vascular attenuation, and optic atrophy.

CANINE SUDDEN ACQUIRED RETINAL DEGENERATION

Sudden acquired retinal degeneration (SARD) is a condition involving acute widespread photoreceptor death in dogs. Vision is lost rapidly—over a few days to weeks—with little obvious evidence of reduced rod versus cone function. Dogs are usually middle aged, of any breed or mix, and often have a history of hyperadrenocorticism-like signs: polyuria-polydipsia and especially polyphagia. The retinal examination is usually normal, but electroretinographic tracings are flat. The condition has no known cause and no known treatment. With time, retinas of dogs with SARD resemble those of dogs with end-stage PRA.

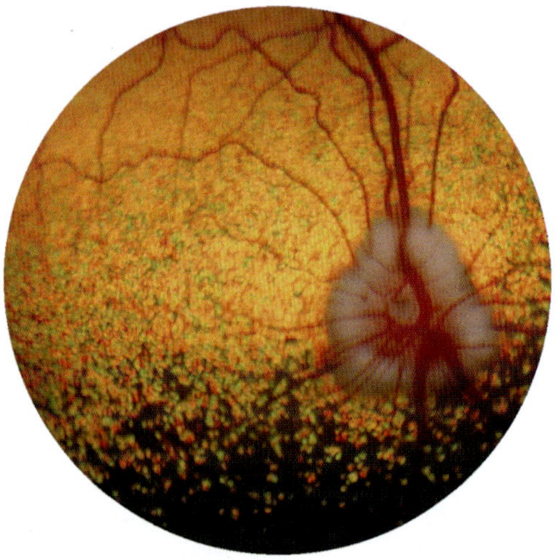

Figure 11-148
Normal-appearing retina in a dog with SARD. The dog was acutely blind with an extinguished electroretinogram.

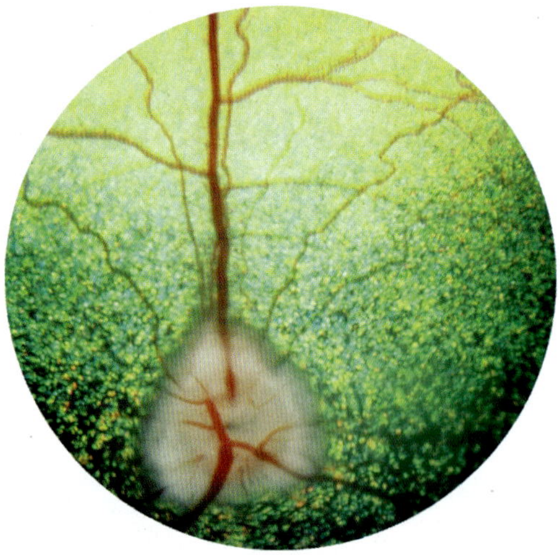

Figure 11-149
Normal looking retina in a dog with SARD. The dog was acutely blind with an extinguished electroretinogram.

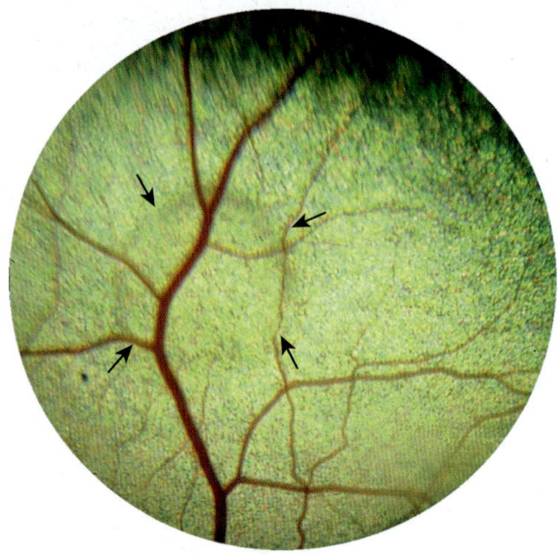

Figure 11-150
Golden retriever with SARD. A focal area of retinal edema and flat detachment *(arrows)*, which is unusual in SARD cases, is shown. The dog went blind 4 days before photographs were taken and was acutely blind with an extinguished electroretinogram. Whether the edema is related to SARD is unclear.

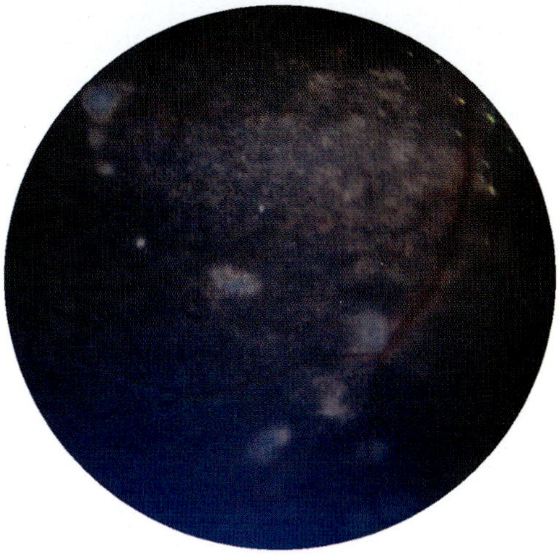

Figure 11-151
Foci of retinal edema in the nontapetum in the same golden retriever as shown in Figure 11-150.

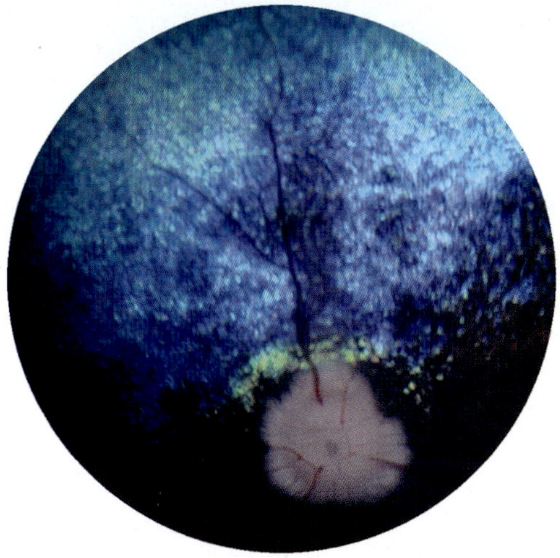

Figure 11-152
Fox terrier with a chronic history of SARD, with optic atrophy and attenuated vessels.

FELINE CENTRAL RETINAL DEGENERATION

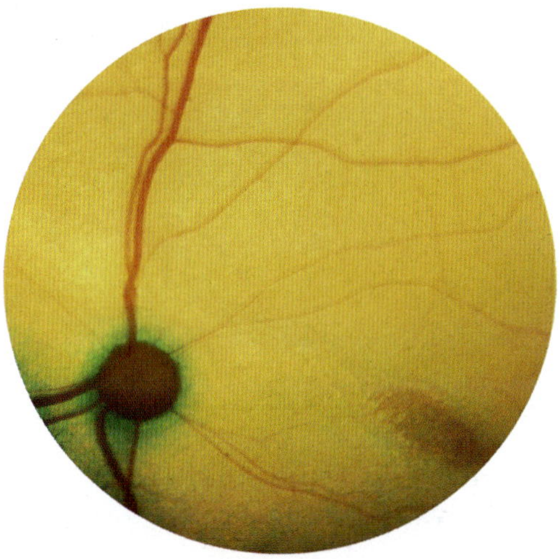

Figure 11-153
Feline central retinal degeneration (FCRD). A hyperreflective zone is visible at this light intensity as a discoloration in the area centralis of a cat with an early FCRD lesion. FCRD is caused by taurine deficiency and involves the loss of cones first, then rods. Because the area centralis has the highest density of cones in the cat, ophthalmoscopic changes are first seen as retinal thinning (hyperreflective tapetum) in this area. With continued taurine deficiency, the entire retina becomes degenerative, resembling end-stage PRA.

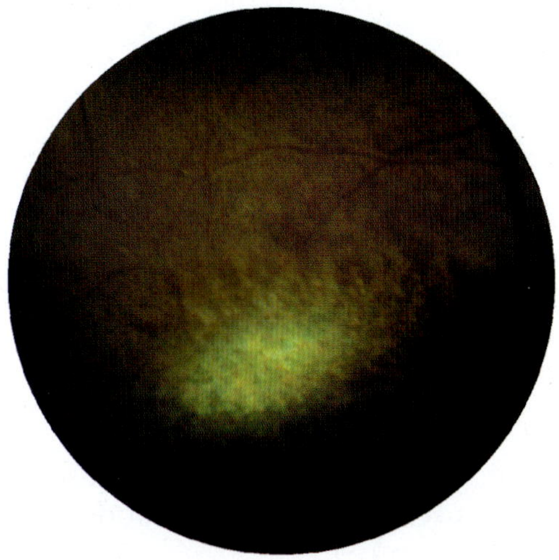

Figure 11-154
Area centralis hyperreflectivity in a cat with FCRD, photographed at low flash intensity to highlight contrast with the surrounding tapetum.

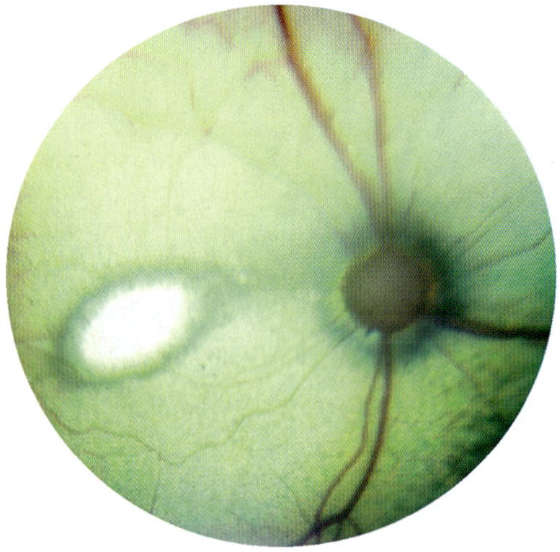

Figure 11-155
Hyperreflective zone in the area centralis of a cat with taurine deficiency.

A 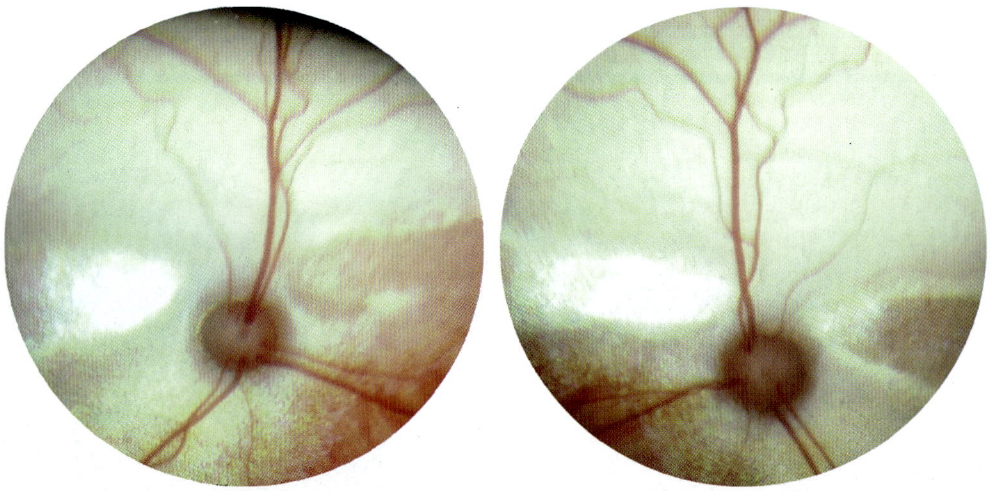 B

Figure 11-156 A-B
Bilateral FCRD in a Siamese cat. Note the nearly symmetric bands of hyperreflectivity that run above the optic disc. **A**, Right eye. **B**, Left eye.

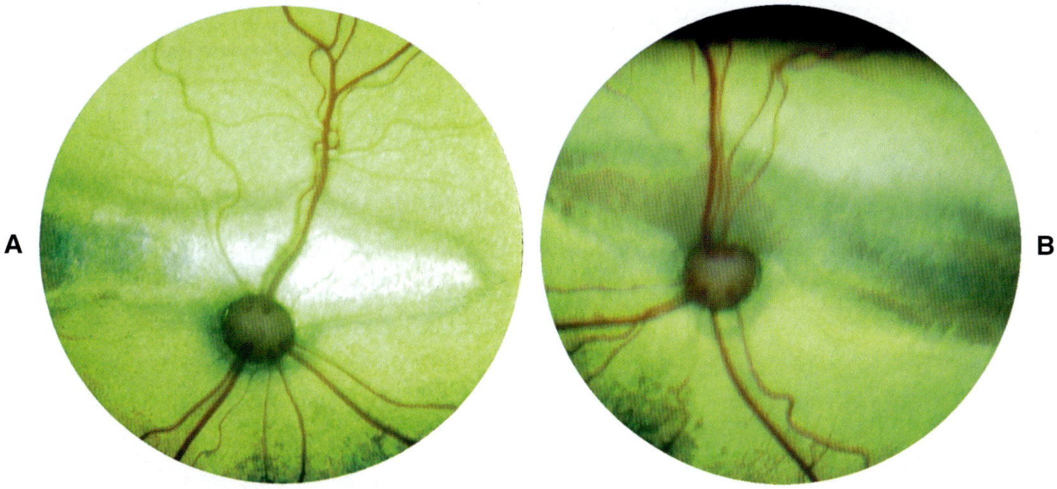

Figure 11-157 A-B
Variation in appearance of central band of retinal degeneration in a cat with FCRD. Depending on the incident lighting from the camera or ophthalmoscope the degenerate central zone may appear light or dark. Photographs are from the **A**, right and **B**, left eyes.

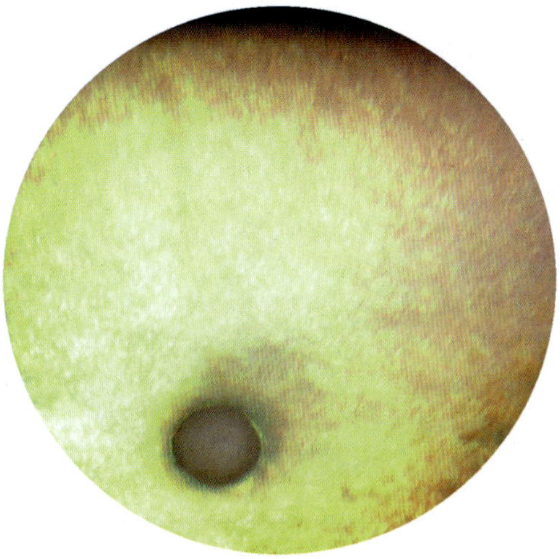

Figure 11-158
Advanced taurine deficiency in a cat. Retinal vessels are totally absent, and the entire tapetal fundus is hyperreflective (retina is degenerate). This cannot be distinguished ophthalmoscopically from any other advanced retinal degeneration.

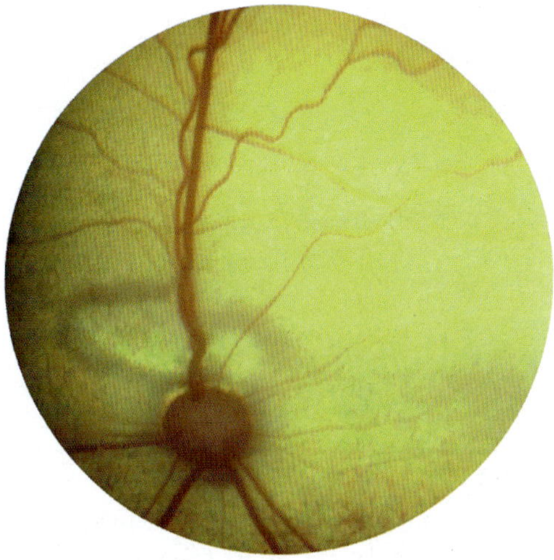

Figure 11-159
Oval hyperreflective chorioretinal scar above the optic nerve of a cat. This condition is not a result of taurine deficiency.

RETINAL DYSPLASIA

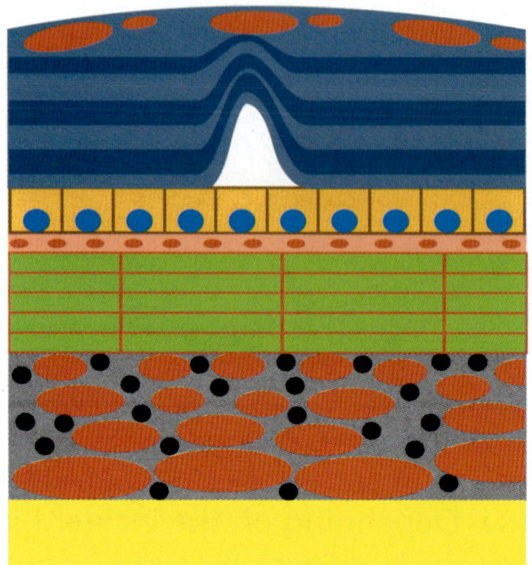

Figure 11-160
Retinal dysplasia. The most typical presentation is of folds in the outer part of the retina that appear as linear or dotlike areas of reduced reflectance in the tapetal fundus and white or gray foci in the nontapetal fundus.

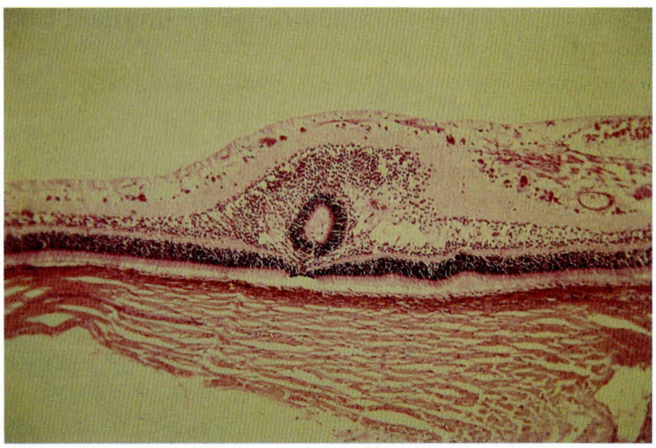

Figure 11-161
Histopathologic specimen of retinal dysplasia (hematoxylin-eosin [H & E] stain). A retinal fold or rosette thickens the retina. Retinal dysplasia is the maldevelopment of the retina in utero or early in life. Retinal dysplasia includes photoreceptor dysplasias, retinal folds, large geographic areas of maldeveloped retina, and retinal nonattachments or detachments. Many retinal dysplasias are inherited in dogs, and clinical signs range from none to blindness. Retinal dysplasia can also result from intrauterine retinal inflammation (canine herpesvirus, feline panleukopenia virus) and damage to the developing retina from radiation (x-rays).

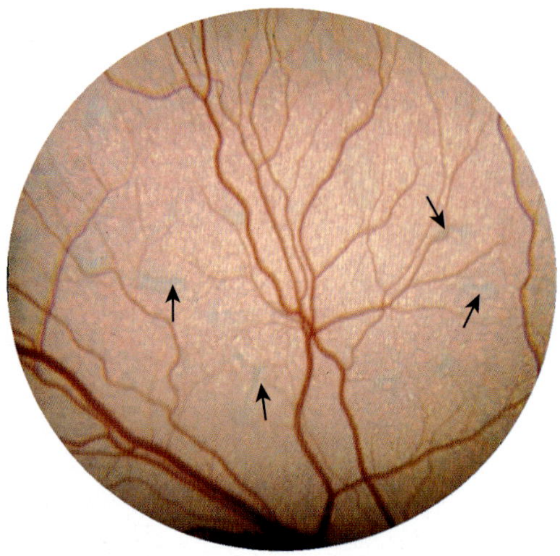

Figure 11-162
Australian shepherd with retinal folds or dysplasia (gray streaks in the tapetal fundus *[arrows]*).

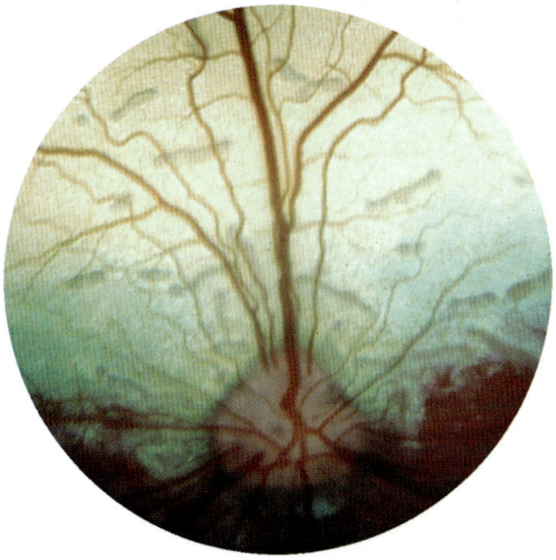

Figure 11-163
Focal retinal folds (retinal dysplasia) visible as linear and Y-shaped streaks.

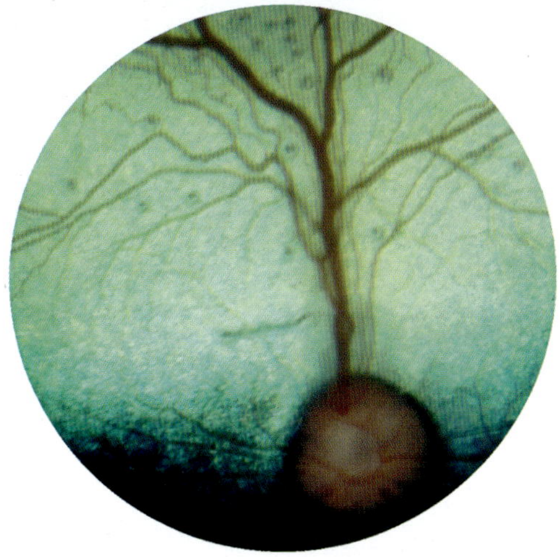

Figure 11-164
Retinal dysplasia. Note dotlike and linear retinal folds.

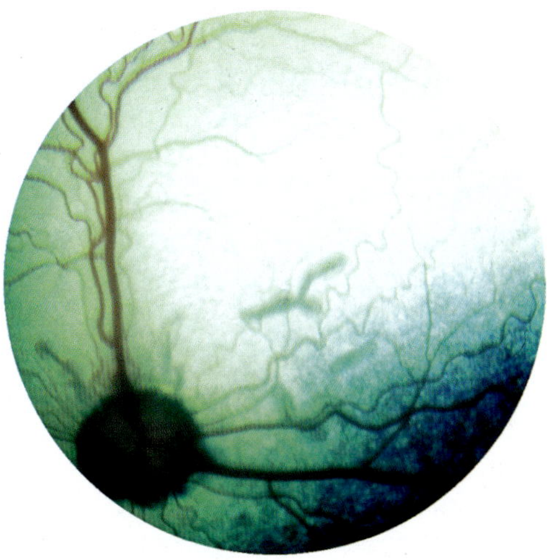

Figure 11-165
Retinal folds, visible as linear and Y-shaped streaks.

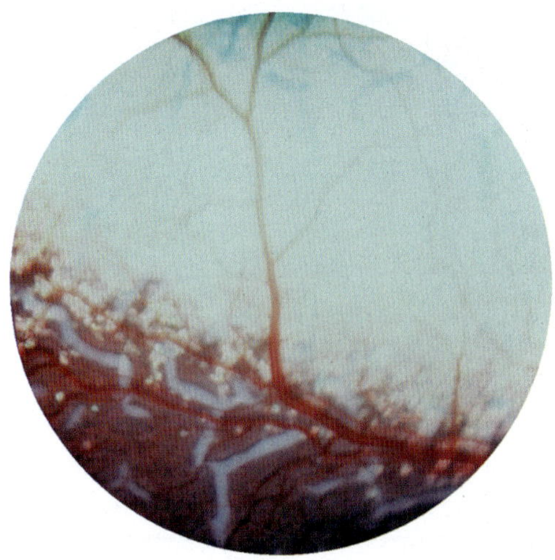

Figure 11-166
Retinal folds, visible as linear and Y-shaped streaks, in tapetal and nontapetal fundus in a springer spaniel.

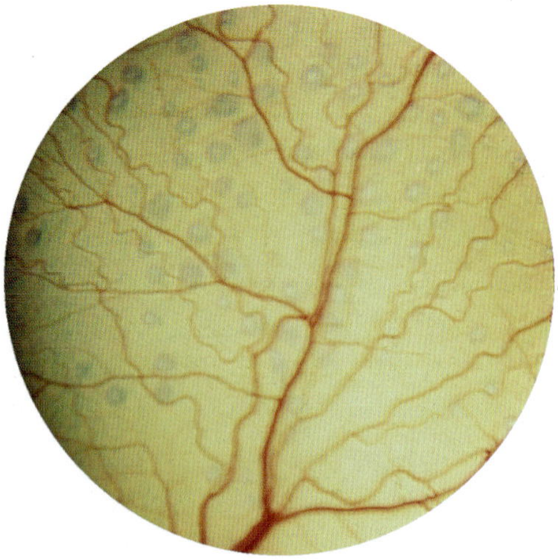

Figure 11-167
Retinal dysplasia in a golden retriever, visible as multifocal circular areas in the tapetum.

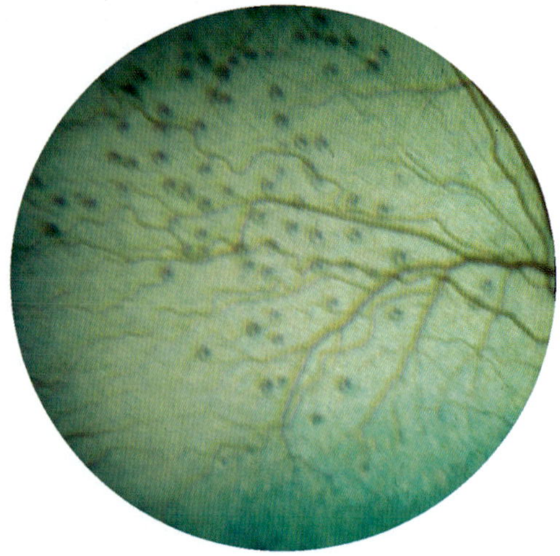

Figure 11-168
Retinal dysplasia, visible as multifocal circular areas in the tapetum.

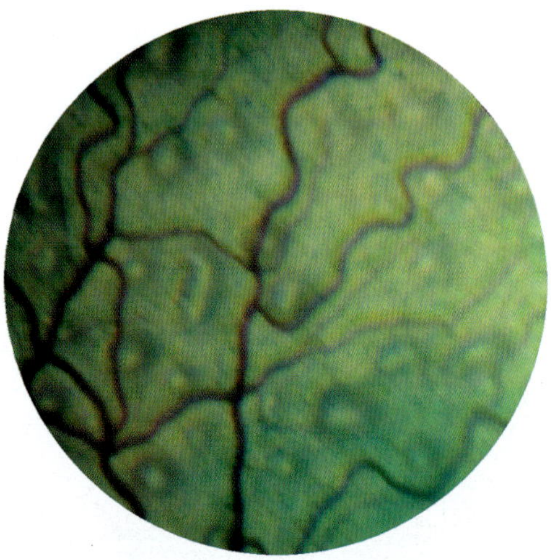

Figure 11-169
Retinal dysplasia in a fox terrier. Multiple circular retinal folds are evident. Vision was not detectably affected.

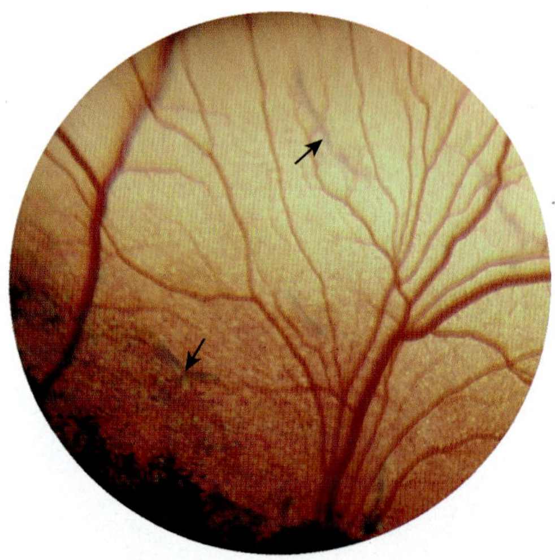

Figure 11-170
Retinal folds, visible as linear and Y-shaped streaks *(arrows)*, in the tapetum of an American cocker spaniel.

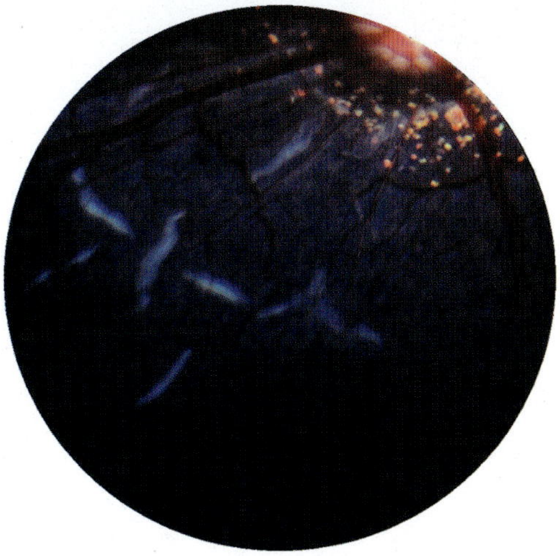

Figure 11-171
Retinal folds, visible as linear and Y-shaped streaks, in the nontapetal fundus of an American cocker spaniel. This is the same dog as shown in Figure 11-170.

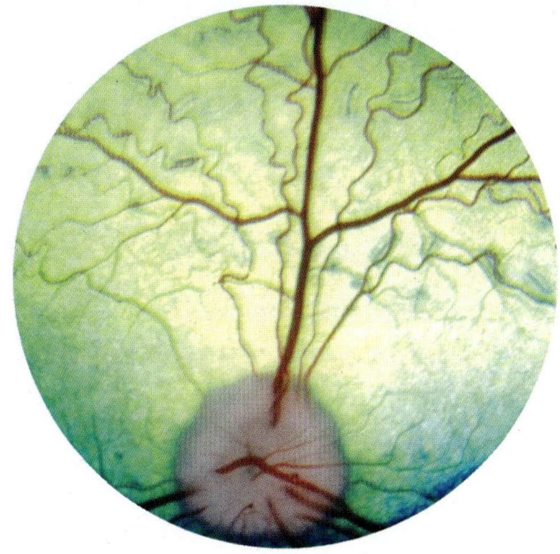

Figure 11-172
Tapetal retinal folds, visible as green dots and linear streaks, in an Akita.

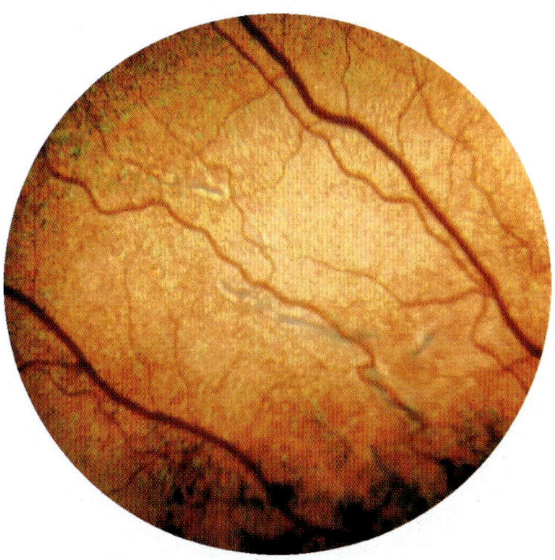

Figure 11-173
Retinal folds, visible as linear streaks, in the tapetum.

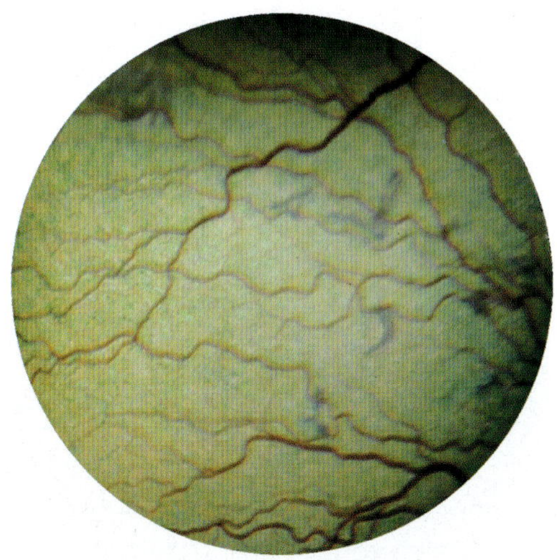

Figure 11-174
Retinal folds, visible as linear and Y-shaped streaks, in the peripheral tapetum.

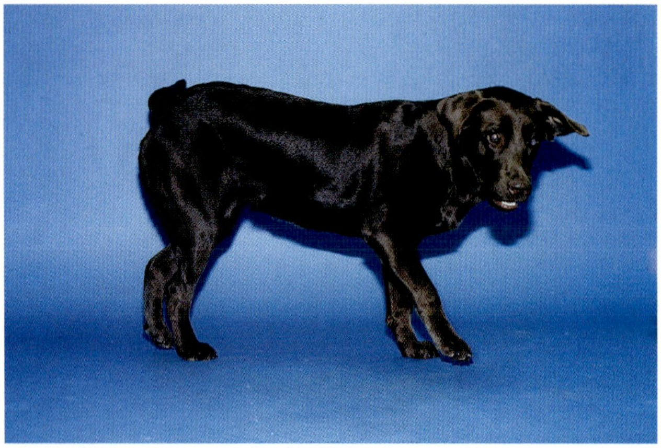

Figure 11-175
Labrador retriever puppy with inherited chondrodysplasia and multiple ocular anomalies. Labrador retrievers often have cataracts and retinal nonattachment or detachment. It is postulated that heterozygotes for this gene have geographic retinal dysplasia and no skeletal abnormalities.

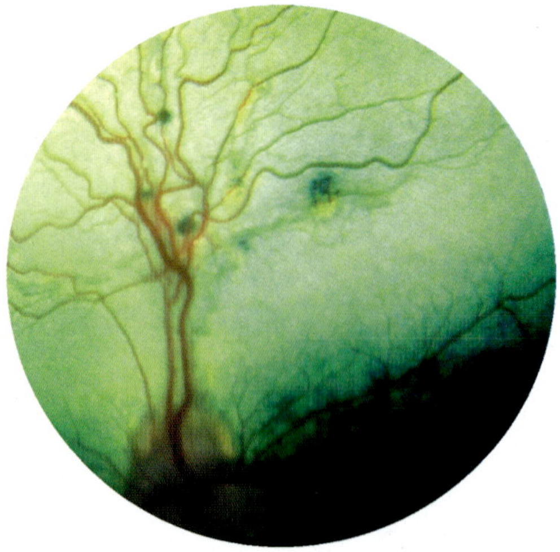

Figure 11-176
Retinal dysplasia in a field-trial Labrador retriever. Lesions are more geographic and usually occur superior to the optic nerve. Retinal folds and foci of degeneration (increased reflectivity, yellow color change, and pigment proliferation in the RPE) are seen.

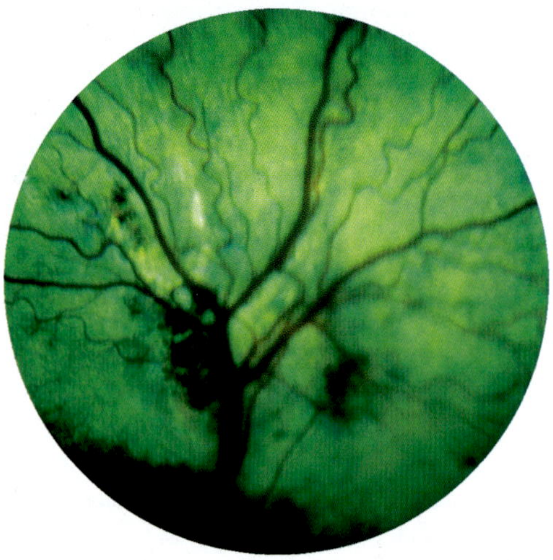

Figure 11-177
Retinal dysplasia superior to disc in a field-trial Labrador retriever.

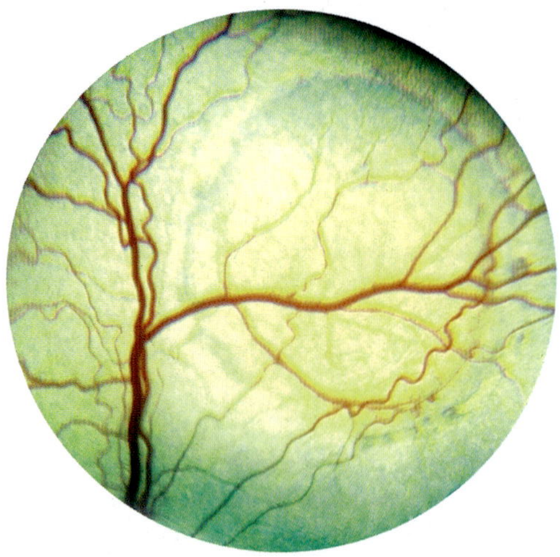

Figure 11-178
Geographic retinal dysplasia in a Labrador retriever. This large circular area was elevated.

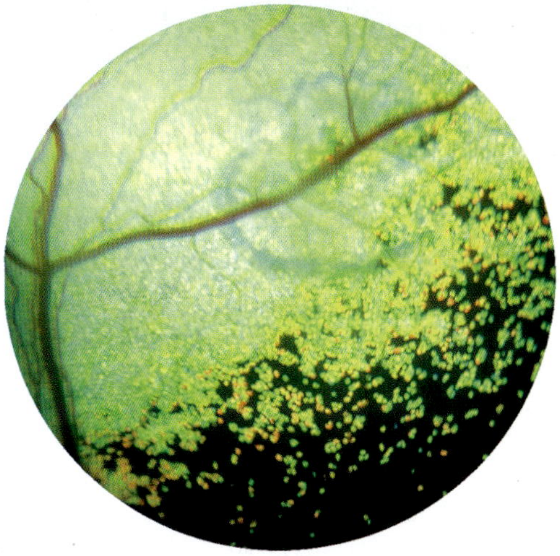

Figure 11-179
Large circular area of retinal dysplasia in a Labrador retriever.

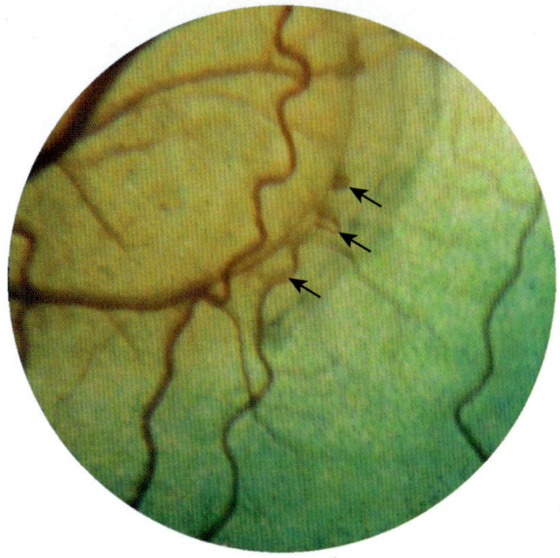

Figure 11-180
Geographic retinal dysplasia with preretinal vascular loops *(arrows)* in a Labrador retriever.

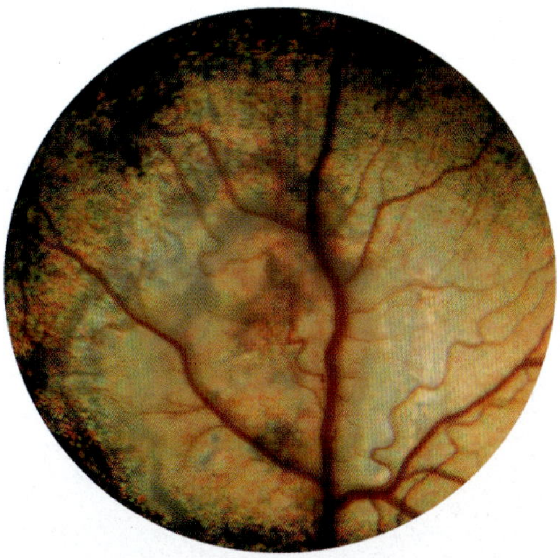

Figure 11-181
Geographic retinal dysplasia in a Labrador retriever.

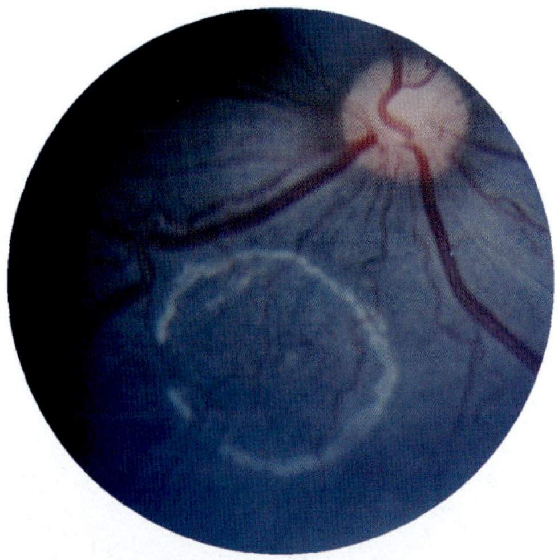

Figure 11-182
Circular area of retinal dysplasia in nontapetum of a 7-week-old Labrador retriever.

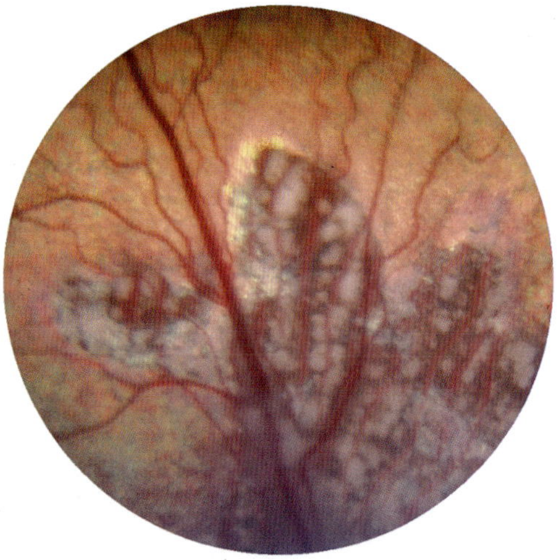

Figure 11-183
Springer spaniel with normal lack of tapetum and choroidal depigmentation secondary to retinal dysplasia.

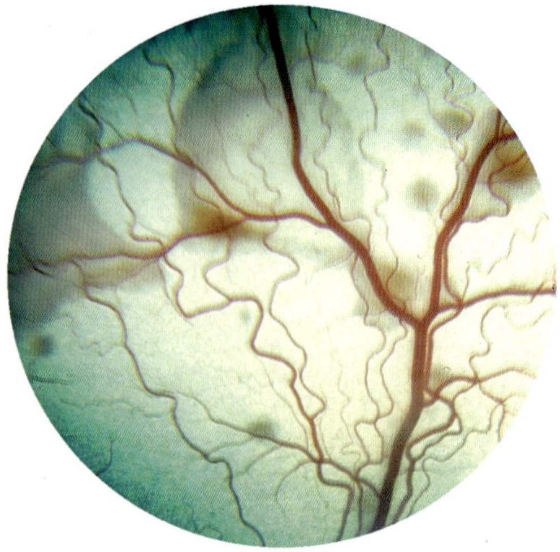

Figure 11-184
Mastiff (2 years old) with retinal dysplasia. Clinically this resembles multifocal retinal detachments with hemorrhage, although the red material settling out in the detached areas is slightly more orange or brown than blood would appear. Similar-looking dysplasias have been described in other giant breeds.

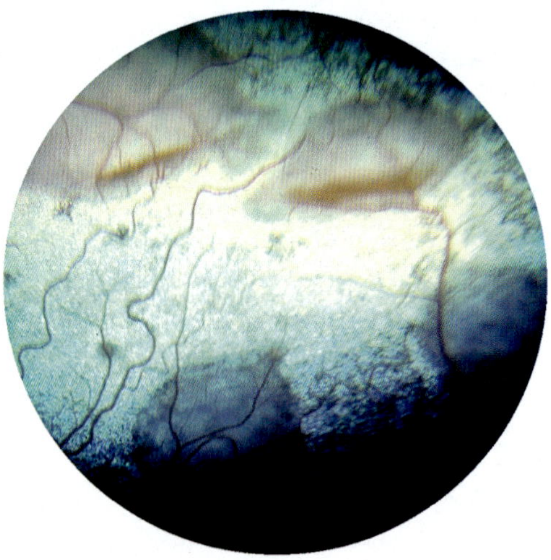

Figure 11-185
Mastiff (2 years old) with retinal dysplasia, with bullous retinal detachments and ventral gravitation of red-colored material. Same dog as shown in Figures 11-184 and 11-186.

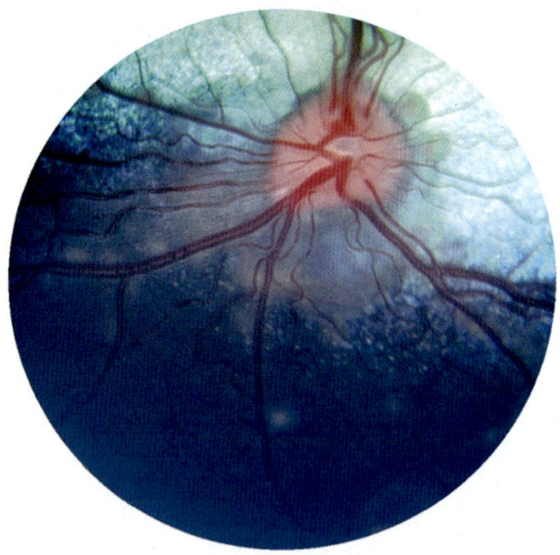

Figure 11-186
Mastiff (2 years old) with retinal dysplasia in the nontapetum. Same dog as shown in Figures 11-184 and 11-185.

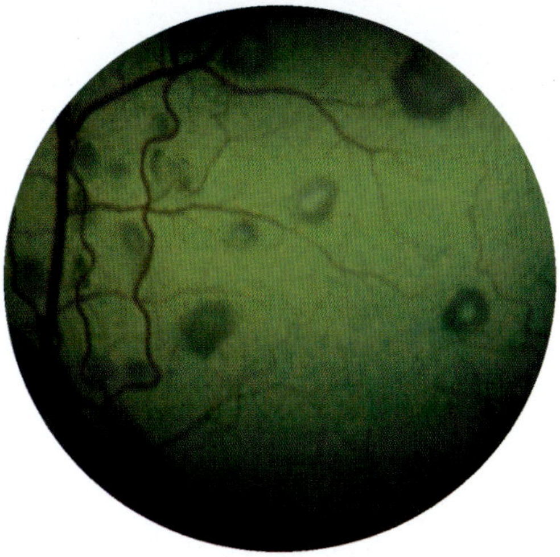

Figure 11-187
Belgian shepherd, 10 weeks old, with degenerative retinopathy. The dog was blind. Note the circular dysplastic foci in the tapetal fundus.

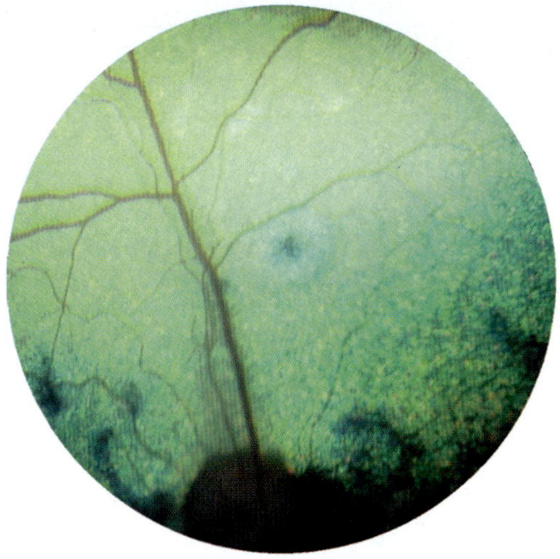

Figure 11-188
Adult Belgian shepherd with areas of tapetal hyperreflectivity, color change, and hyperpigmentation in areas of previous dysplasia. The dog was blind as a result of inherited degenerative retinopathy.

COLLIE EYE ANOMALY

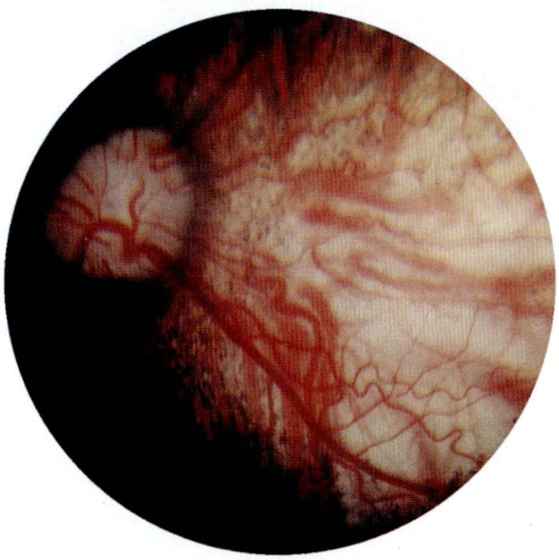

Figure 11-189
Collie eye anomaly (CEA) in a rough collie. CEA is an inherited disease that occurs in collies and related dogs such as Shetland sheepdogs. Affected dogs are homozygotes. Lesions include choroidal hypoplasia, colobomas of the optic disc or other parts of the fundus, and retinal nonattachments or detachments. Clinical signs range from none to blindness. This dog has choroidal hypoplasia visible as a pale area temporal to the optic disc in the left eye.

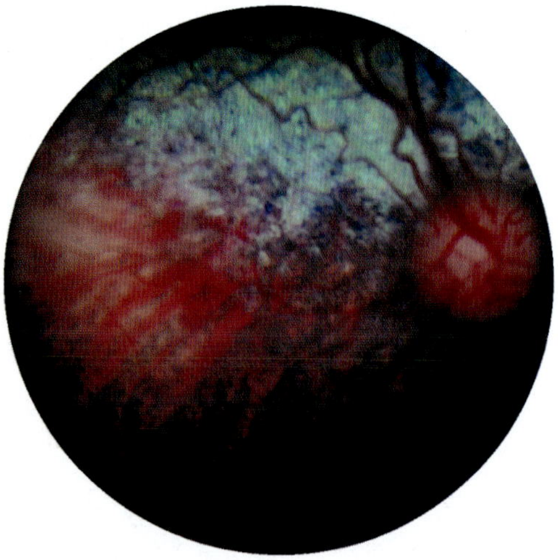

Figure 11-190
Choroidal hypoplasia is present temporal to the optic nerve in the right eye.

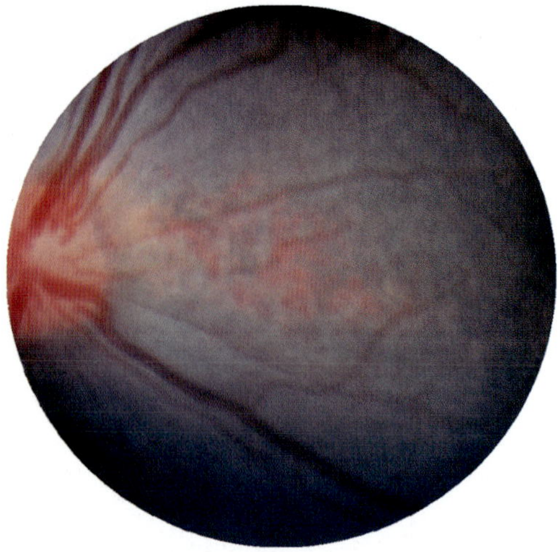

Figure 11-191
CEA with choroidal hypoplasia in the left eye of a 7-week-old puppy. With lesions this small, it is possible for the dog to pigment the affected area as it ages; a genetically affected dog may therefore appear phenotypically normal as an adult.

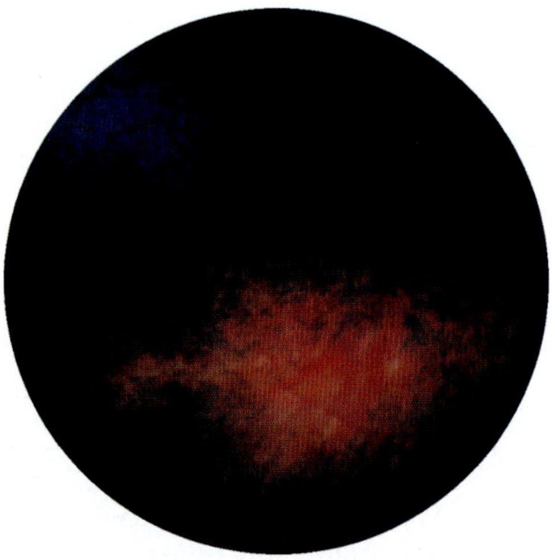

Figure 11-192
CEA with choroidal hypoplasia in a 6-week-old puppy.

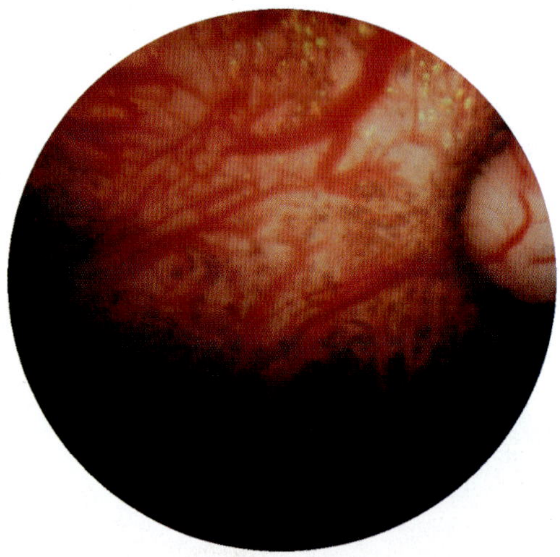

Figure 11-193
Choroidal hypoplasia in a Shetland sheepdog.

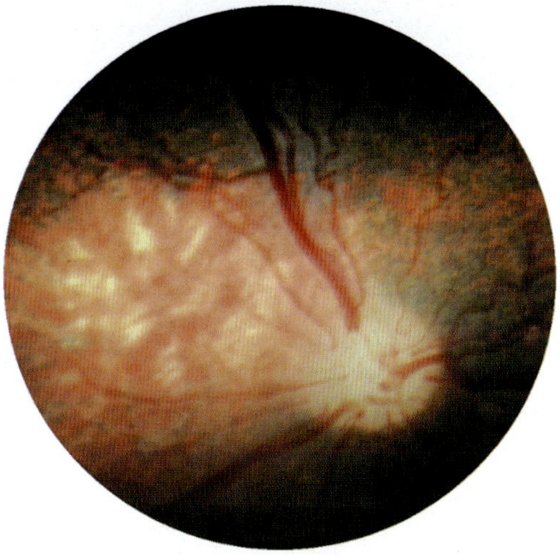

Figure 11-194
CEA with choroidal hypoplasia in a collie.

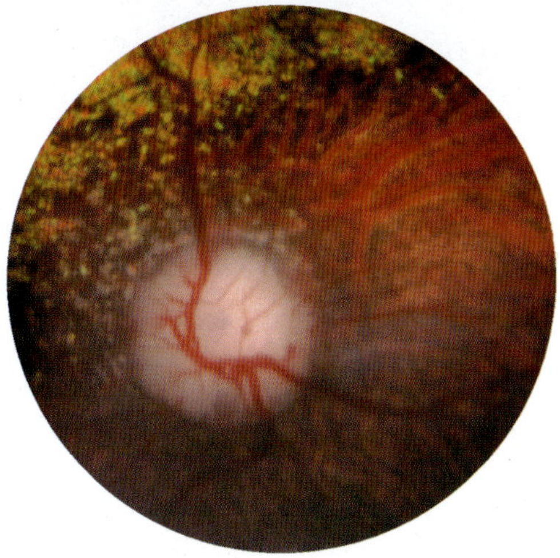

Figure 11-195
A bichon frise with bilateral depigmentation over the temporal area of the fundus next to the optic nerve, which resembles choroidal hypoplasia in CEA (also, a suspicious, small, circular, gray area at the 6 o'clock position in the optic nerve resembles a coloboma).

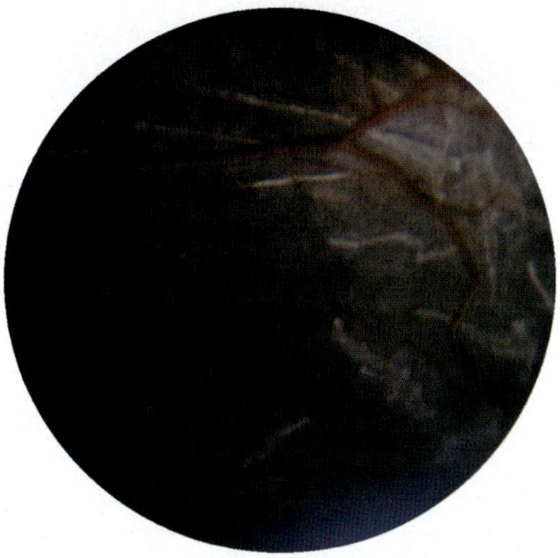

Figure 11-196
CEA with retinal folds in the nontapetum of a collie puppy.

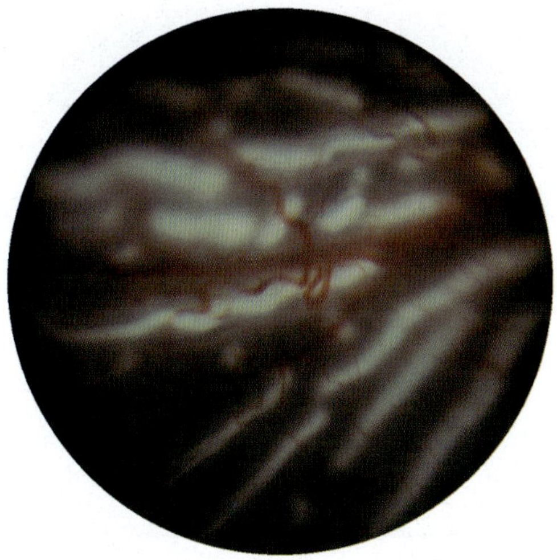

Figure 11-197
CEA with severe retinal folds in a 6-week-old collie puppy.

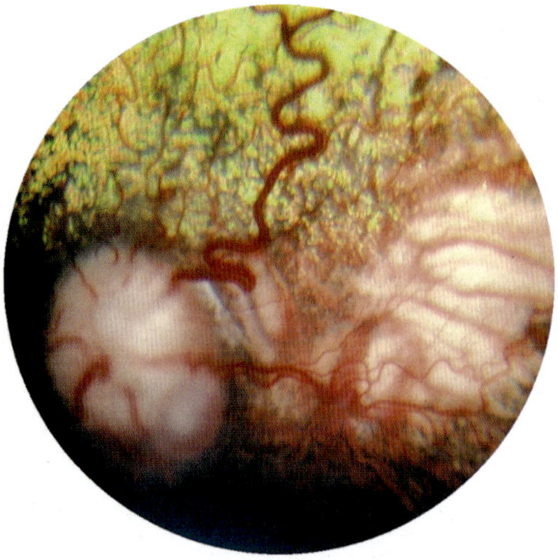

Figure 11-198
CEA with choroidal hypoplasia and coloboma (gray, unfocused area) at the inferotemporal area (at the 5 o'clock position) of the optic nerve in the left eye.

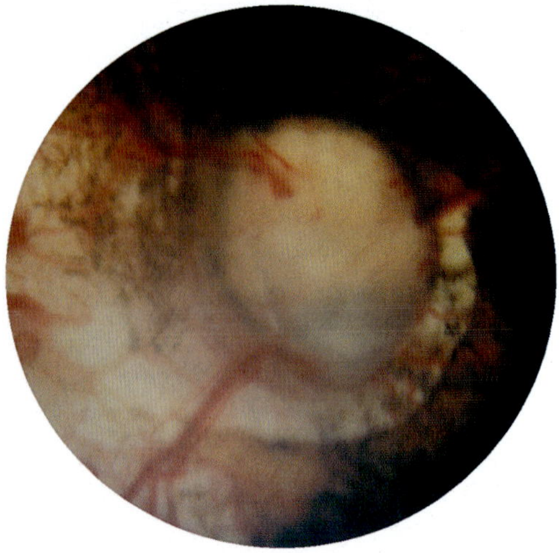

Figure 11-199
CEA with choroidal hypoplasia and large coloboma of the optic nerve with peripapillary depigmentation.

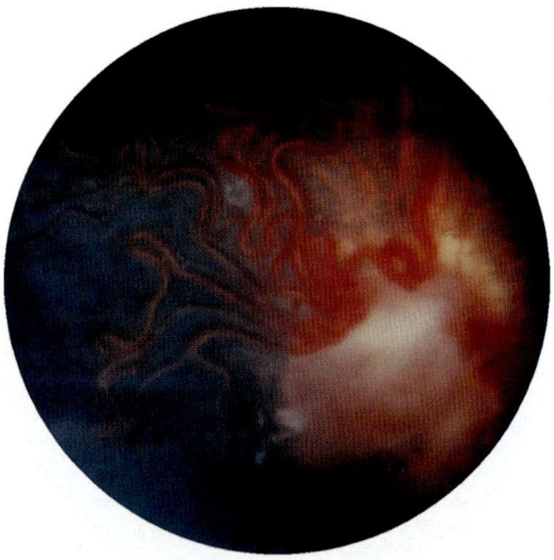

Figure 11-200
CEA with optic nerve coloboma, abnormally tortuous retinal vessels, and retinal folds.

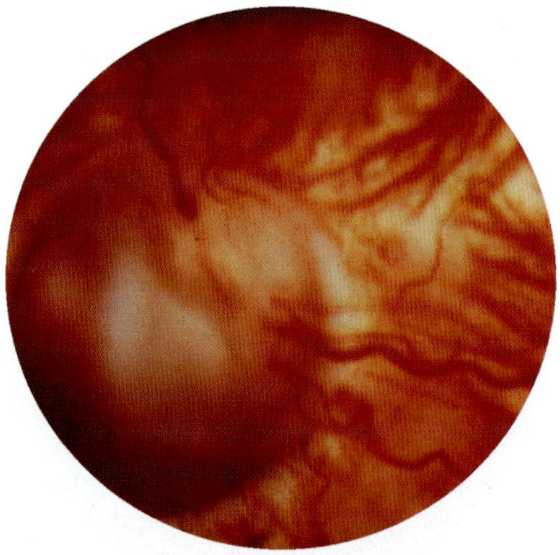

Figure 11-201
CEA with large coloboma of the optic nerve and choroidal hypoplasia.

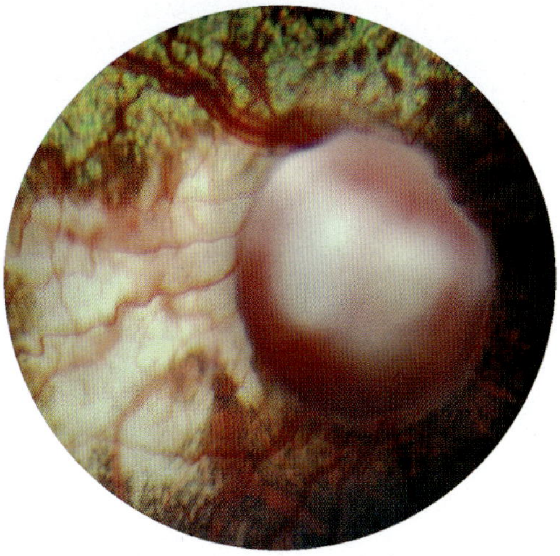

Figure 11-202
Collie with CEA with optic nerve coloboma and choroidal hypoplasia. The dog had reduced vision in this eye but, surprisingly, was not totally blind.

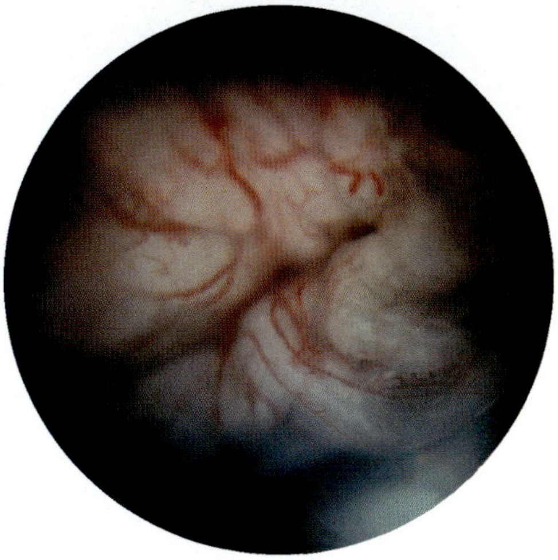

Figure 11-203
CEA with retinal nonattachment.
(Courtesy Dr. E. Dan Wolf.)

ACTIVE CHORIORETINITIS

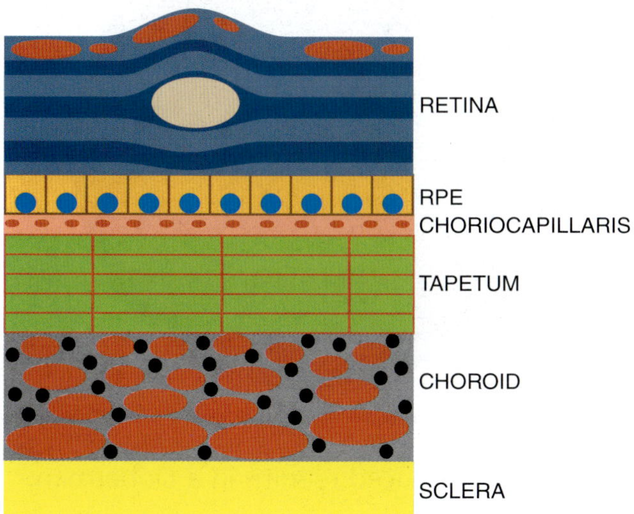

Figure 11-204
Inflammation in the retina can cause exudate (tan oval) that obscures the view of the tapetum, because more light is absorbed by the thickened area of retina and less light is reflected back from the tapetum to an observer. This results in tapetal hyporeflectivity.

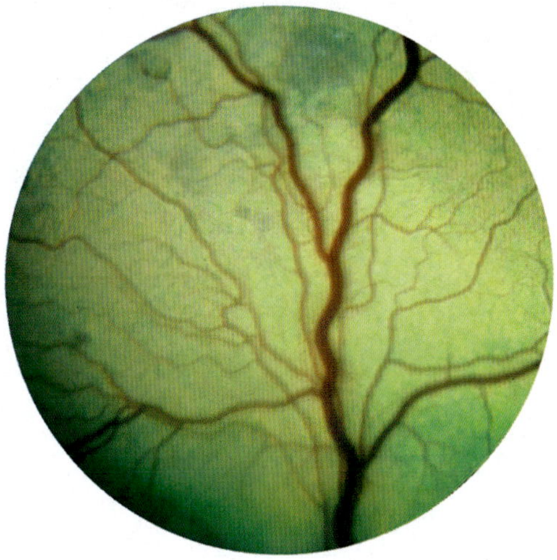

Figure 11-205
Focal areas of active chorioretinitis in the superior tapetum. The focal areas are duller or grayer (hyporeflective) than the surrounding normal tapetum.

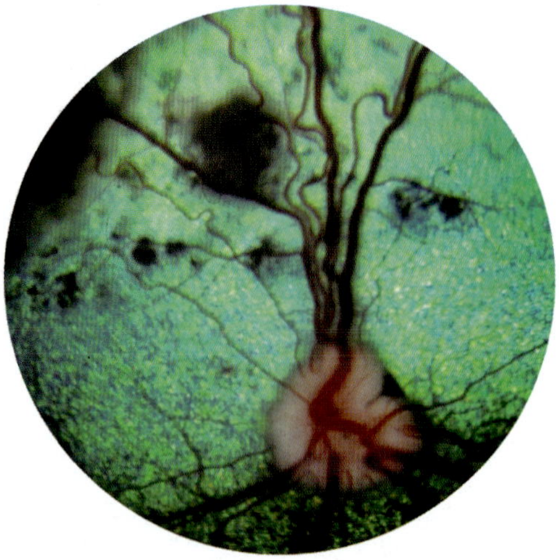

Figure 11-206
German shepherd dog with active chorioretinitis resulting from aspergillosis. Chorioretinitis is visible as multifocal dark areas in the tapetum.

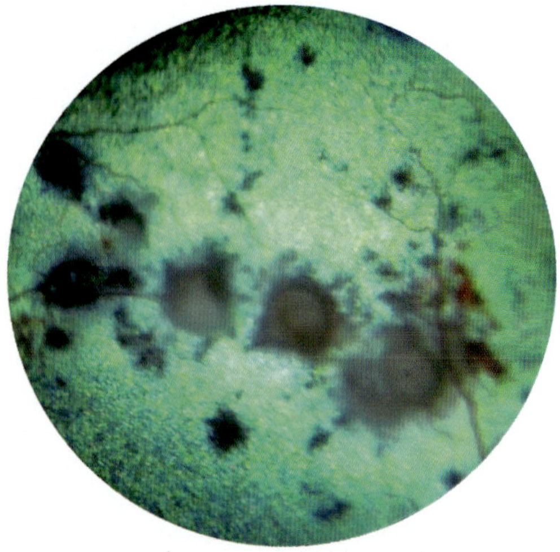

Figure 11-207
German shepherd dog with active chorioretinitis resulting from aspergillosis after treatment with itraconazole. This is the same dog as shown in Figure 11-206. Note the change in color of the lesions after treatment.

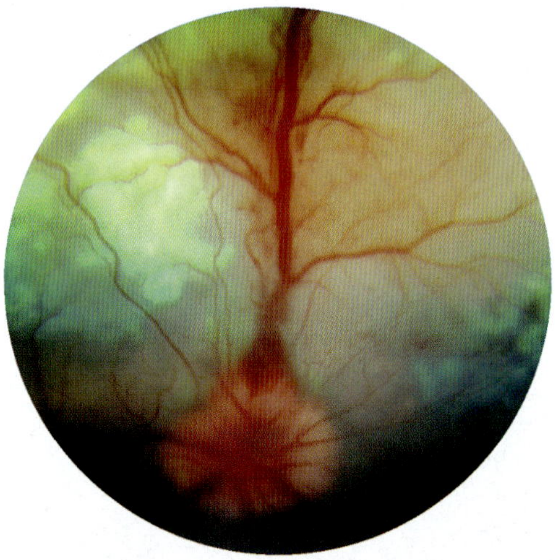

Figure 11-208
Dog with chorioretinitis, optic neuritis, and areas of retinal hemorrhage resulting from coccidioidomycosis.

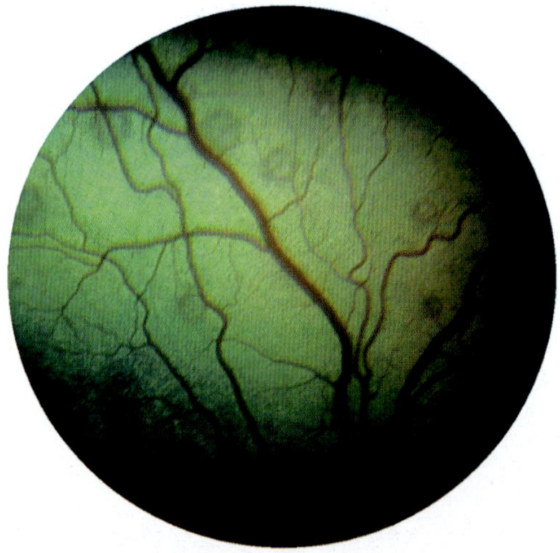

Figure 11-209
Sulfonamide-induced retinitis in a Doberman.

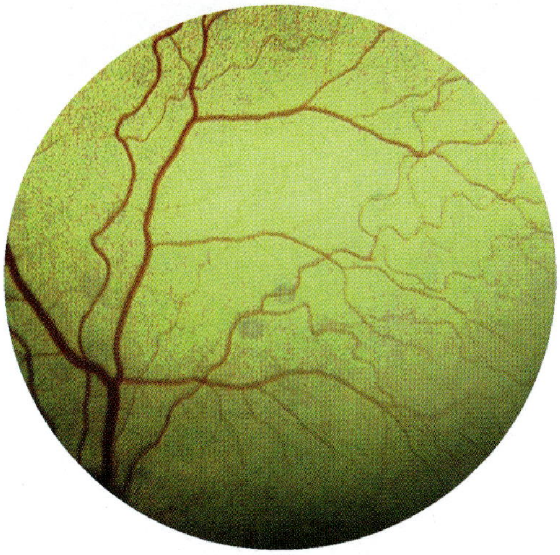

Figure 11-210
Dog with multifocal areas of retinal edema resulting from acute retinitis caused by distemper.

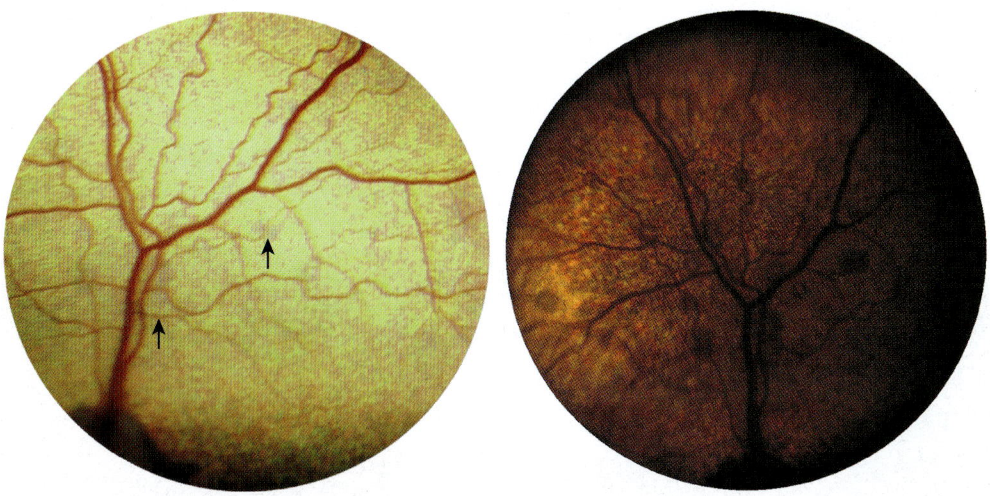

Figure 11-211
Dog with multifocal areas of retinal edema resulting from distemper. Photograph on right was taken with low flash light intensity, which highlights the lesions, compared with the brighter left-hand photograph. Indirect ophthalmoscopy at low light intensity improves contrast for both hyperreflective and hyporeflective tapetal lesions.

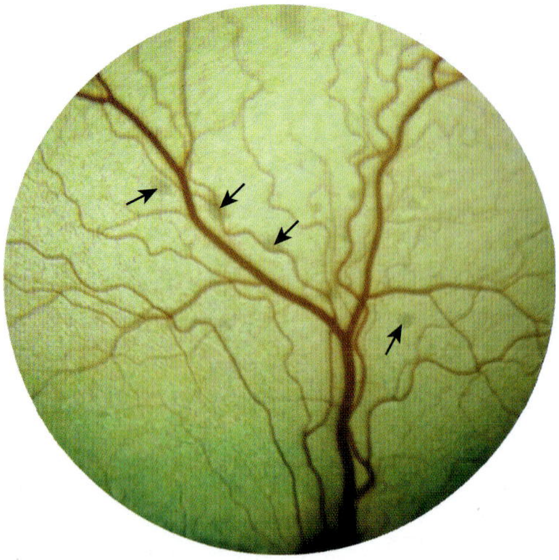

Figure 11-212
Dog with distemper and focal areas of retinal edema *(arrows)*.

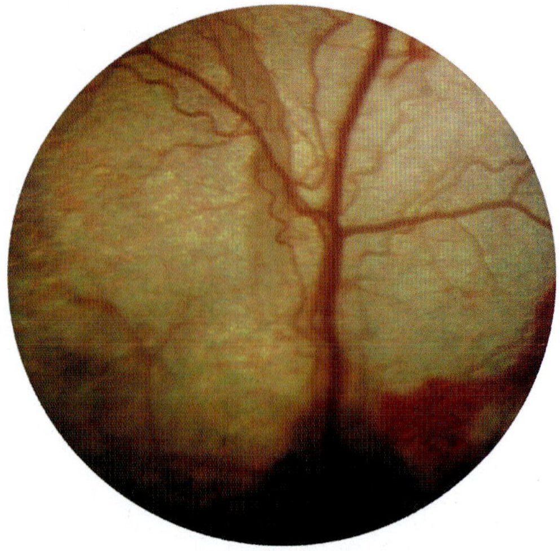

Figure 11-213
Fold of retinal edema superior to the optic nerve and retinal hemorrhage secondary to a retrobulbar abscess.

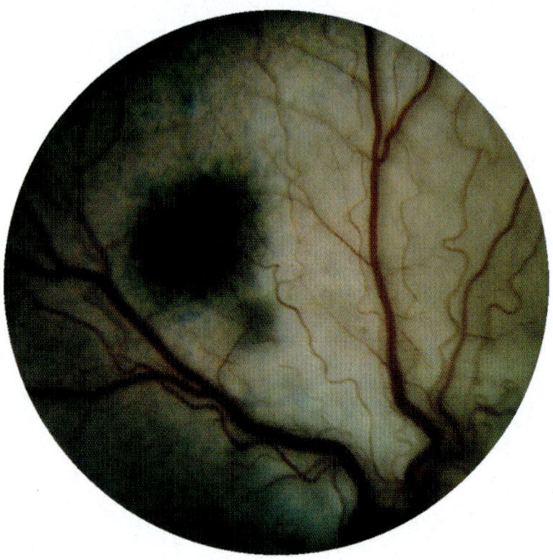

Figure 11-214
Doberman with granulomatous meningoencephalitis (GME). Retinal and tapetal edema is present throughout most of the fundus. The dark area results from chorioretinal exudate.

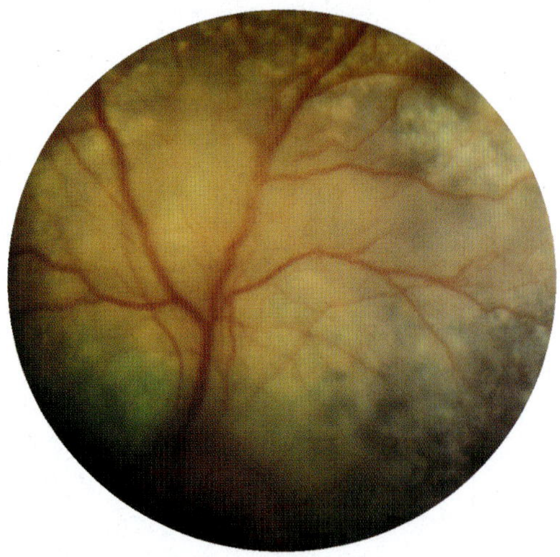

Figure 11-215
Active choroiditis and retinal effusion in a rottweiler with episcleritis and chorioretinitis. All of this part of the fundus is abnormal.

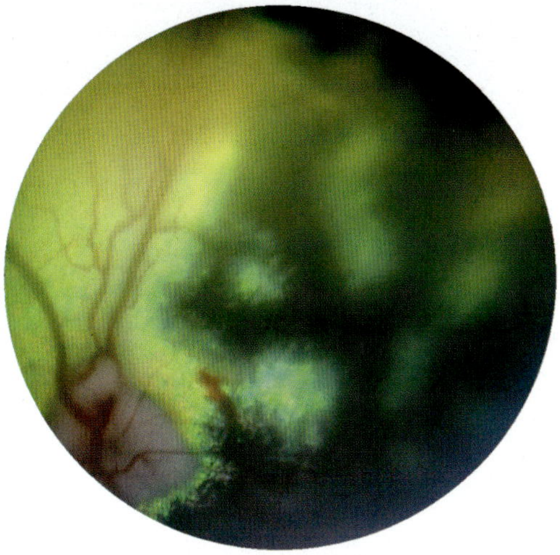

Figure 11-216
Dog with retinal edema, choroiditis (dark areas in the tapetum), and retinal hemorrhage.

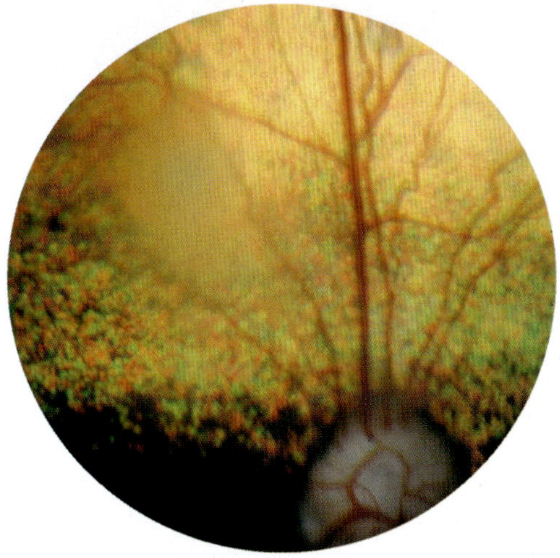

Figure 11-217
Miniature poodle with focal area of retinal edema of undetermined cause at the 10 o'clock position in the tapetum.

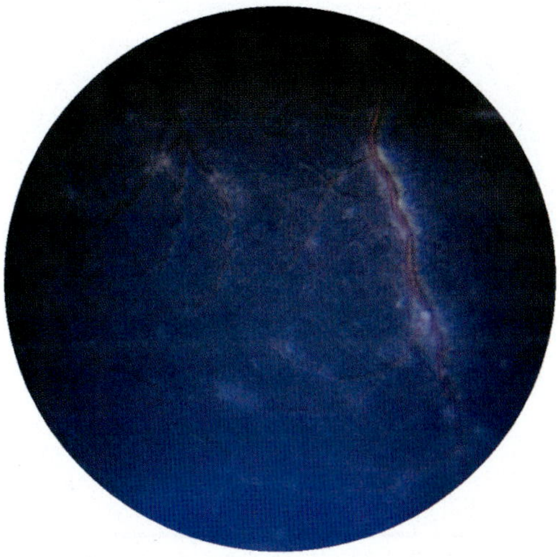

Figure 11-218
Acute perivascular cuffing (vasculitis) caused by *Ehrlichia canis* in the nontapetum of a dog.

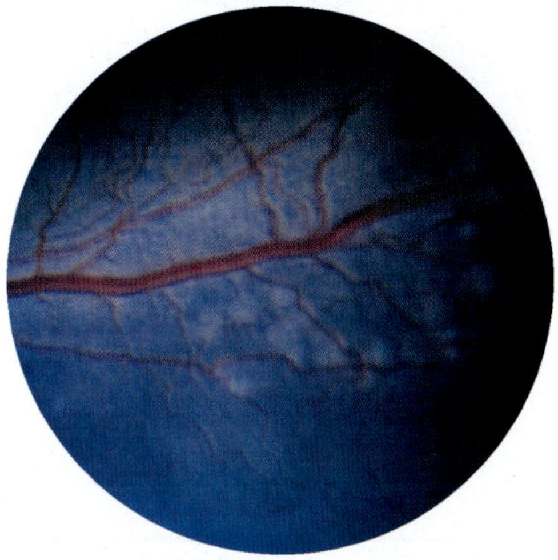

Figure 11-219
Infiltrates in the nontapetal retina of dog with distemper virus infection.

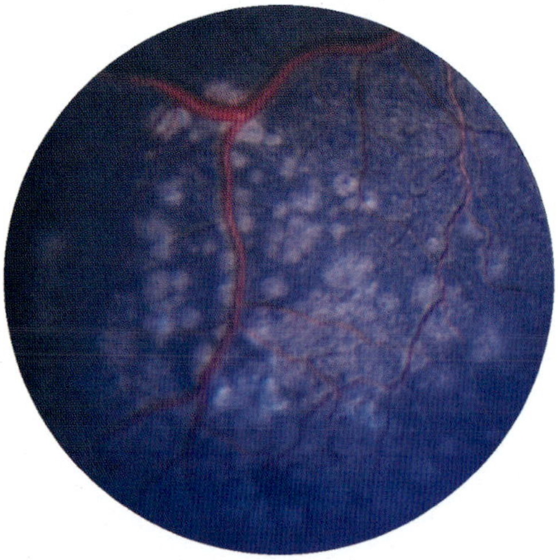

Figure 11-220
Chronic and active chorioretinitis. Active lesions are gray and fuzzy; inactive, scarred lesions are bright white.

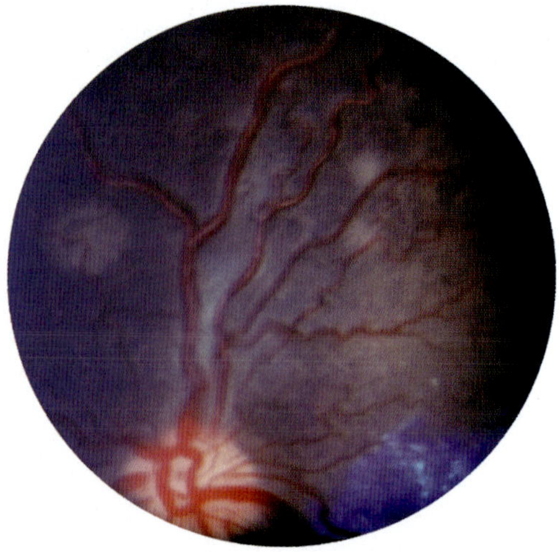

Figure 11-221
Puppy with focal areas of retinal edema associated with distemper infection.

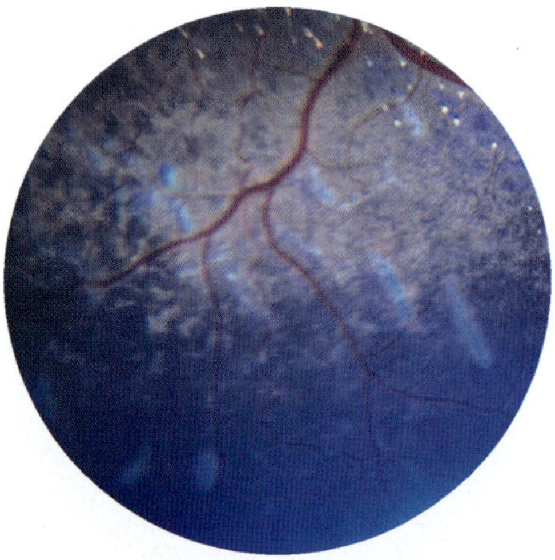

Figure 11-222
Striate retinopathy secondary to trauma. The linear gray opacities in the nontapetal fundus are the result of retinal edema.

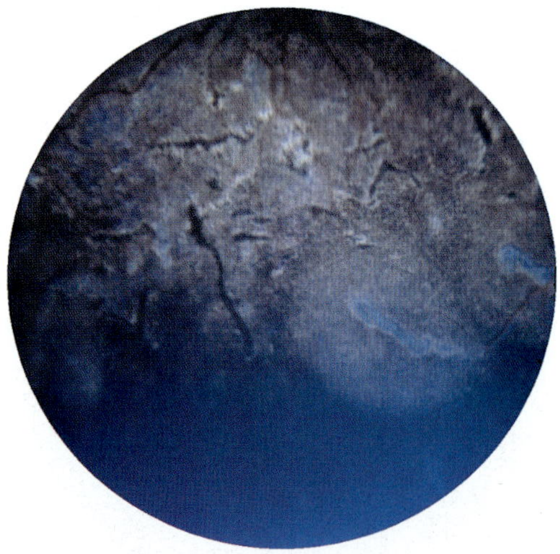

Figure 11-223
Dog with chronic and active chorioretinitis. Areas of retinal edema and areas of depigmentation and hyperpigmentation are present.

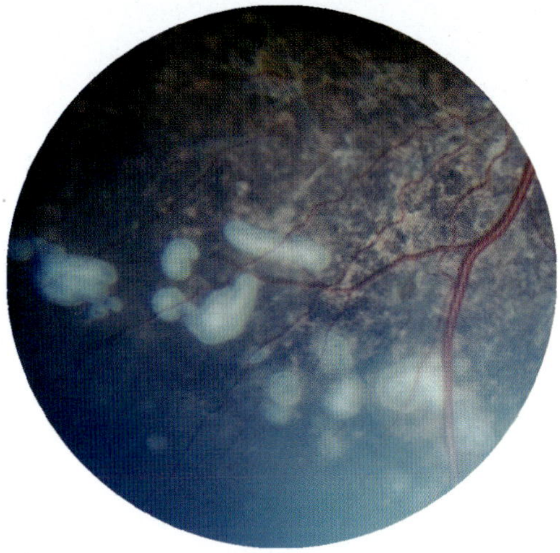

Figure 11-224
Active chorioretinal lesions resulting from *Ehrlichia* infection. Multifocal areas of retinal edema with or without cellular infiltrate. Some retinal vessels are elevated by the retinal edema.

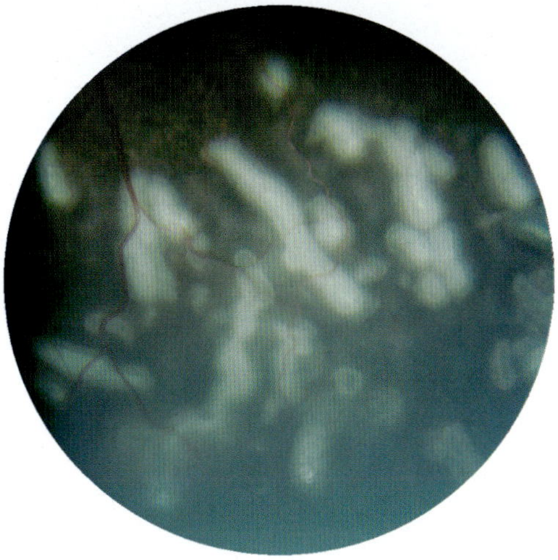

Figure 11-225
Retinal folds and edema resulting from ehrlichiosis.

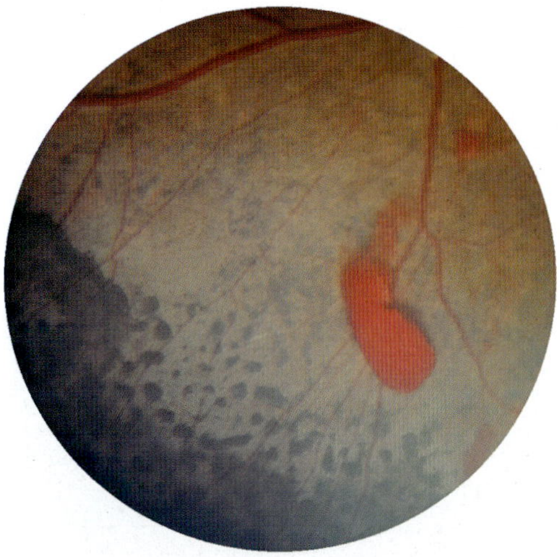

Figure 11-226
Dog with preretinal hemorrhage resulting from *E. canis* infection.

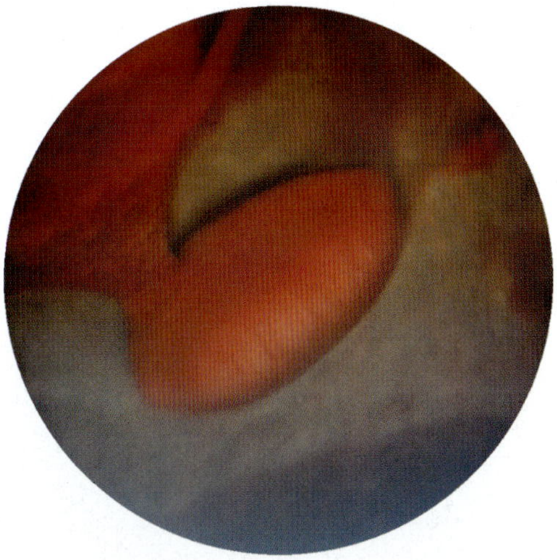

Figure 11-227
Dog with *E. canis* infection with retinal, preretinal, and vitreal hemorrhage in the nontapetal fundus.

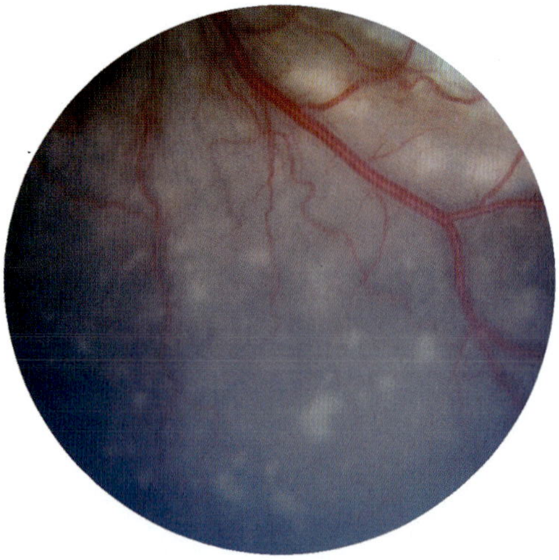

Figure 11-228
Dog with focal areas of retinal infiltrate and hemorrhage in the nontapetal fundus resulting from coccidioidomycosis.

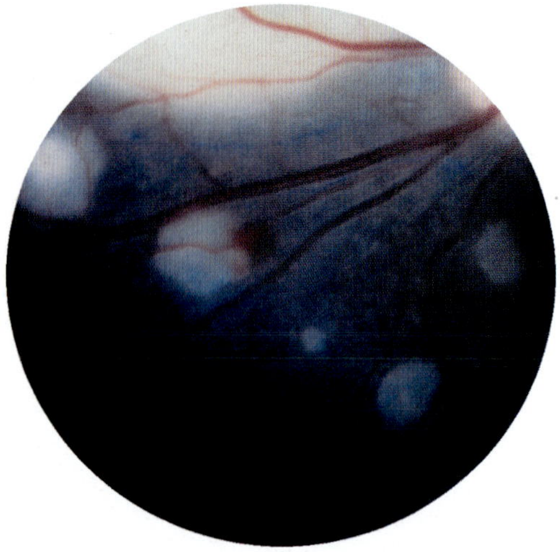

Figure 11-229
Dog with focal areas of retinal infiltrates and hemorrhage resulting from coccidioidomycosis after 4 weeks of itraconazole treatment.

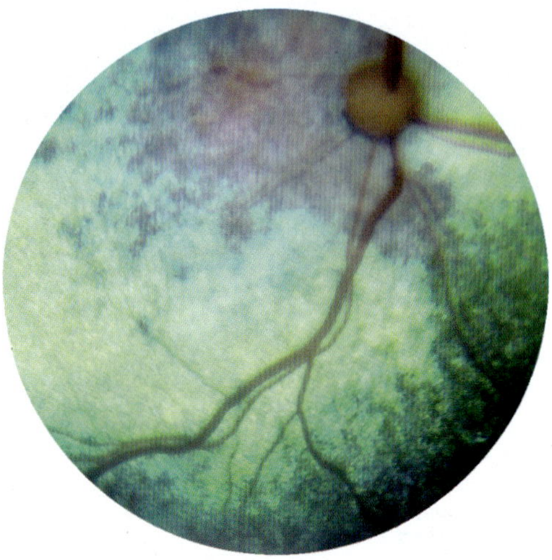

Figure 11-230
Large area of active chorioretinitis adjacent to the optic nerve in a cat that also had anterior uveitis of undiagnosed cause. The tapetum in these areas is dark; the red-pink area is retinal infiltrate.

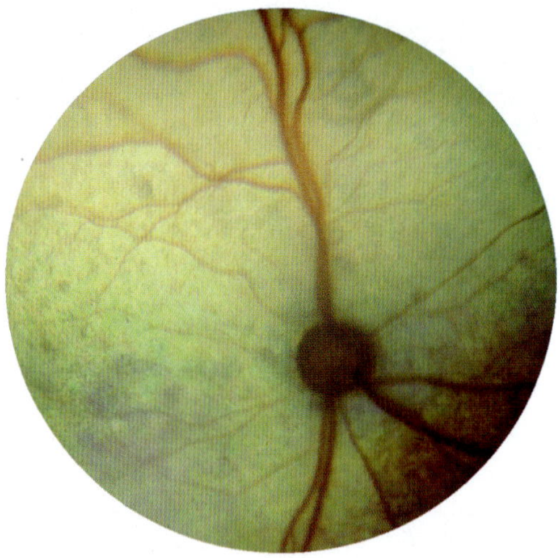

Figure 11-231
Active chorioretinitis adjacent to the disc and in the superior tapetum, visible as a color change in these areas.

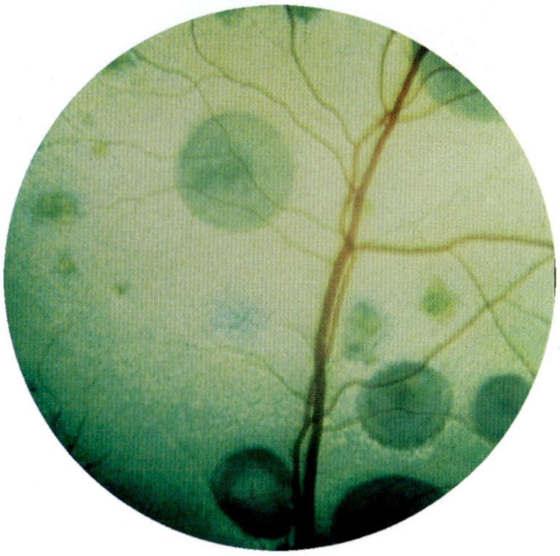

Figure 11-232
Cat with multifocal granulomatous lesions resulting from cryptococcosis.
(Courtesy Dr. E. Dan Wolf.)

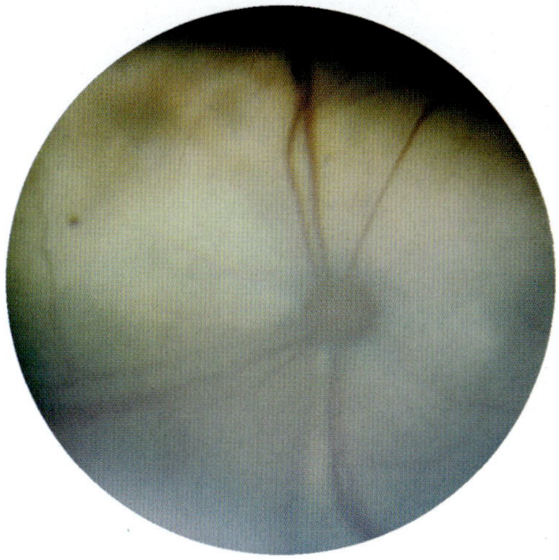

Figure 11-233
Chorioretinitis in a cat. The entire retina is edematous and detached with subretinal cellular infiltrates.

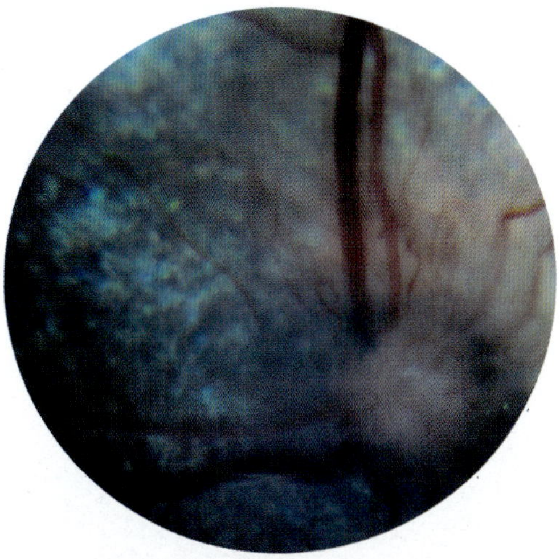

Figure 11-234
Cat with chorioretinitis and optic neuritis resulting from lymphosarcoma. The entire fundus is abnormal.

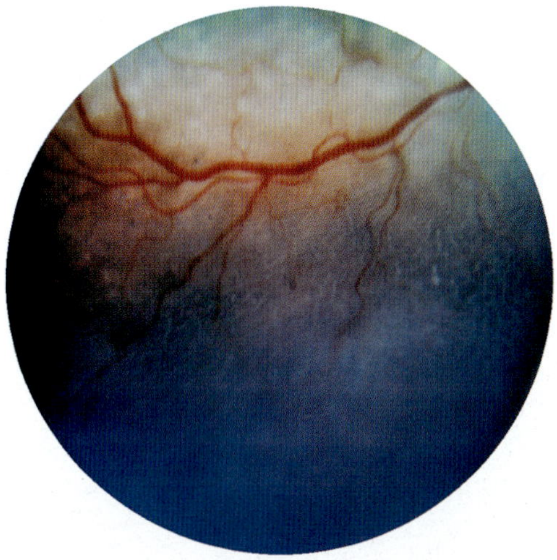

Figure 11-235
Retinal infiltrates with retinal edema and folding resulting from histoplasmosis in a cat.

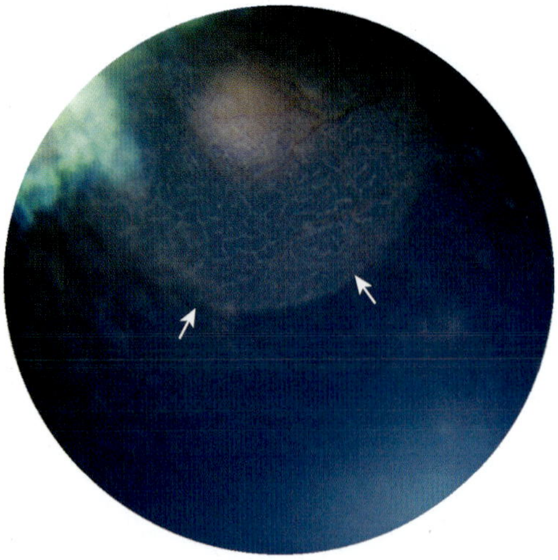

Figure 11-236
An area of flat retinal detachment *(arrows)* with folds and a choroidal granuloma occurring centrally in a cat with histoplasmosis. Small focal areas of chorioretinitis are present inferiorly.

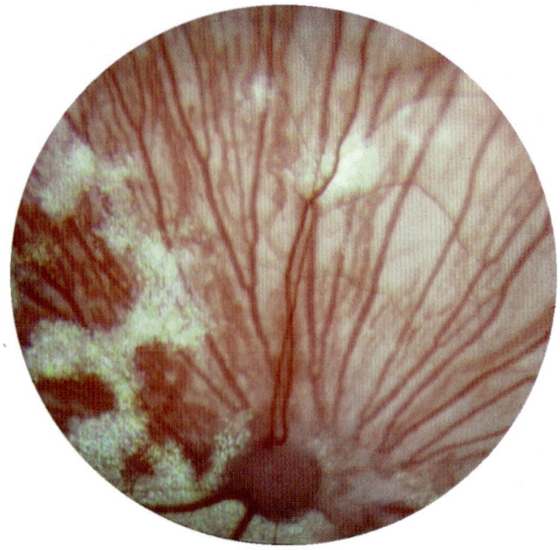

Figure 11-237
Cat with chorioretinitis and destruction of tapetum resulting from feline infectious peritonitis.

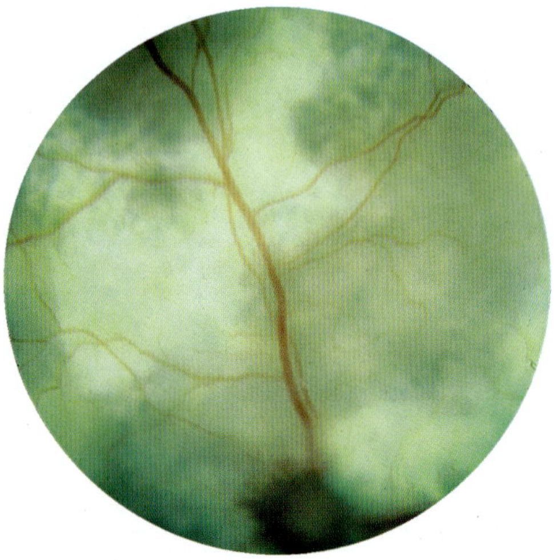

Figure 11-238
Cat with chorioretinitis involving the entire tapetum and optic neuritis.

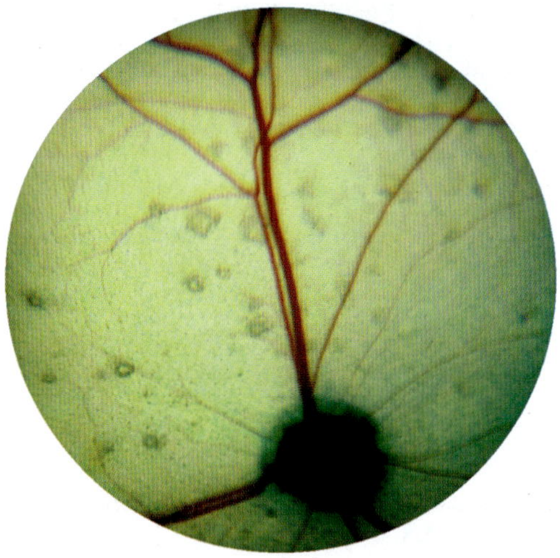

Figure 11-239
Cat with chronic and active chorioretinitis associated with toxoplasmosis. The tapetum looks discolored and mottled, indicating active inflammation; the multifocal circular lesions are hyperreflective in their centers, indicating inactive scars.

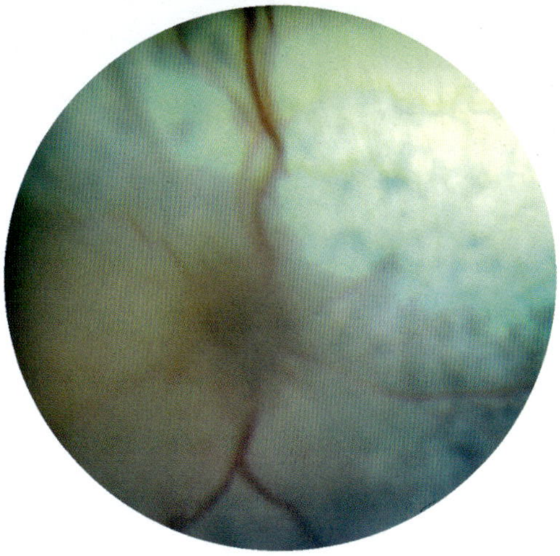

Figure 11-240
Cat with active chorioretinitis and optic neuritis resulting from toxoplasmosis.

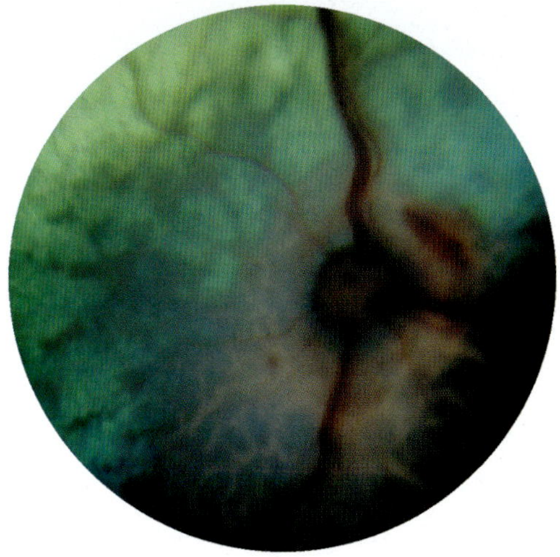

Figure 11-241
Cat with retinal hemorrhage, optic nerve hemorrhage, and linear areas of retinal edema.

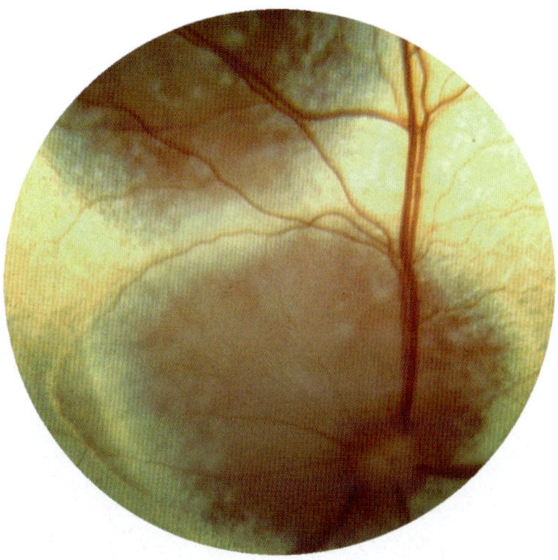

Figure 11-242
Cat with active chorioretinitis resulting from cryptococcosis.
(Courtesy Dr. Robert Playter.)

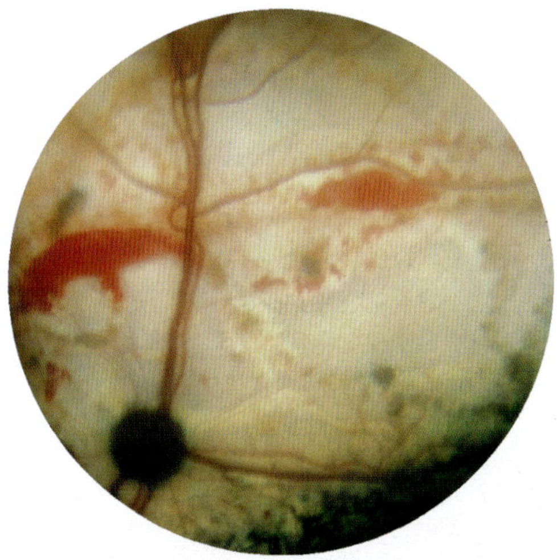

Figure 11-243
Cat with ophthalmomyiasis (parasitic invasion of the eye) with retinal hemorrhage and linear tracks in tapetum.

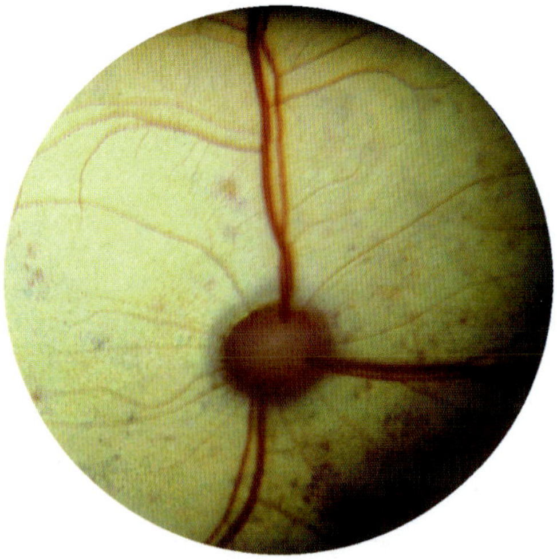

Figure 11-244
Multifocal small foci of inflammation and pigmentary abnormalities in the tapetal fundus of a cat, visible as small dark dots.

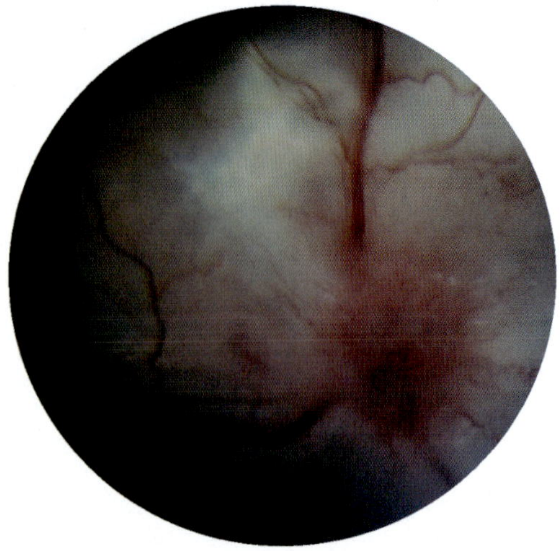

Figure 11-245
Cat with severe chorioretinitis and optic neuritis. The appearance of the disc is very abnormal.

RETINAL DETACHMENT

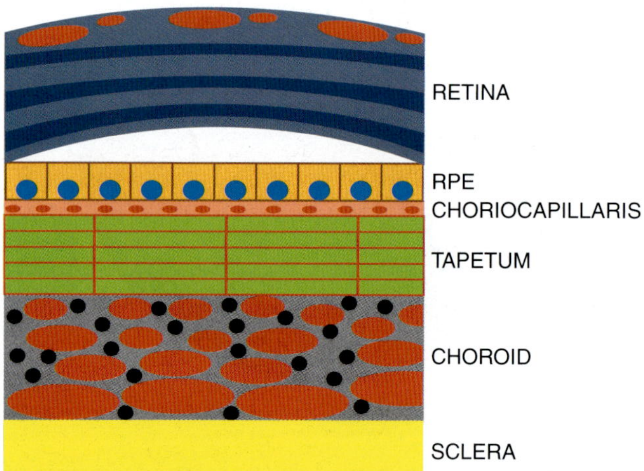

Figure 11-246
In retinal detachment the neural layers of the retina become separated from the underlying RPE. The retina is usually detached by exudate from the choroid or by the penetration of vitreous between the retina and RPE.

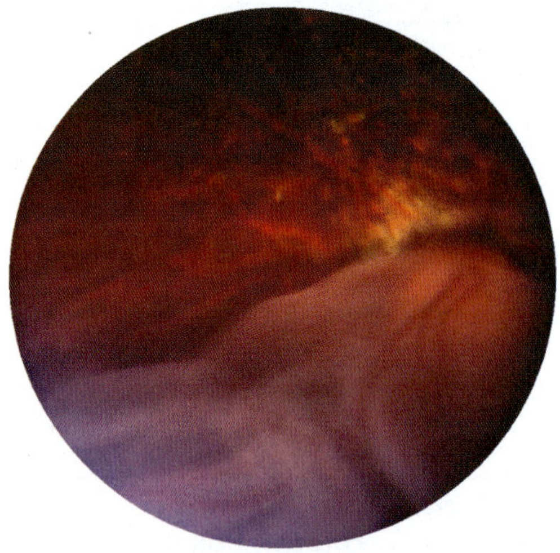

Figure 11-247
Dog with retinal dialysis (giant tear of the retina at the ora ciliaris retinae) and retinal detachment. The retina usually stays attached at the optic nerve but folds over the nerve, hiding it. Note the presence of retinal vessels in the detached retina, but no retinal vessels superiorly. (Courtesy Dr. Robert Playter.)

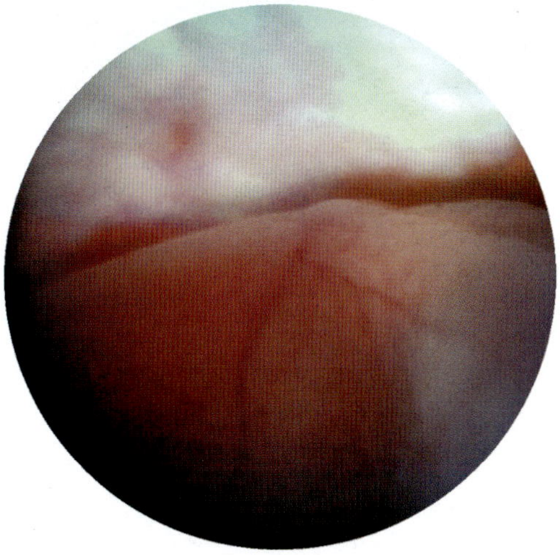

Figure 11-248
Giant retinal dialysis. The retina is folded over, obscuring the optic nerve.

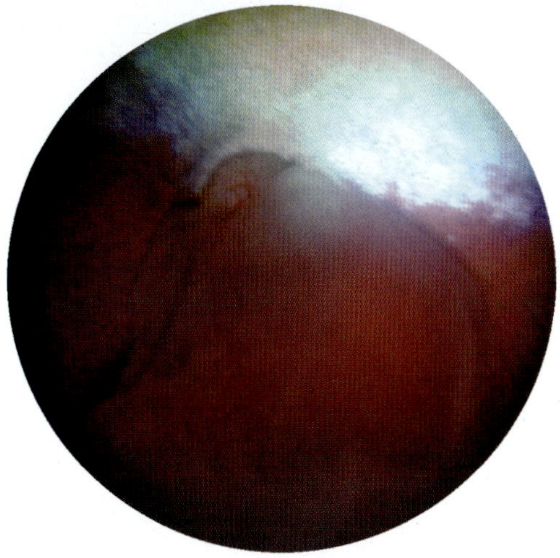

Figure 11-249
A complete retinal detachment with dialysis in a dog. The tapetum is hyperreflective because no overlying retina is present to absorb light.

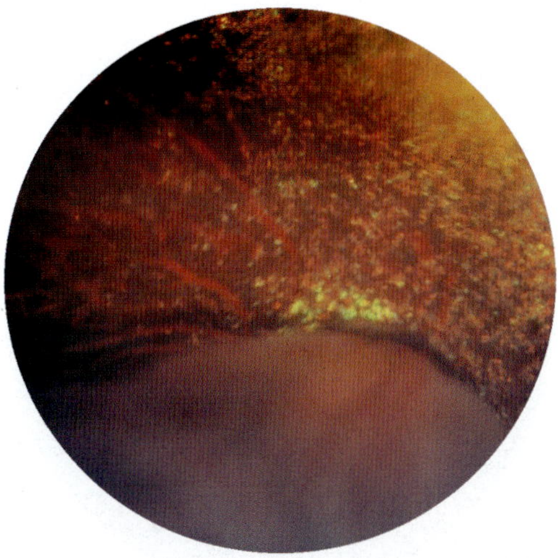

Figure 11-250
Giant retinal dialysis. The retina is folded over, obscuring the optic nerve.

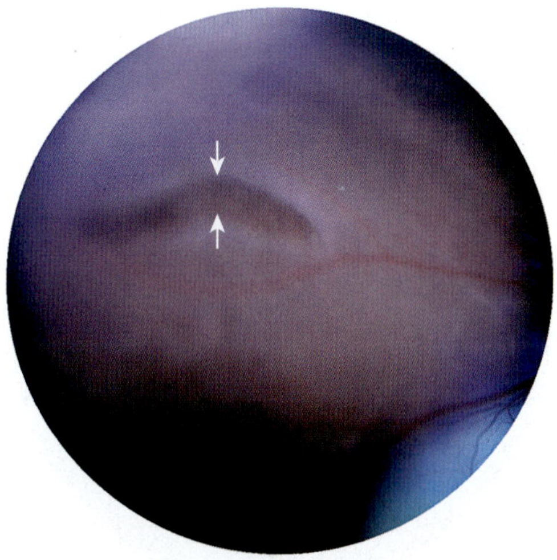

Figure 11-251
Retinal detachment with retinal tear and retinal holes.

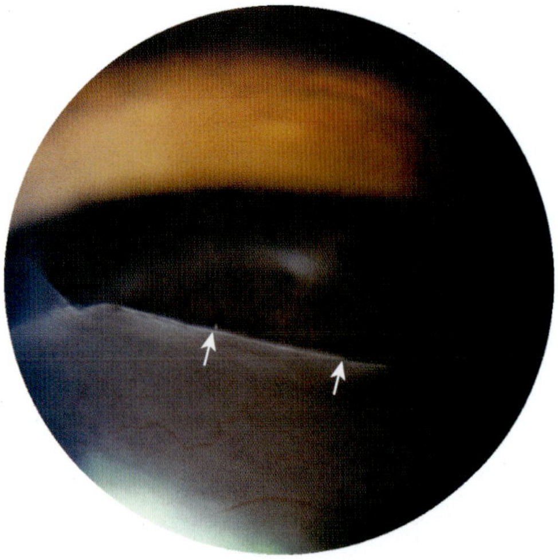

Figure 11-252
Labrador retriever with peripheral retinal tear *(arrows)* after intracapsular lens removal.

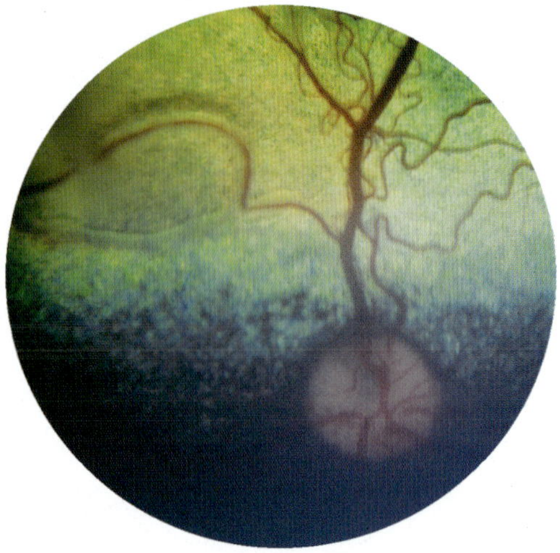

Figure 11-253
Dog with focal retinal detachment in the upper left of this photograph. A retinal vessel runs through the detachment and is casting a shadow on the tapetum.

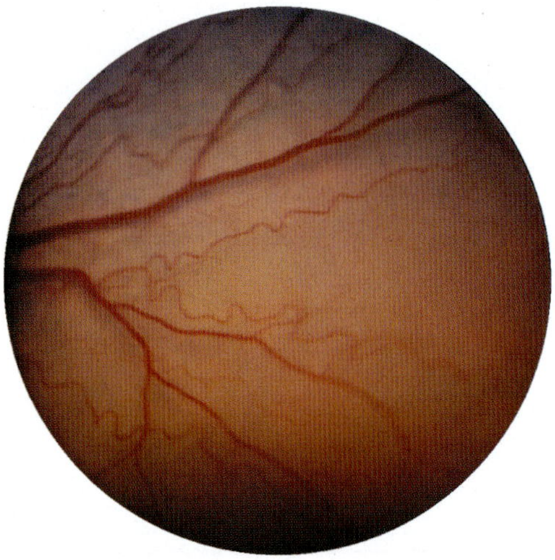

Figure 11-254
Flat retinal detachment in a dog with *E. canis* infection. Note the shadowing of retinal vessels. Also note the absence of retinal hemorrhage, which often accompanies the thrombocytopenia that occurs with this disease.

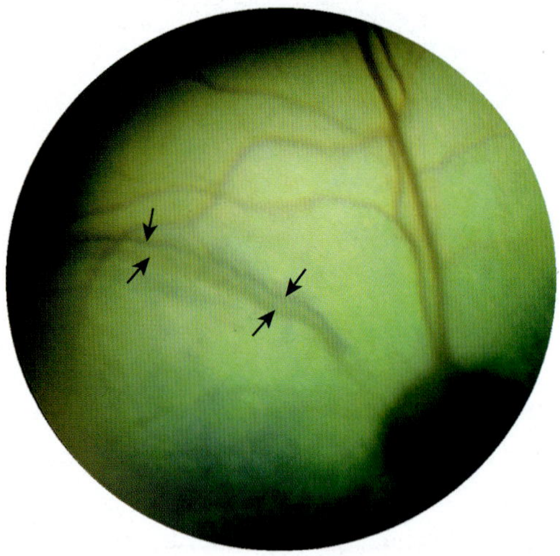

Figure 11-255
Retinoschisis (a splitting of the retina *[arrows]* that usually occurs in one of the nuclear layers) in a cat.

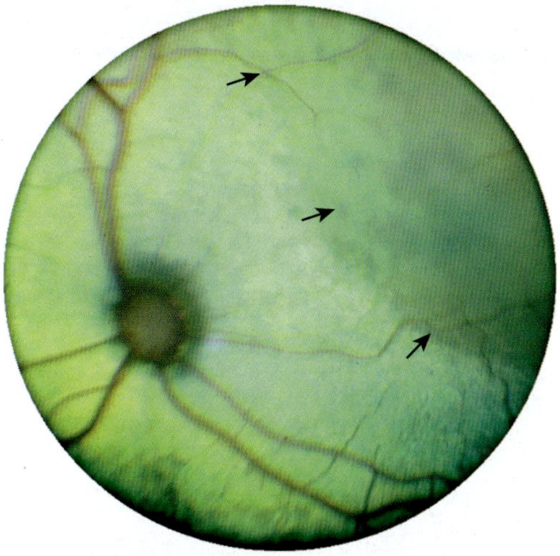

Figure 11-256
Superior bullous retinal detachment in a cat.

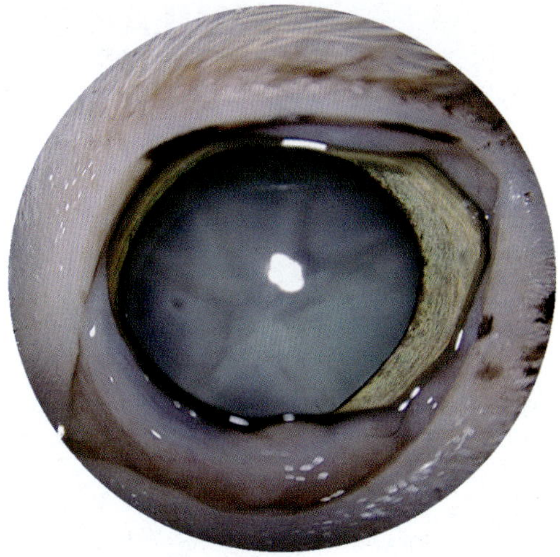

Figure 11-257
Leukocoria (a white pupil) resulting from a total retinal detachment in a cat. The gray retina abuts the posterior lens capsule.

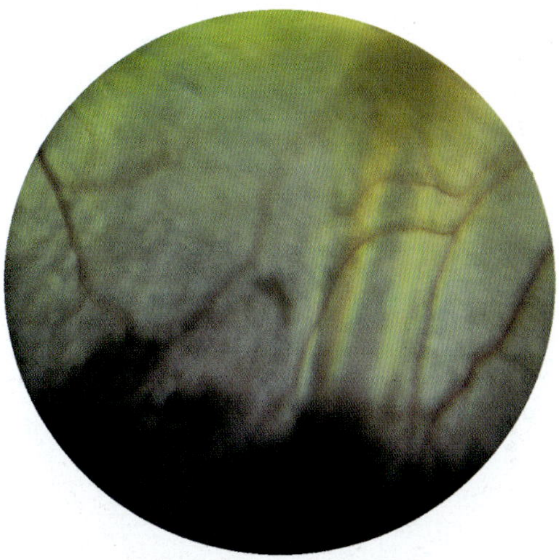

Figure 11-258
Retinal photograph of an exophthalmic cat. The exophthalmia was the result of a melanoma in the medial orbit and caused focal retinal detachment, visible as retinal folds.

VASCULAR DISEASE

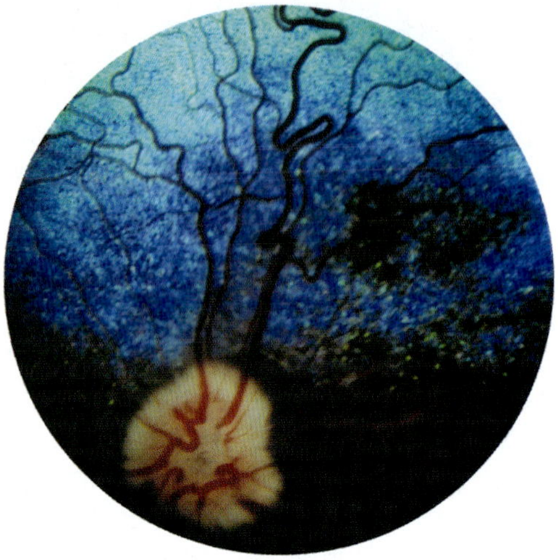

Figure 11-259
Congenital tortuous venules. The rest of the fundus is normal.

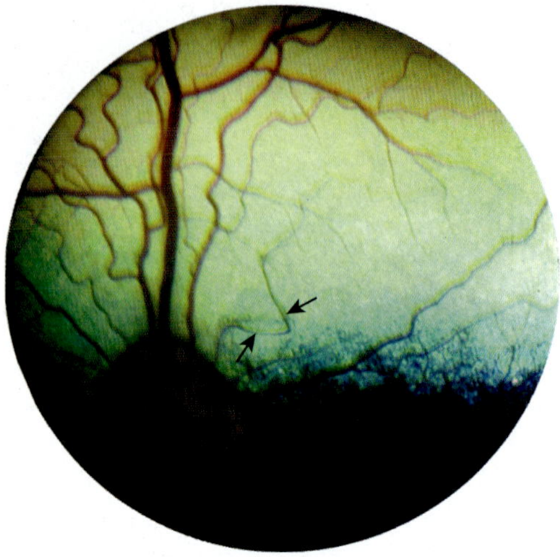

Figure 11-260
Preretinal arteriolar loop with shadow *(arrows)* in a giant schnauzer.

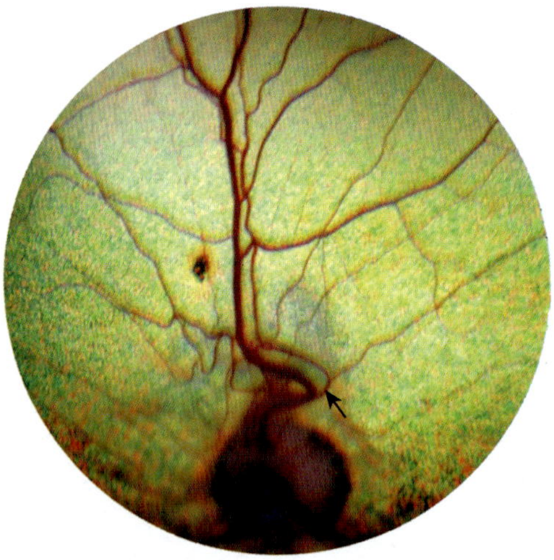

Figure 11-261
Vascular anomalies: preretinal venous loops *(arrow)*, possible hyaloid remnants at the optic disk.

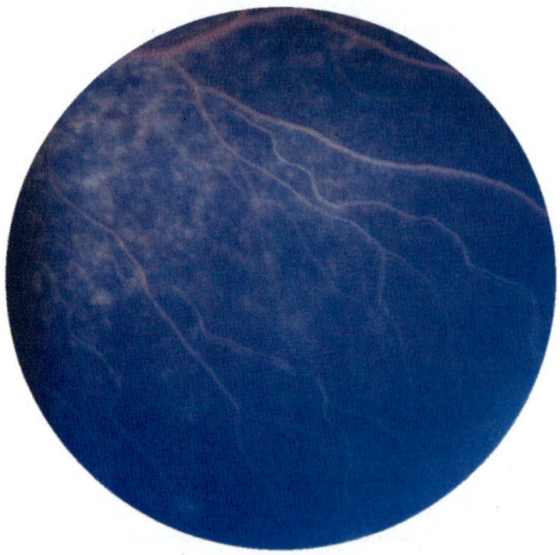

Figure 11-262
Lipemia retinalis in a dachshund with toxoplasmosis. Lipemia retinalis makes blood vessels look pink (red blood with white lipid added). There are multifocal gray opacities indicative of active chorioretinitis.

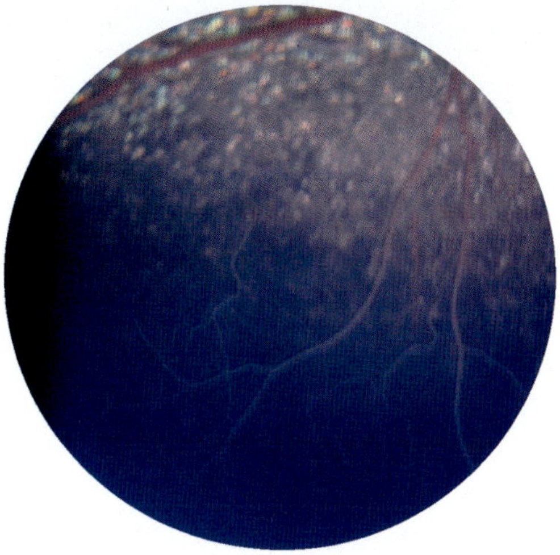

Figure 11-263
Lipemia retinalis.

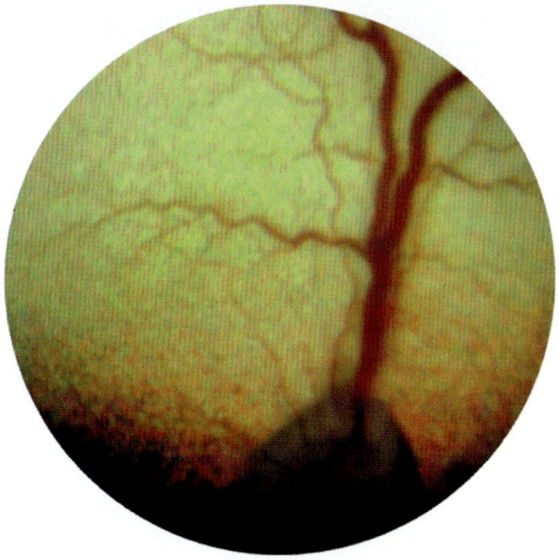

Figure 11-264
Engorged vessels in a dog with cardiac anomaly.

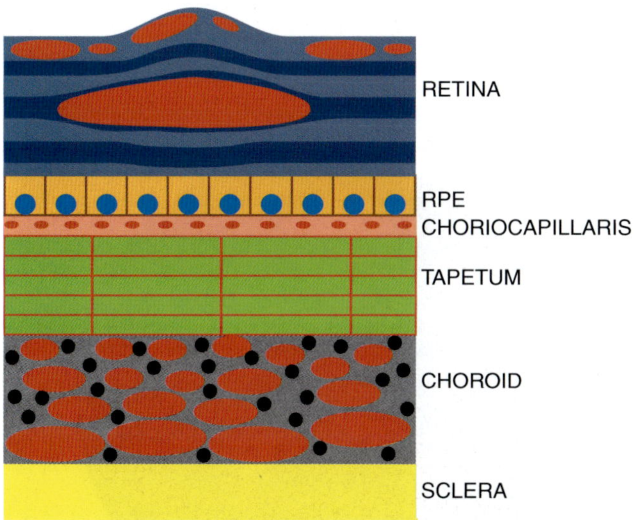

Figure 11-265
In cases of hypertensive retinopathy or bleeding from trauma or coagulopathies, hemorrhage may be seen at various levels in the retina or in front of the retina in the vitreous. The level of the hemorrhage may be determined by its appearance relative to retinal vessels (which are obscured if the hemorrhage is in the nerve fiber layer or the vitreous). The shape of small hemorrhages can also indicate depth; flame-shaped hemorrhages tend to lie in the nerve fiber or plexiform layers, whereas "dot and blot"–shaped focal hemorrhages may be located in the nuclear layers.

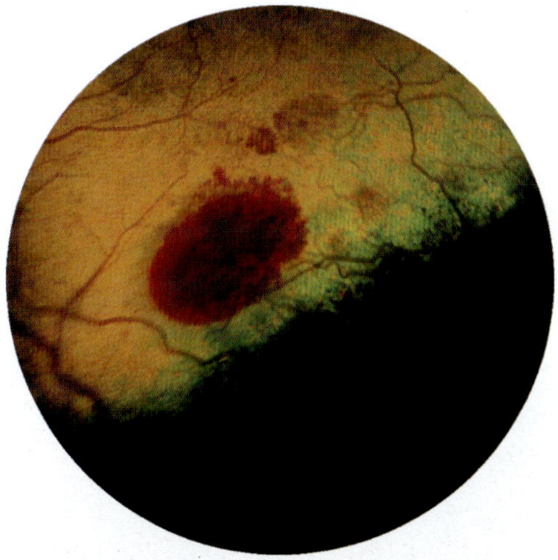

Figure 11-266
Retinal hemorrhage.

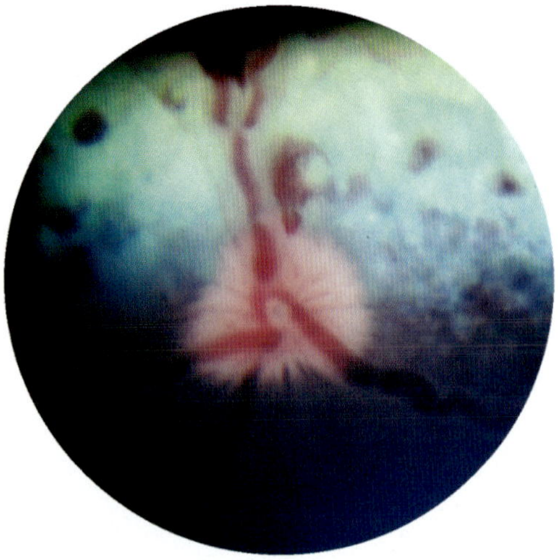

Figure 11-267
Hyperviscosity syndrome in a dog, with engorged venules, retinal petechiae, and hemorrhage.

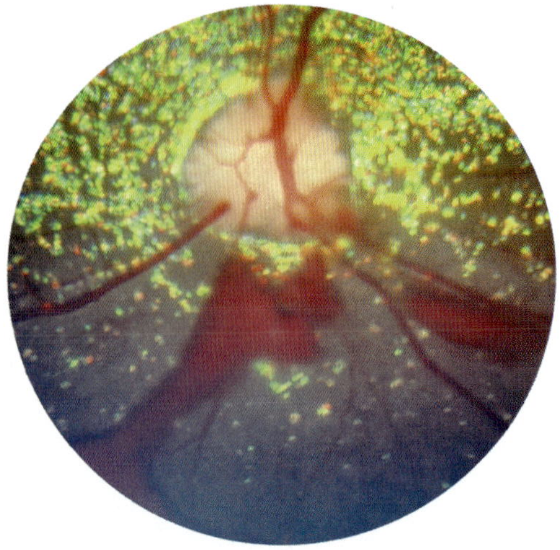

Figure 11-268
Retinal hemorrhage associated with a compressive injury to the chest in a dog.

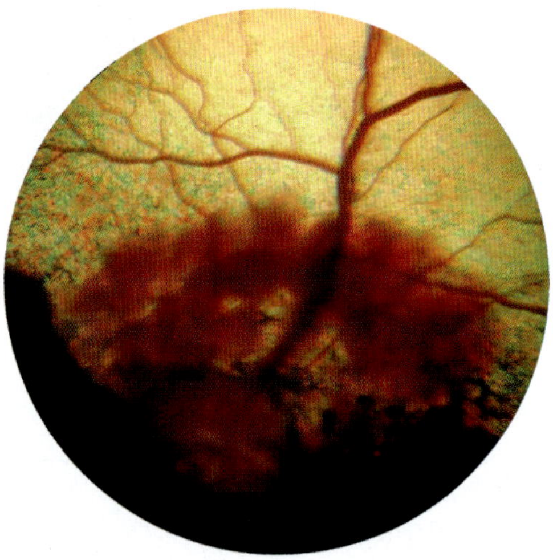

Figure 11-269
Retinal hemorrhage in a dog.

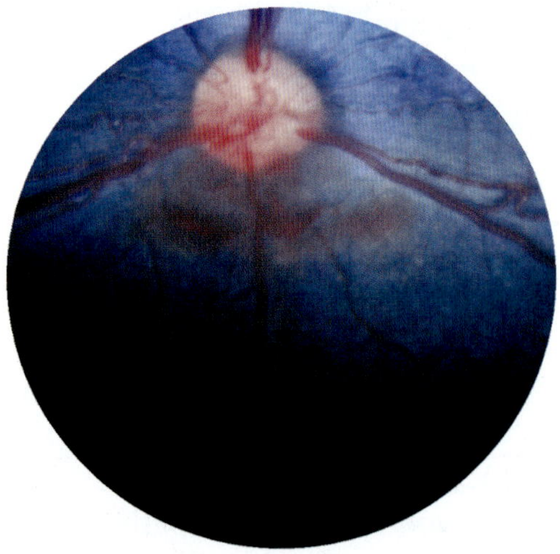

Figure 11-270
Preretinal hemorrhage in a sheltie.

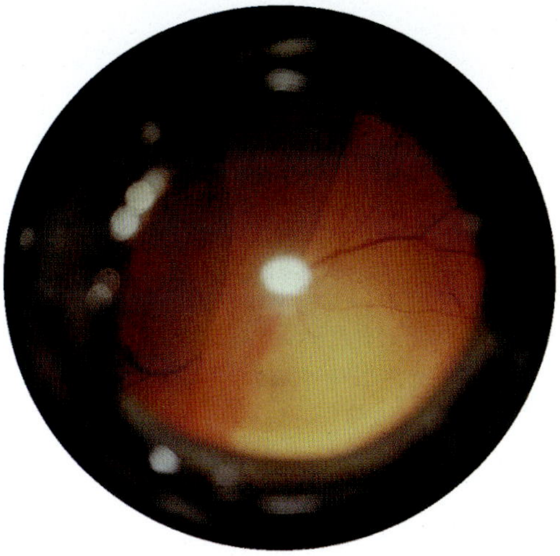

Figure 11-271
External photograph of retinal detachment resulting from Waldstrom's macroglobulinemia.

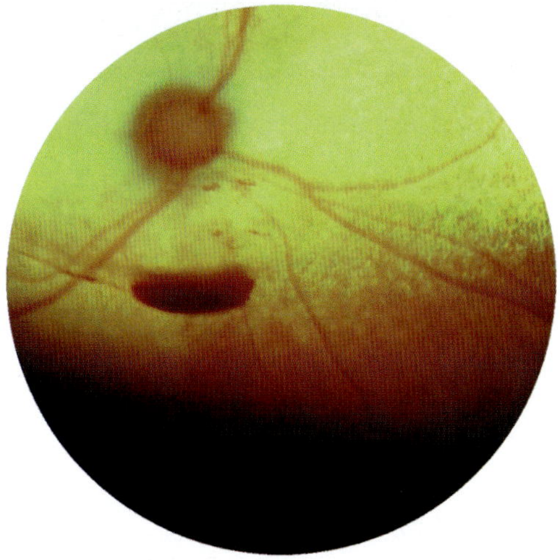

Figure 11-272
Preretinal hemorrhage in a cat in feline leukemia virus–associated anterior uveitis and anemia.

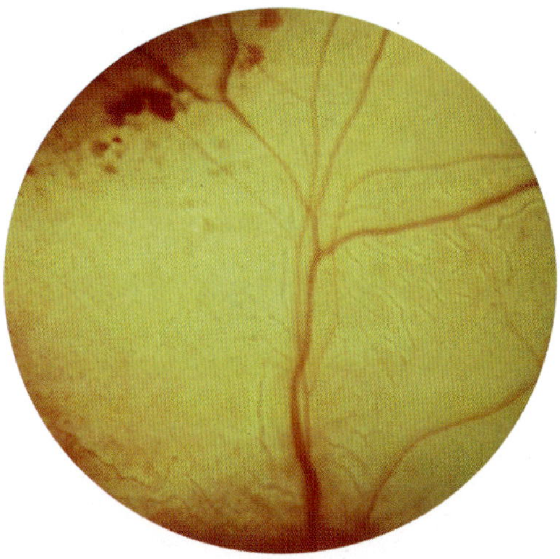

Figure 11-273
Cat with retinal folds and retinal hemorrhage resulting from hypertension.

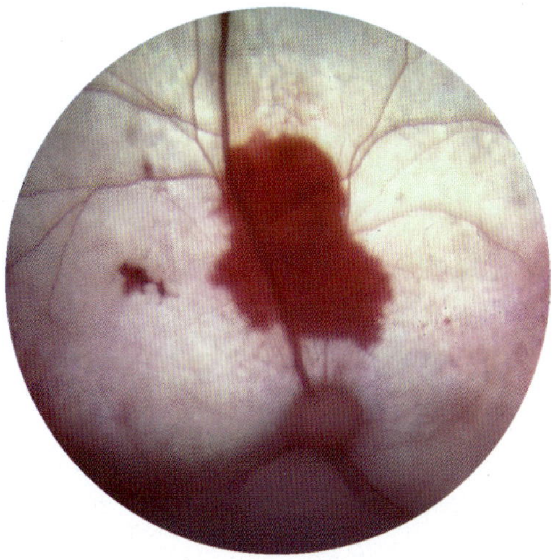

Figure 11-274
Cat with retinal edema and retinal and subretinal hemorrhage.

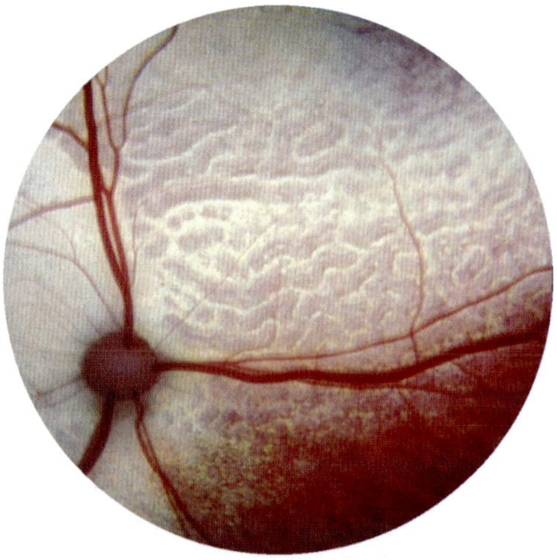

Figure 11-275
Hypertensive cat with retinal folds caused by subretinal serous exudate.

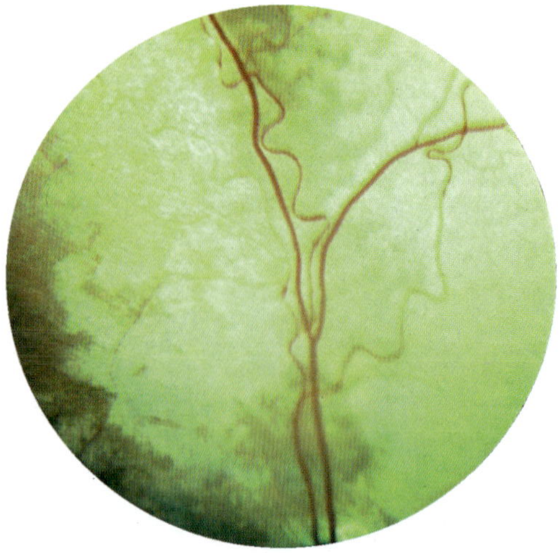

Figure 11-276
"Boxcar" lesions in the vessel of a cat with diffuse tapetal hyperreflectivity (retinal degeneration) secondary to systemic hypertension.

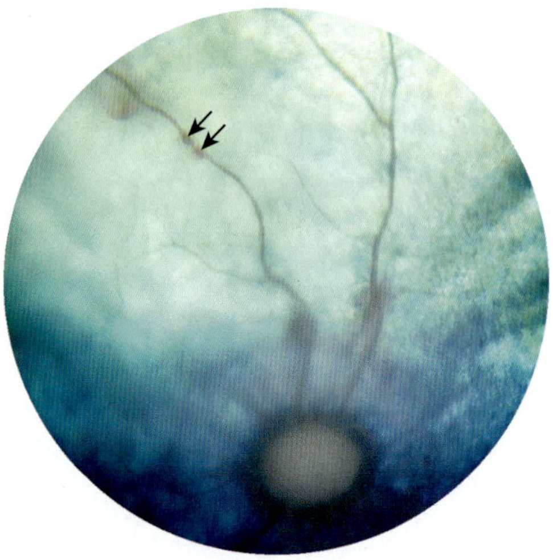

Figure 11-277
Hypertensive cat with aneurysms *(arrows)*, small petechiae, retinal degeneration, and optic atrophy.

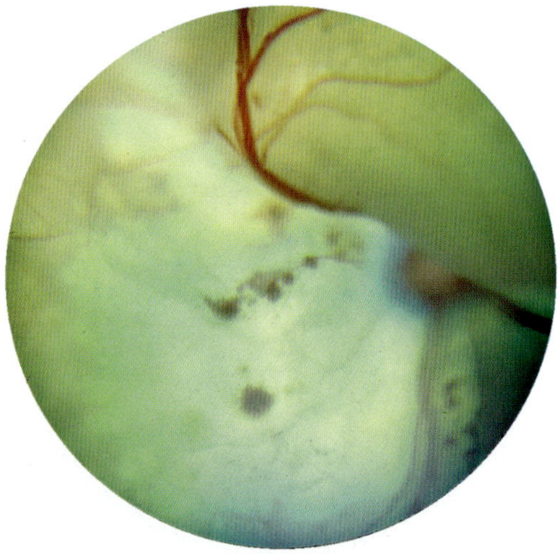

Figure 11-278
Hypertensive cat with bullous retinal detachment and retinal hemorrhage.

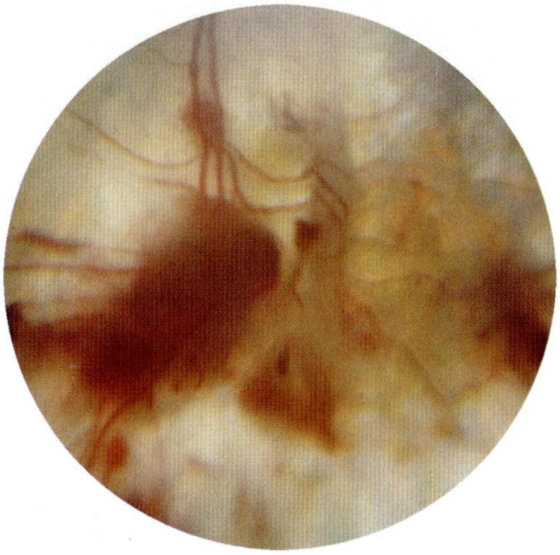

Figure 11-279
Hypertension in a cat. Total retinal detachment and retinal and preretinal hemorrhage are present.

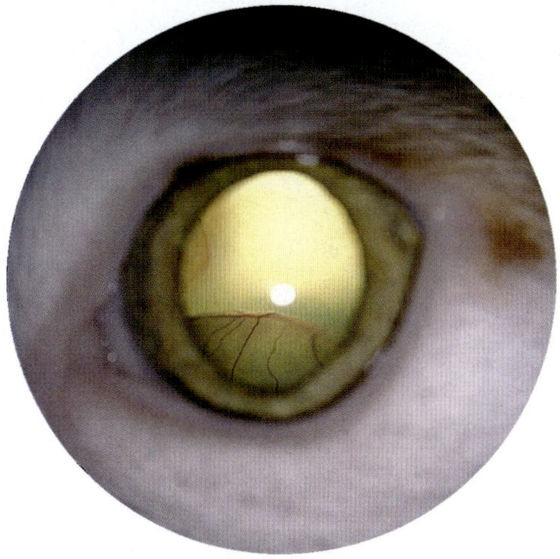

Figure 11-280
External photograph of hypertensive cat with retinal detachment. Retinal blood vessels usually cannot be seen clearly without an ophthalmoscope.

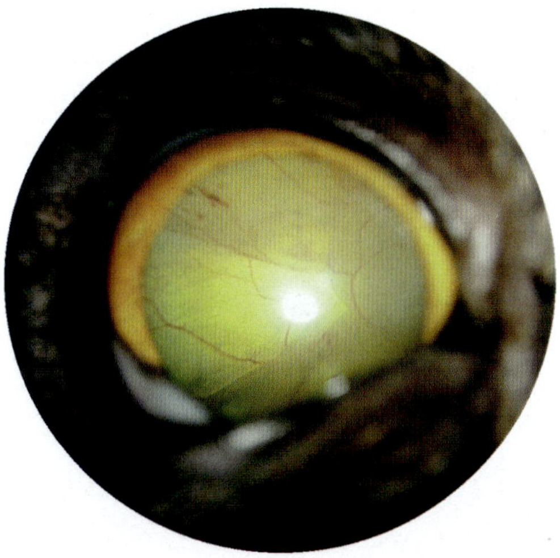

Figure 11-281
External photograph of hypertensive cat with retinal detachment and retinal hemorrhage.

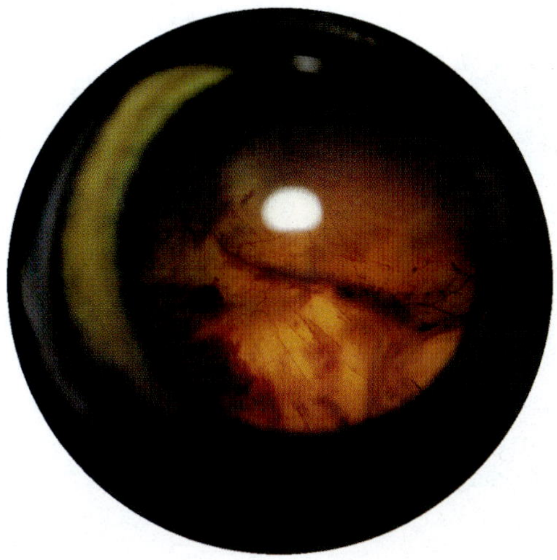

Figure 11-282
External photograph of hypertensive cat with bullous retinal detachment and retinal hemorrhage.

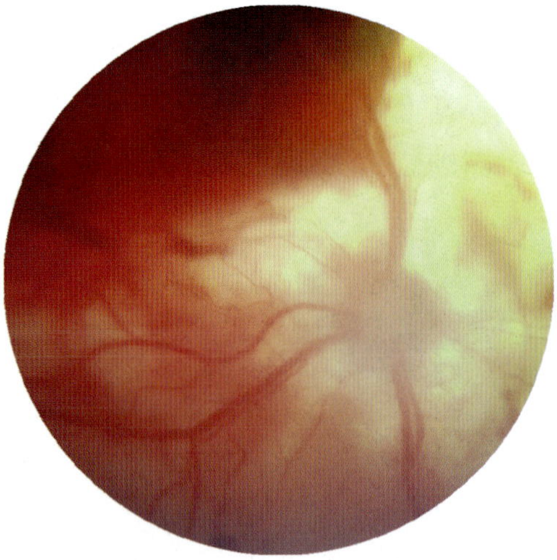

Figure 11-283
Cat with hypertension. Retinal detachment and hemorrhage are present.

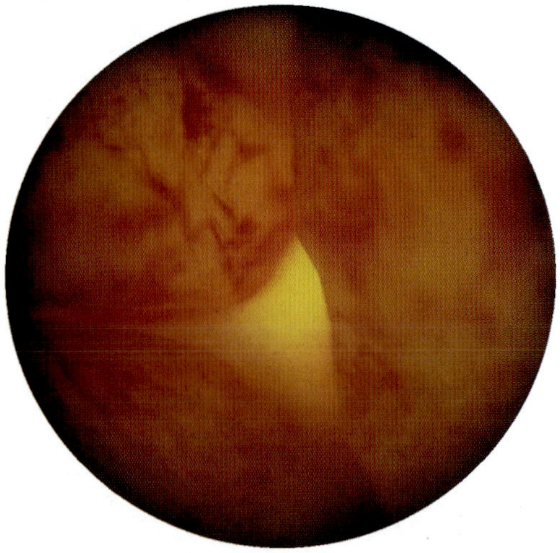

Figure 11-284
Hypertensive cat with total bullous detachment and retinal hemorrhage.

INACTIVE CHORIORETINITIS

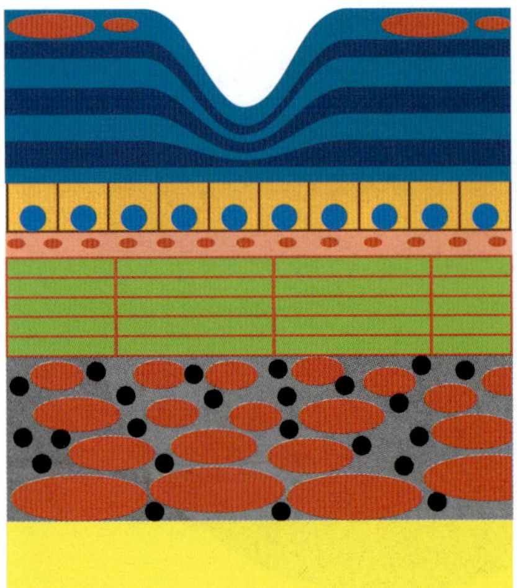

Figure 11-285
Retinal degeneration and atrophy. This figure shows a focal lesion with localized thinning of the retina. The normal retina absorbs some light, but when its thickness is reduced less light is absorbed, and in the tapetal fundus more light entering the eye from an ophthalmoscope is reflected back to the observer. This results in the characteristic tapetal hyperreflectivity visible when a retinal degeneration in the tapetal fundus is viewed.

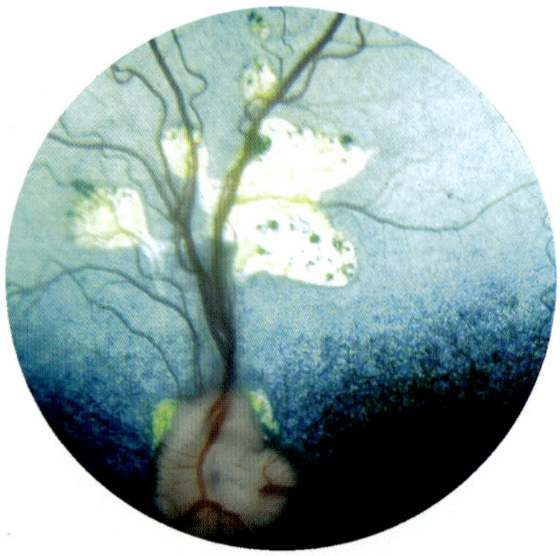

Figure 11-286
Multifocal hyperreflective areas above the disc in a dog recovering from inflammatory disease.

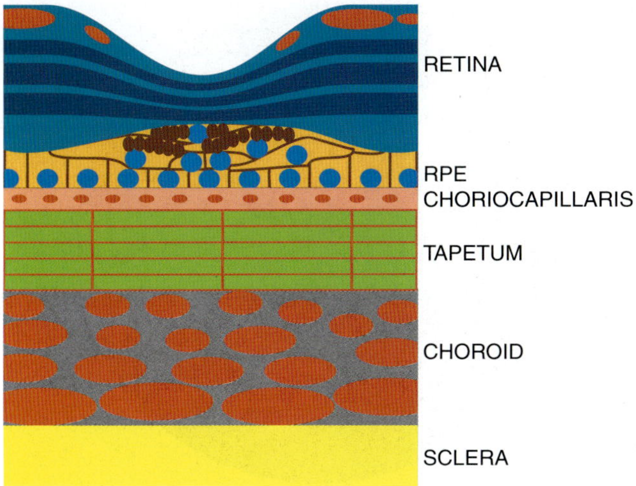

Figure 11-287
Retinal atrophy. In the nontapetal fundus the RPE reacts to degeneration of the overlying retina by undergoing depigmentation, migration, and hyperplasia and hypertrophy of cells, with focal areas becoming more pigmented than the surroundings. Similar pigmentary changes are visible in the tapetal and nontapetal fundus.

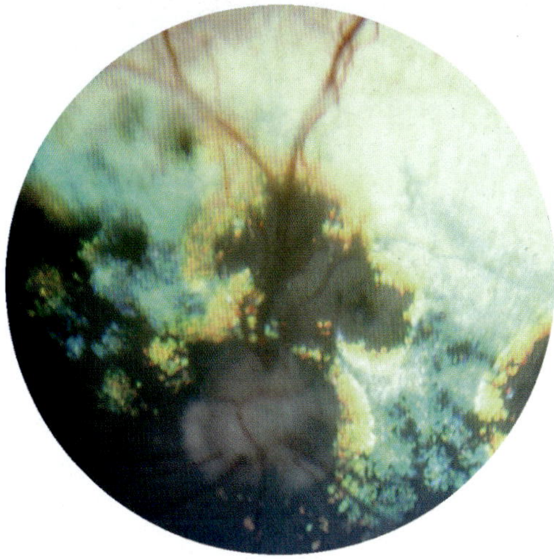

Figure 11-288
Massive chorioretinal scarring (hyperpigmented areas surrounded by hyperreflective areas in the tapetum) and optic atrophy (disc is gray and demyelinated) in a dog recovered from ehrlichiosis.

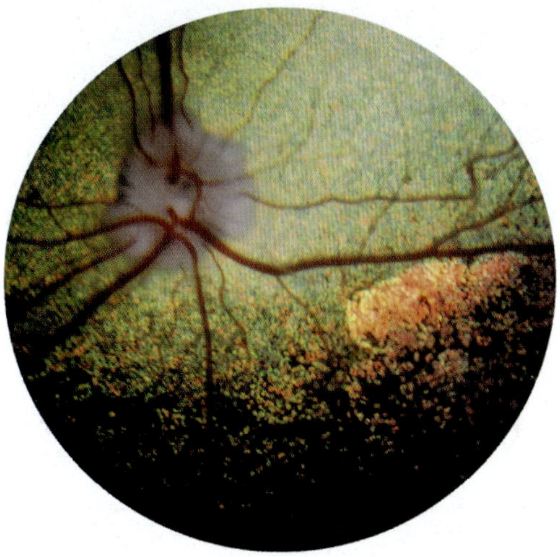

Figure 11-289
Focal chorioretinal scar of unknown cause in a dog.

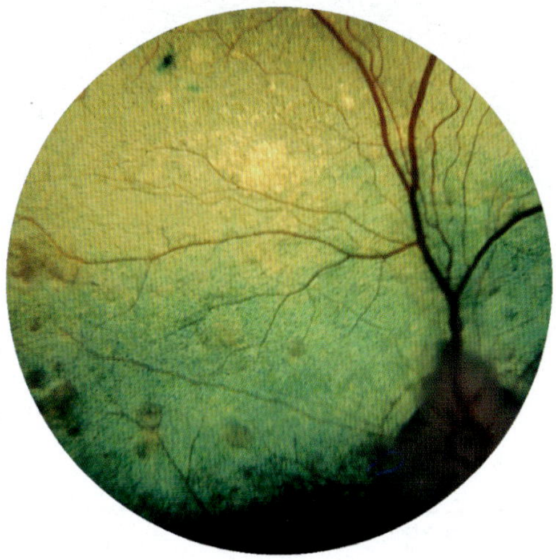

Figure 11-290
Multifocal chorioretinal scars in the tapetum secondary to distemper virus in a dog.

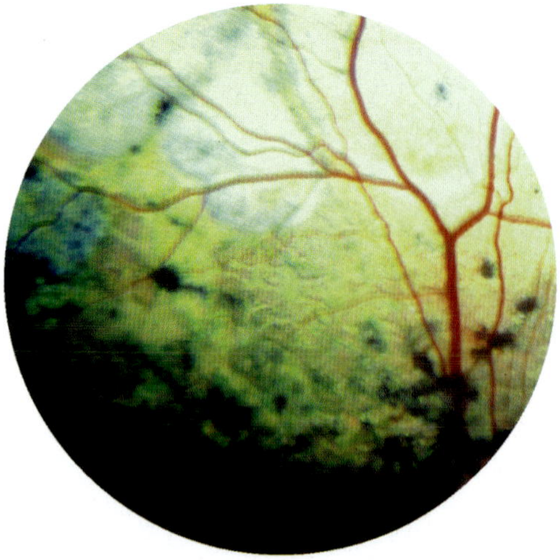

Figure 11-291
Ophthalmomyiasis in a dog, with focal areas of tapetum hyperreflectivity, color change, and secondary pigmentation.

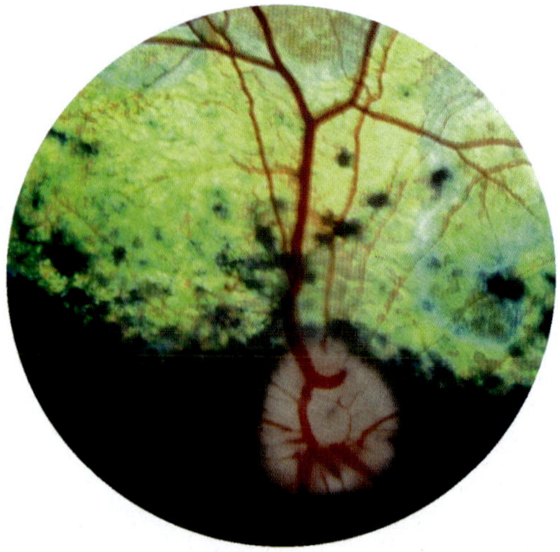

Figure 11-292
Ophthalmomyiasis in the tapetum of the same dog as shown in Figure 11-291. Note the hyper-reflective tracks and pigment spots.

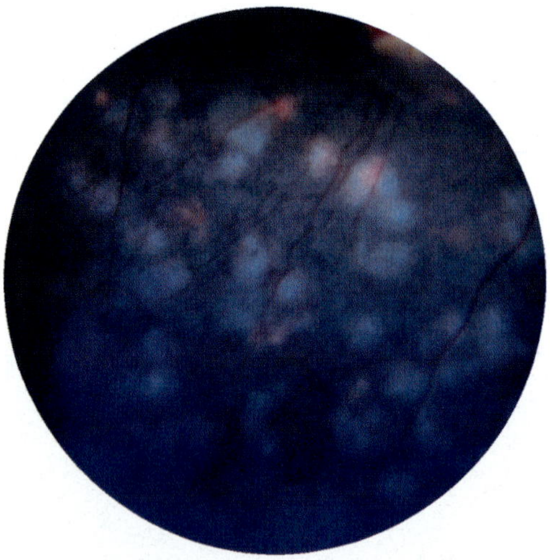

Figure 11-293
Chronic chorioretinitis in a dachshund, with multifocal gray-white areas (retinal edema and exudate) in the nontapetum. Choroidal vessels are visible in some areas in which inflammation has been succeeded by focal retinal atrophy.

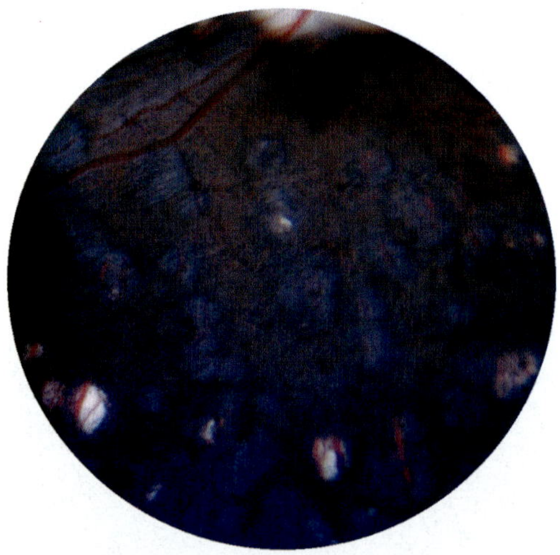

Figure 11-294
Depigmented lesions in the nontapetum of the same dog as in Figure 11-293.

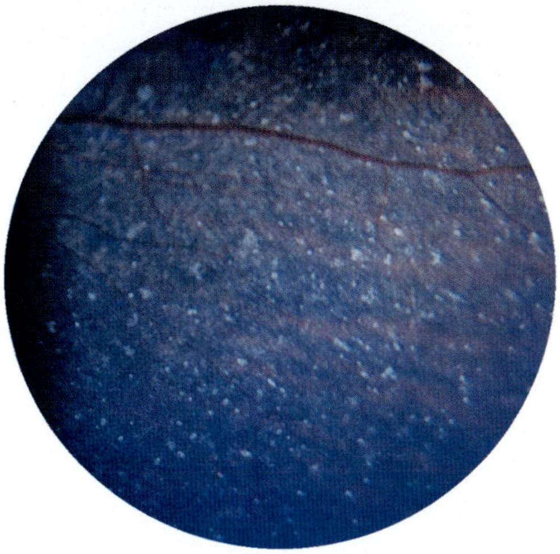

Figure 11-295
Multifocal white opacities in the nontapetum of a dog. The dog had active chorioretinitis and retinal detachment, which resolved with corticosteroid treatment. Normal choroidal vasculature (pink horizontal streaks) can just be seen through the pigment epithelium.

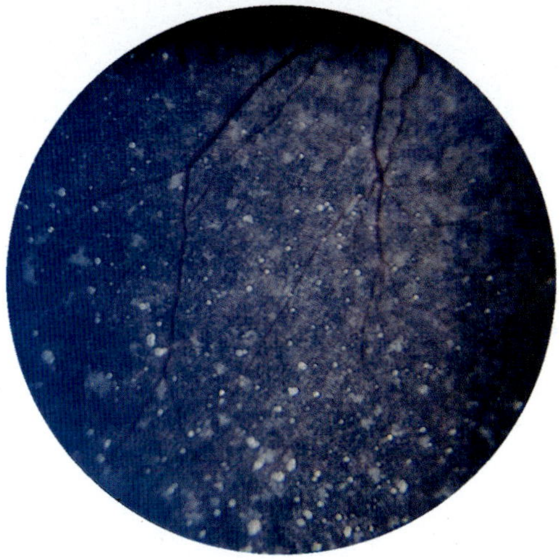

Figure 11-296
Multifocal white opacities in the nontapetum of an American cocker spaniel. The dog had active chorioretinitis and retinal detachment, which resolved with corticosteroid treatment.

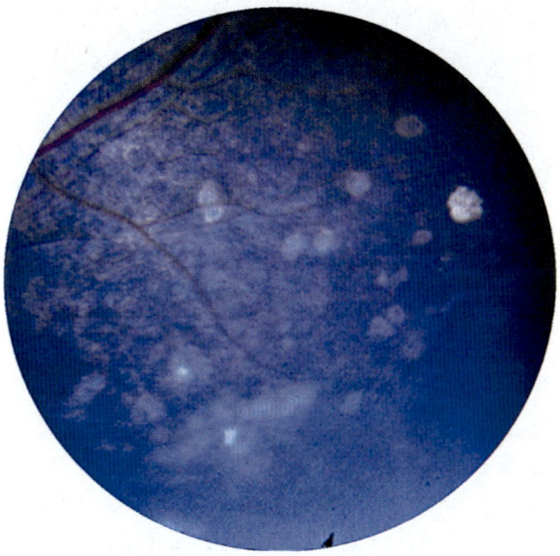

Figure 11-297
Multifocal pigmentary abnormalties and hard exudates in canine eye with resolving chorioretinitis.

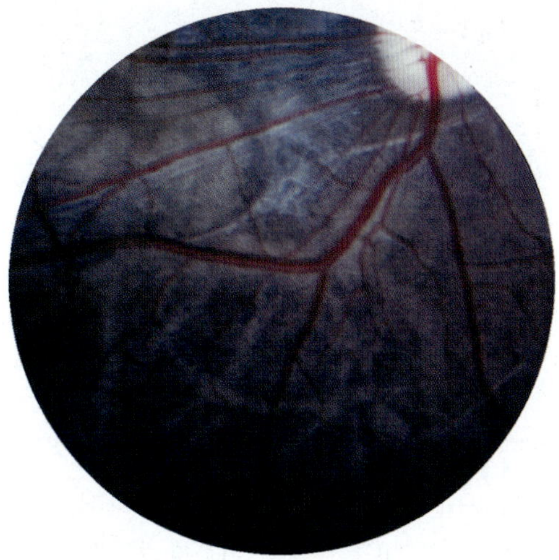

Figure 11-298
Internal ophthalmomyiasis in a dog. Note the pale tracks in the nontapetum and scarring below the optic disc.

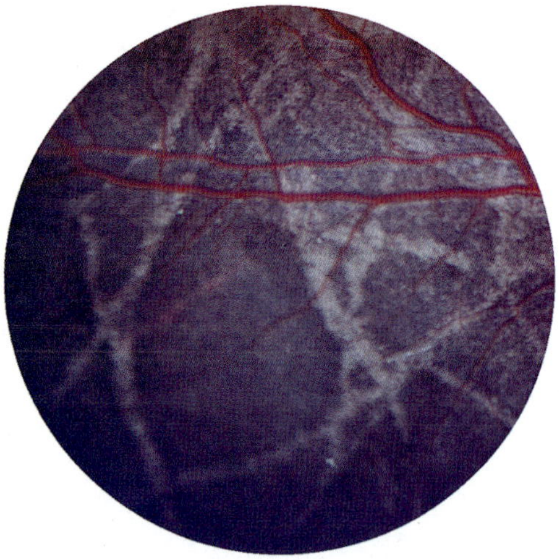

Figure 11-299
Internal ophthalmomyiasis in the same dog as in Figure 11-298. This is a more peripheral view. Note the pale tracks in the nontapetum.

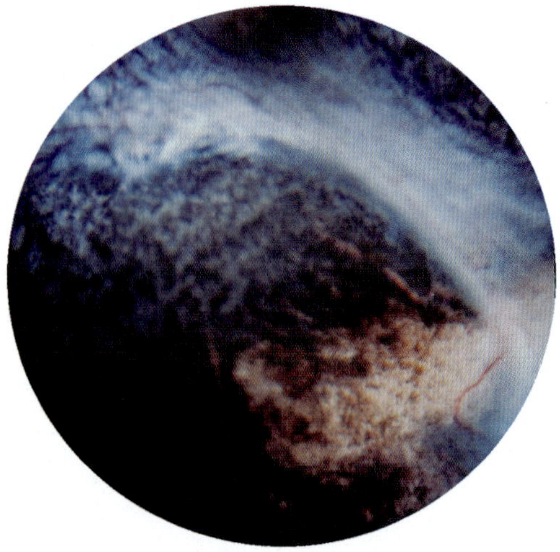

Figure 11-300
Vitreal fibrosis and retinal scarring in a dog.

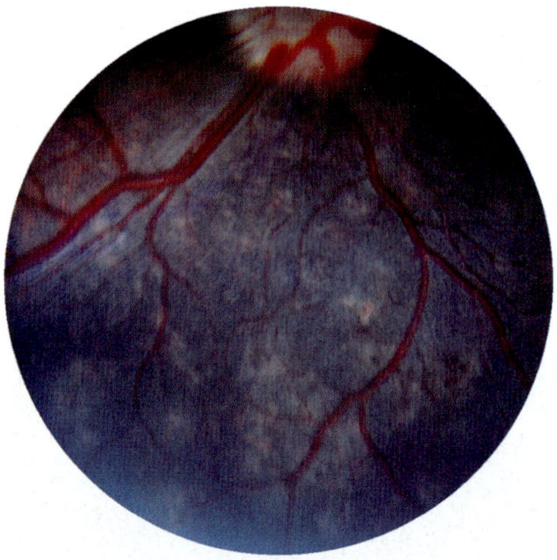

Figure 11-301
Multifocal chorioretinal scars in the nontapetum, visible as depigmented areas resulting from distemper virus infection in a poodle.

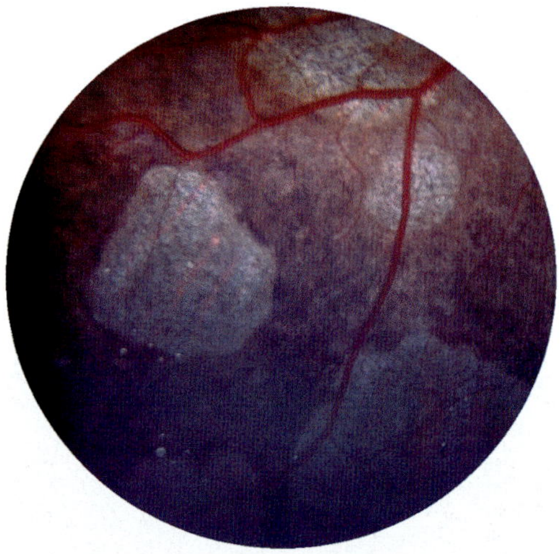

Figure 11-302
Multifocal retinal degeneration secondary to chorioretinitis that had been controlled with corticosteroids. Large areas of RPE depigmentation are present.

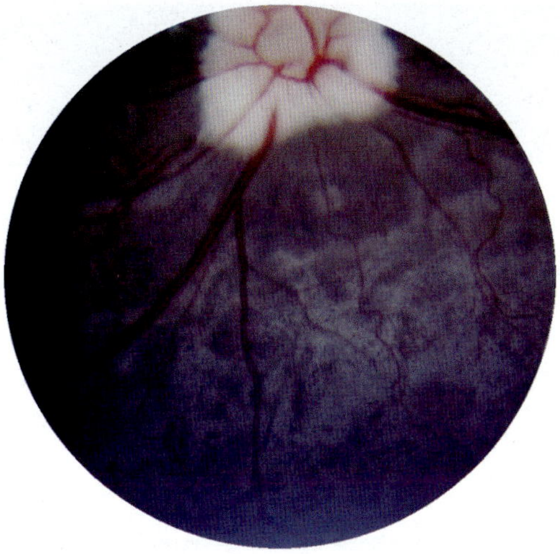

Figure 11-303
Depigmentation (degeneration) in the nontapetal retina of a dog with a pituitary tumor. A recordable electroretinogram was present in this eye.

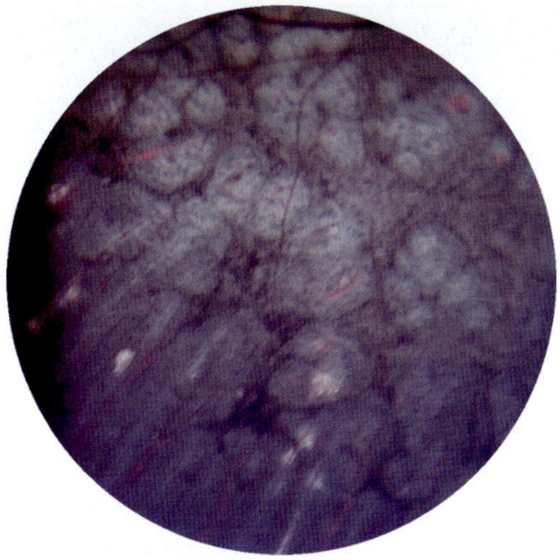

Figure 11-304
Chronic chorioretinitis of unknown cause in the nontapetum of a dachshund. The condition was responsive to corticosteroids. This is the same dog as in Figures 11-293 and 11-294, but later in the disease process. Depigmentation focally reveals choroidal vessels, underlying sclera, and hyperpigmentation.

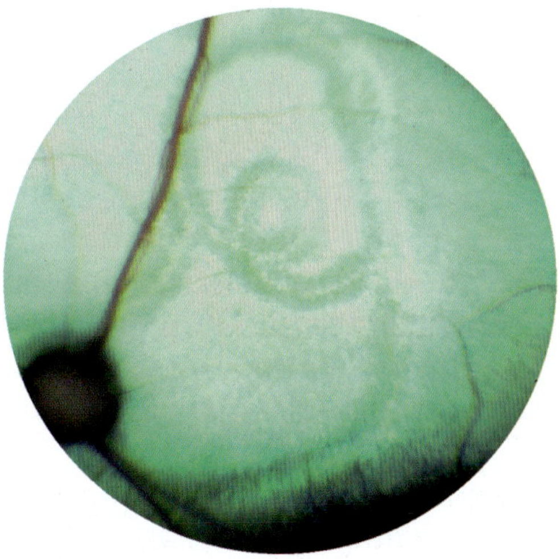

Figure 11-305
Cat with ophthalmomyiasis, with inactive lesions from previous migrating parasite.
(Courtesy Dr. E. Dan Wolf.)

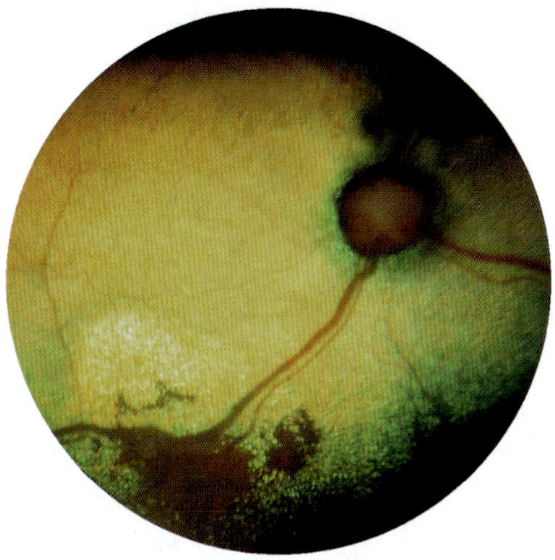

Figure 11-306
Cat with multifocal hyperreflective and hyperpigmented chorioretinal scars secondary to treated histoplasmosis.

Chapter 12

Optic Nerve

INTRODUCTION

The optic nerve enters the eye through the lamina cribrosa of the sclera. In cats the normal optic nerve loses its myelination as it enters the eye. In dogs the nerve retains some degree of myelination as it passes through the sclera and loses the myelin as it radiates into the nerve fiber layer of the retina. The shape of the optic nerve in cats is normally fairly circular, whereas in dogs the extent of myelination determines the shape—which may be quite irregular, especially in some breeds.

Lesions of the nerve may be developmental or acquired. The most common developmental conditions are optic nerve hypoplasia (aplasia is rare), in which the nerve leaving the eye has reduced or absent nerve fibers and retinal ganglion cells (resulting most often in blindness), and coloboma, in which a defect of fusion of the developing optic cup results in a deep fissure or hole in the nerve head (which may be abnormally large) and occasionally adjacent sclera, choroid, and retina. The extent of visual impairment depends on the size of the defect. Colobomas are most frequently seen in dogs with collie eye anomaly.

Acquired lesions of the optic nerve include papilledema or optic disc edema, optic neuritis, and optic atrophy. These conditions can be divided by clinical appearance into those in which the disc appears swollen (papilledema, disc edema, and neuritis) and optic atrophy, in which the disc loses its myelination and vascularity and develops a dark gray color. The various entities in which the disc is swollen may be difficult to differentiate clinically.

Optic disc edema is swelling of the optic nerve head and may be associated with conditions such as acute glaucoma, uveitis, and very low intraocular pressure after surgery or optic nerve tumors. The disc appears fluffier and raised, with indistinct edges and with edema that radiates into the peripapillary retina. Vision may or may not be affected, depending on the cause.

Papilledema implies bilateral edema of the optic nerve head seen in the funduscopic view. It develops from stasis of axoplasmic flow, often resulting from elevated cerebrospinal fluid pressure associated with central nervous system (CNS) tumors. The eyes retain sight unless central blindness occurs because of the lesion in the brain.

Optic neuritis is inflammation of the optic nerve that may be associated with infectious diseases (e.g., distemper or cryptococcosis) or may be idiopathic and presumedly an autoimmune disease. The optic nerve head and disc appear edematous and raised with irregular indistinct borders and edema that radiates into the retina. Hemorrhage may be present in the nerve and peripapillary retina or preretinal vitreous, and vitreal exudate may partially obscure the nerve. Optic neuritis results in loss of vision in the affected eye.

Optic atrophy most commonly develops secondarily to optic neuritis, glaucoma, and retinal degenerations.

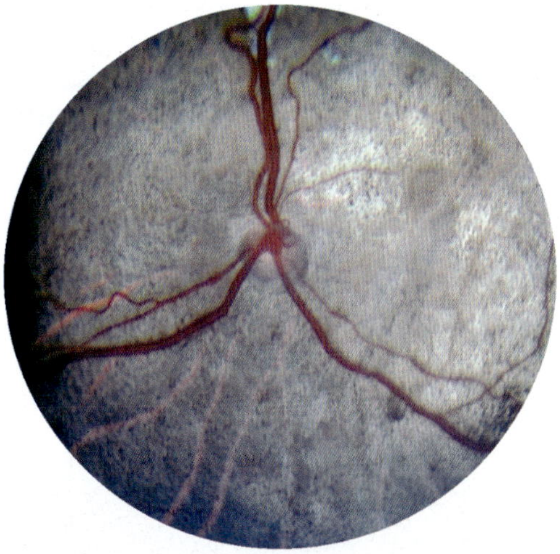

Figure 12-1
Optic nerve hypoplasia in a Samoyed. The retina is severely degenerate. This extent of degeneration is not necessarily seen in association with optic nerve hypoplasia.

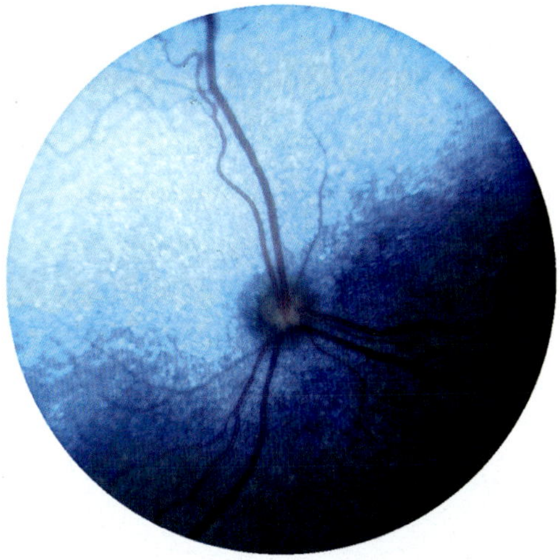

Figure 12-2
Optic nerve hypoplasia in a Labrador retriever cross-breed.

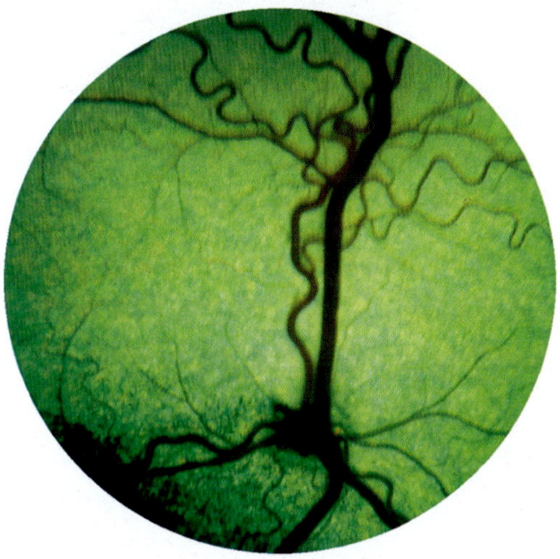

Figure 12-3
Optic nerve hypoplasia in a Russian wolfhound. (Courtesy Dr. Robert Playter.)

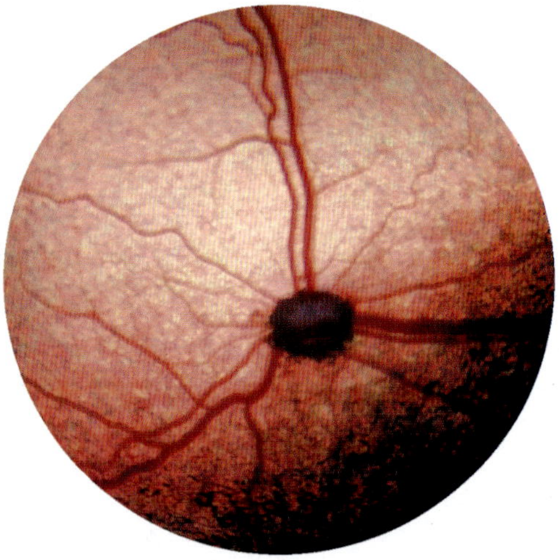

Figure 12-4
Optic nerve hypoplasia in a poodle.

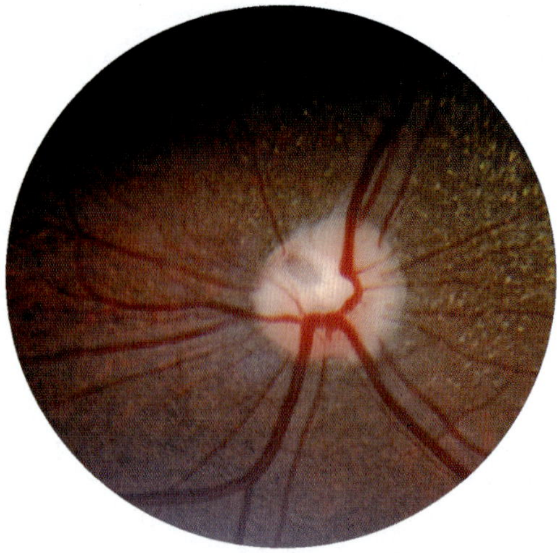

Figure 12-5
A focal coloboma at the 10 o'clock position in the optic nerve of an Australian shepherd.

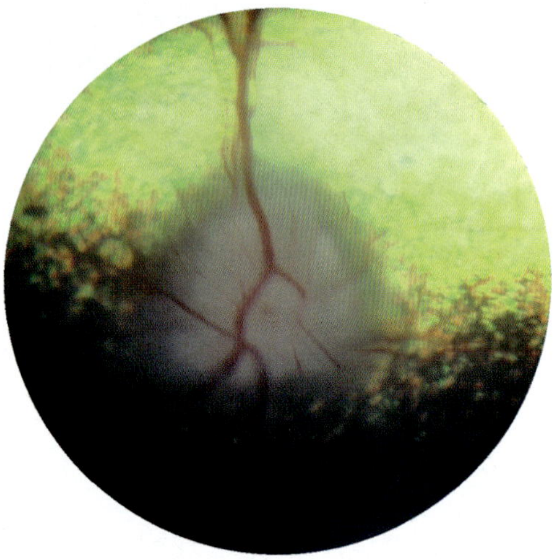

Figure 12-6
Papilledema secondary to CNS neoplasia that is affecting the cerebral cortex. Edema of the optic nerve can occur in association with mass lesions of the orbit or optic nerve (pressure on or in the nerve) or because of elevations in cerebrospinal fluid pressure associated with brain tumors.

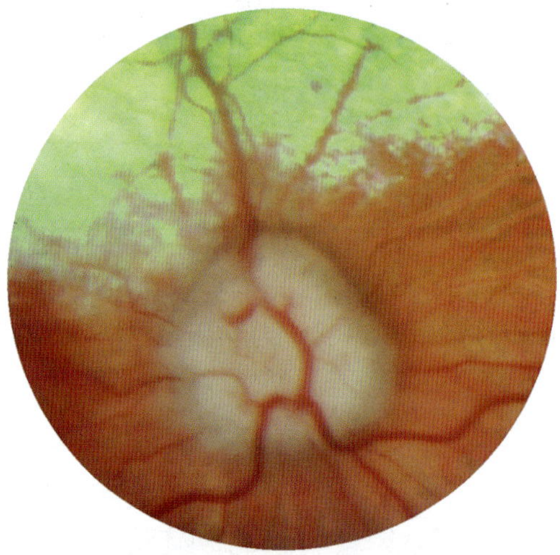

Figure 12-7
Papilledema in a poodle with a frontal lobe tumor.

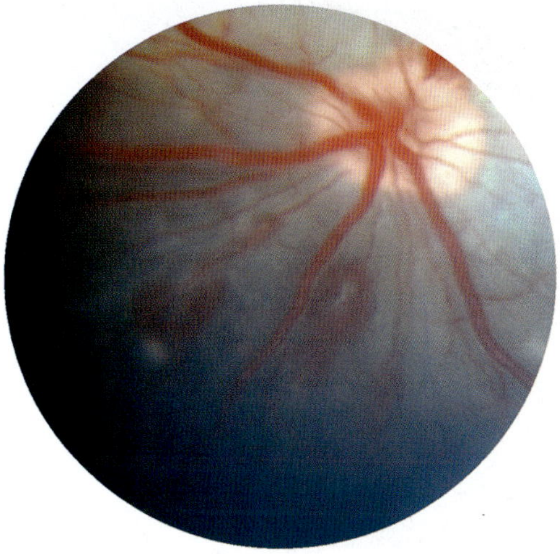

Figure 12-8
Papilledema, optic nerve, and retinal hemorrhages secondary to ehrlichiosis and coccidioidomycosis.

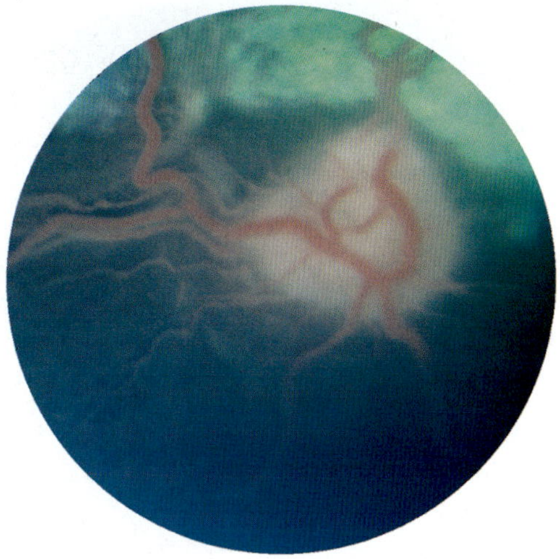

Figure 12-9
Lipemia retinalis and papilledema in a mixed-breed dog with a retrobulbar meningioma.

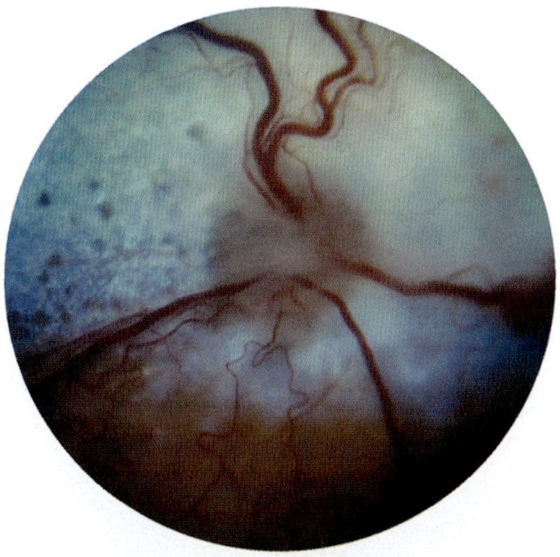

Figure 12-10
Doberman with granulomatous meningoencephalomyelitis (GME), with optic neuritis, chorioretinitis, and retinal hemorrhage.

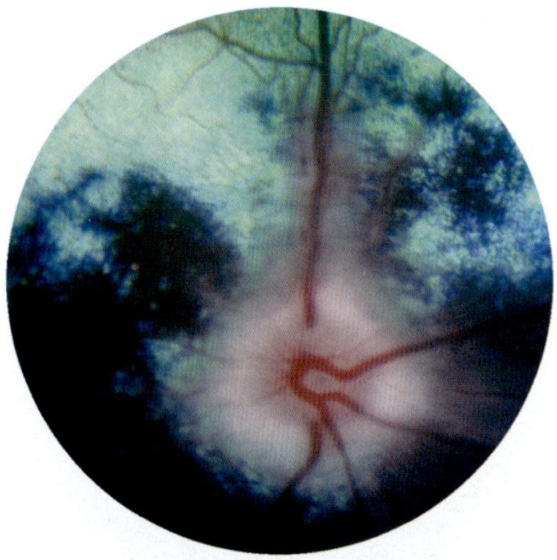

Figure 12-11
Optic neuritis with peripapillary edema and retinal hyperpigmentation in a cocker spaniel.

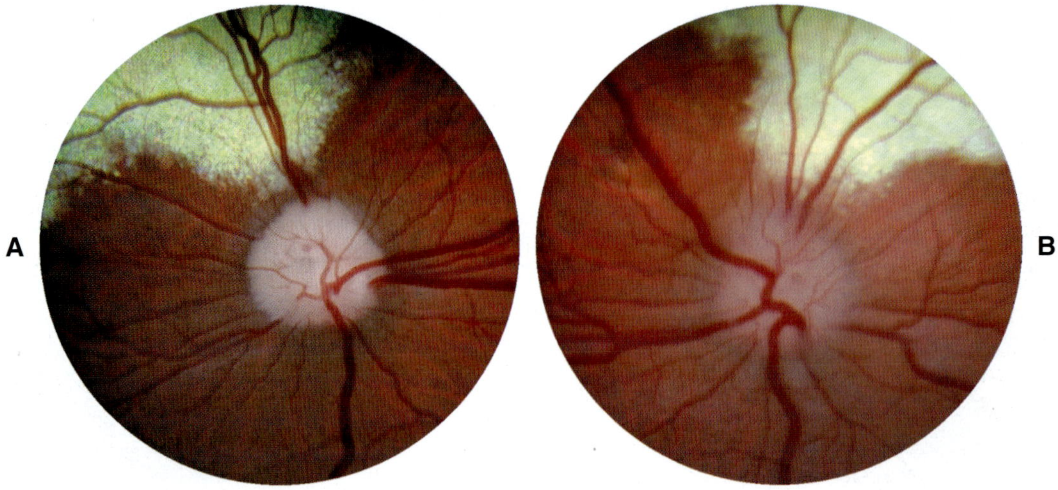

Figure 12-12 A-B
A, Normal optic nerve in the right eye in a Chihuahua with retrobulbar optic neuritis. **B,** Optic neuritis in the left eye of the same dog with retrobulbar optic neuritis. Note the pinker color (vascular hyperemia) and the indistinct margin of the nerve compared with the normal right eye.

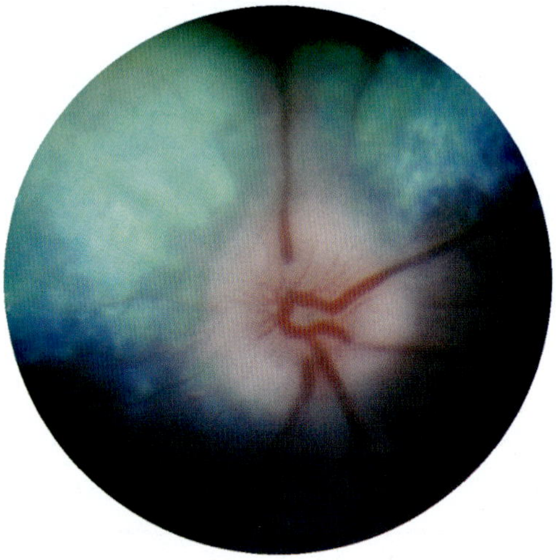

Figure 12-13
Optic neuritis with chorioretinitis and retinal detachment.

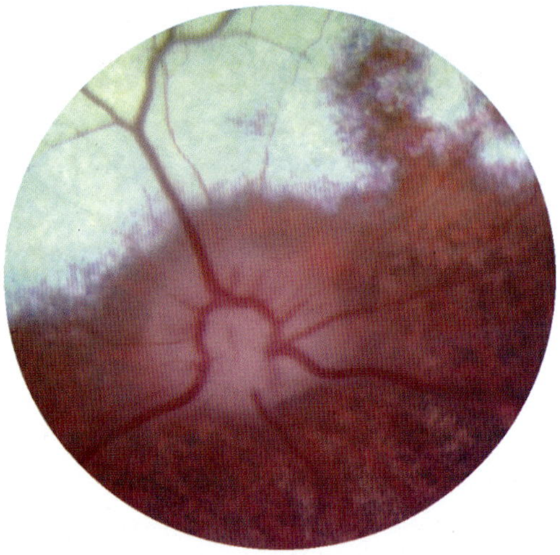

Figure 12-14
Optic neuritis, peripapillary edema.

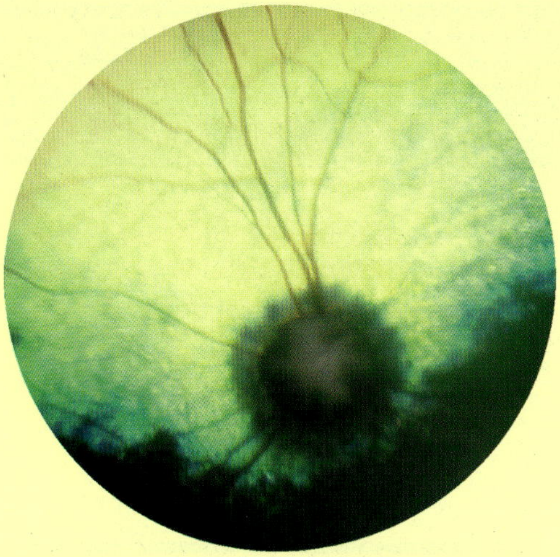

Figure 12-15
Optic atrophy and retinal atrophy after proptosis in a Lhasa apso.

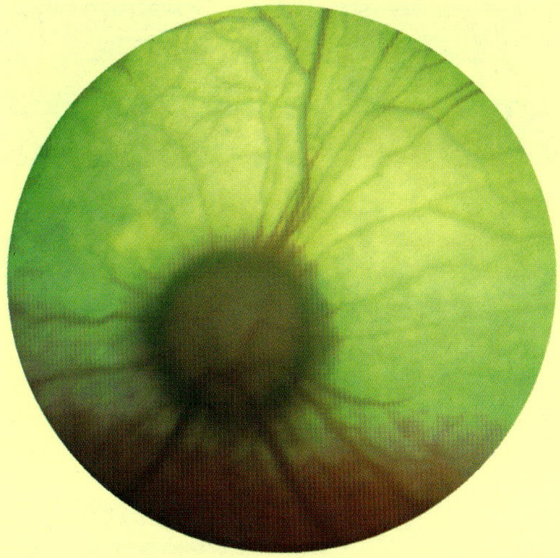

Figure 12-16
Advanced optic nerve cupping and atrophy in a basset hound with chronic glaucoma.

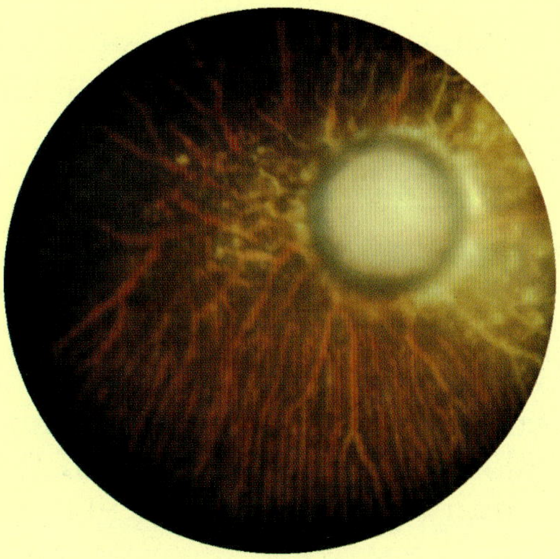

Figure 12-17
Retinal and optic nerve atrophy secondary to glaucoma and Vogt-Koyanagi-Harada–like syndrome in a golden retriever.

Chapter 13

Orbit

INTRODUCTION

The conditions involving the eye and orbit essentially can be divided into those in which the eye itself is abnormally sized (e.g., microphthalmos, phthisis bulbi, glaucoma) and those in which the position of the eye in the orbit is abnormal because of either an increase or decrease in other orbital contents or a traumatic displacement of the eye from the orbit (proptosis). Microphthalmos is a developmental condition often associated with other congenital ocular lesions that may be inherited or may result from some physical or inflammatory insult to the developing eye. The globe looks smaller and more recessed into the orbit. Phthisis bulbi is a shrinking of the globe resulting from reduced aqueous humor production secondary to chronic inflammation or glaucoma.

Enophthalmos is recession of the normally sized eye within the orbit. The condition may result from loss of other ocular contents (fat) or from scarring caused by inflammation. Enophthalmos is also seen as a component of Horner's syndrome, because of sympathetic denervation of the circumferentially arranged muscle fibers in the orbital cone that help maintain the normal position of the globe.

Exophthalmos is a protrusion of the globe resulting from the presence of a space-occupying lesion in the orbit (inflammation or infection, neoplasia, zygomatic salivary gland enlargement, vascular malformation, or myositis).

Proptosis is usually traumatic and results in forward displacement of the globe from the orbit. The proptosed globe may undergo varying degrees of injury—most notably, avulsion of extraocular muscles or the optic nerve.

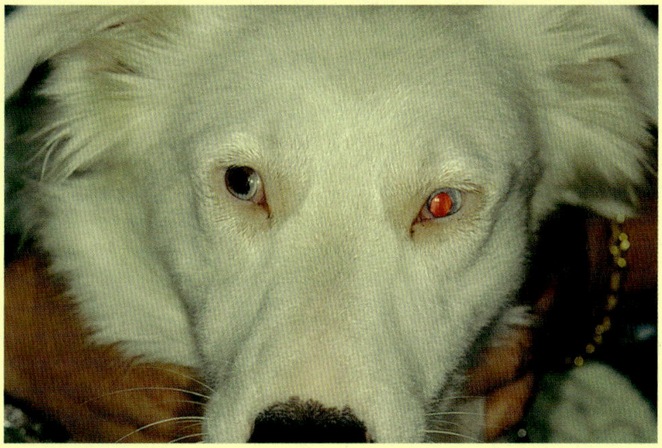

Figure 13-1
Microphthalmia in a blind and deaf Australian shepherd.

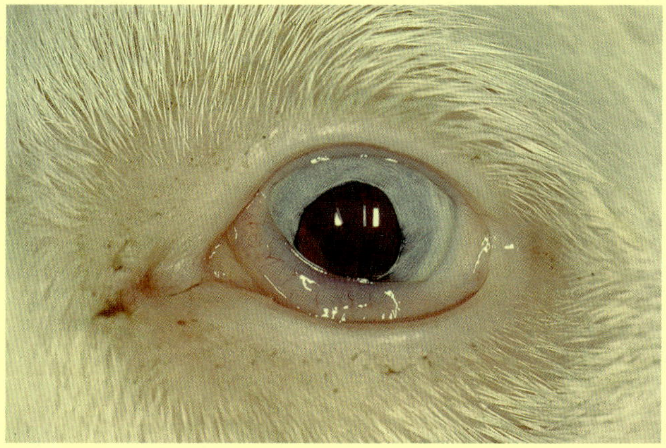

Figure 13-2
Coloboma of the iris associated with hereditary multiple ocular anomalies in an Australian shepherd.

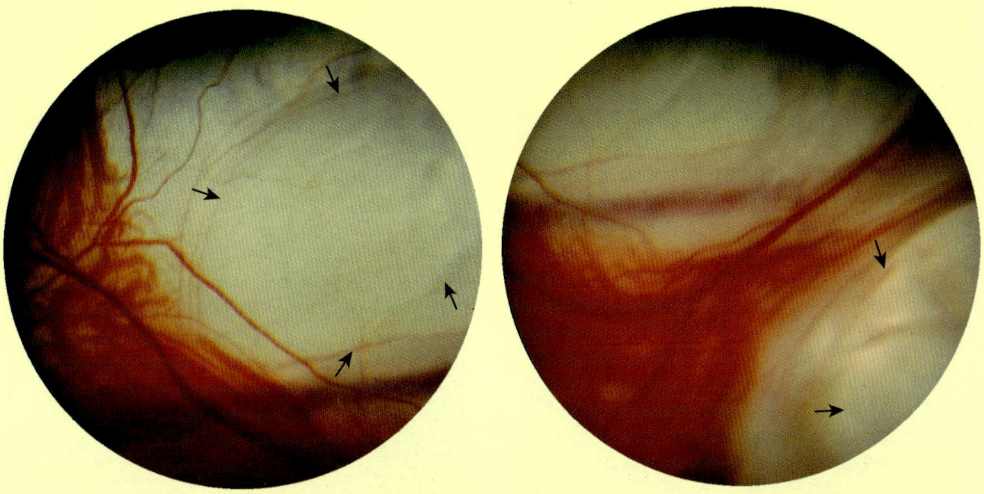

Figure 13-3
Two views of the same eye of the dog shown in Figure 13-2. This Australian shepherd has hereditary multiple ocular anomalies. A large staphyloma *(arrows)* is present in the peripheral fundus, with choroidal dysplasia (choroidal vessels not formed). The purple streak is the long posterior ciliary artery.

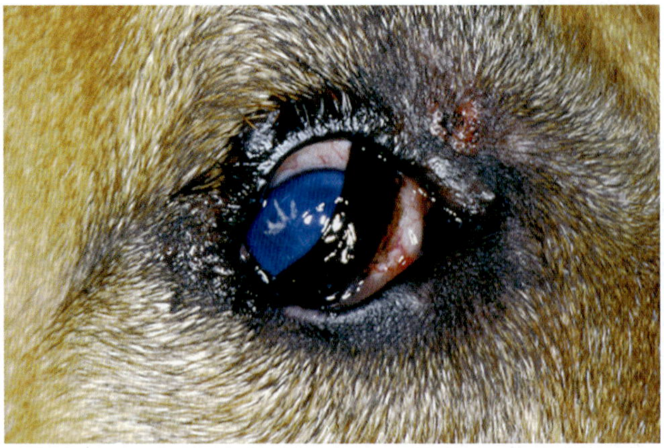

Figure 13-4
A German shepherd dog with phthisis bulbi, apparent enophthalmos, and corneal edema secondary to traumatic uveitis.

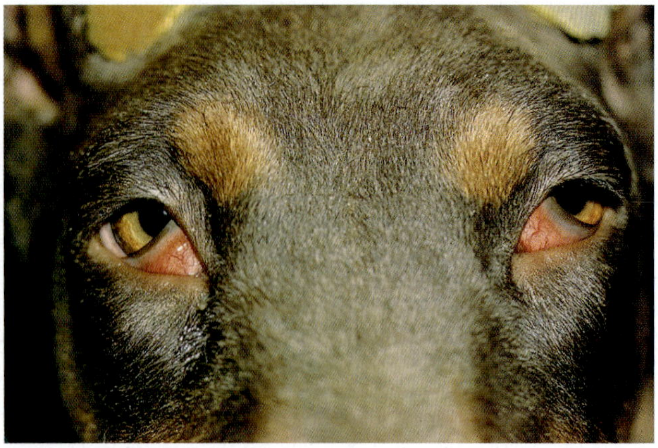

Figure 13-5
Enophthalmos in both eyes resulting from emaciation.

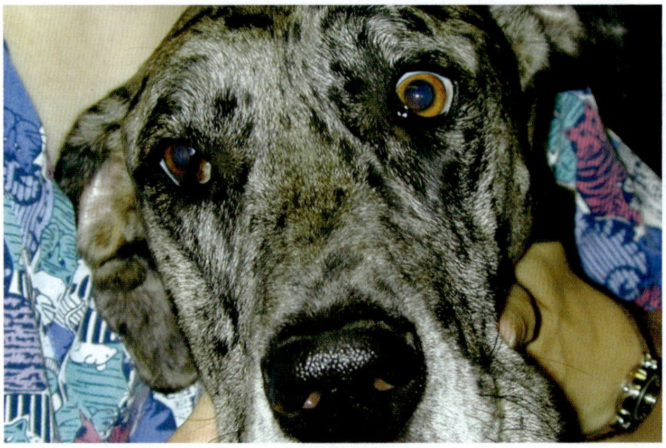

Figure 13-6
Enophthalmos of the right eye in a Great Dane.

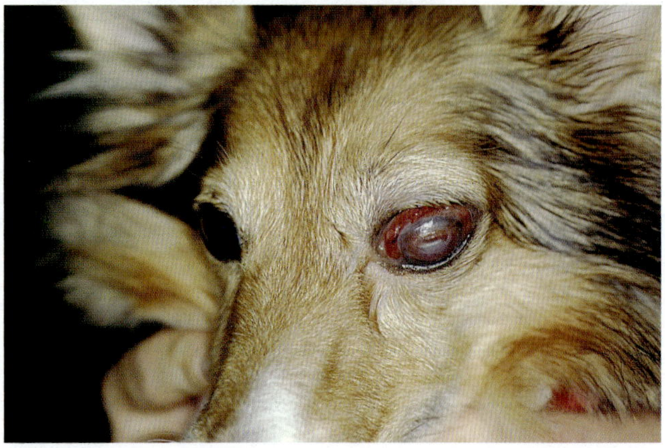

Figure 13-7
Dog with multiple myeloma. Exophthalmos of the left eye causing exposure keratitis, "red eye," and chemosis.

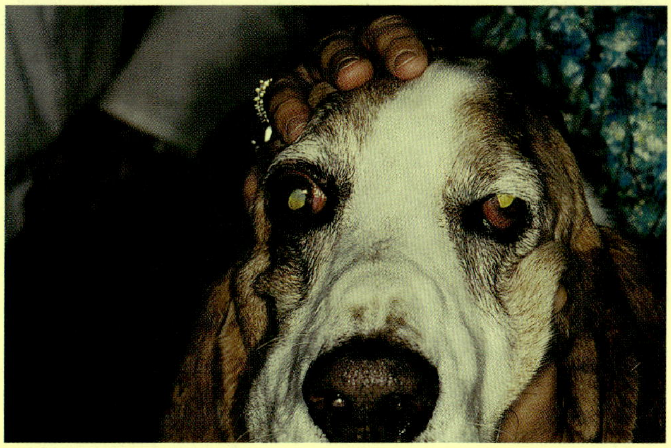

Figure 13-8
Exophthalmos in the right eye in a bassett hound.

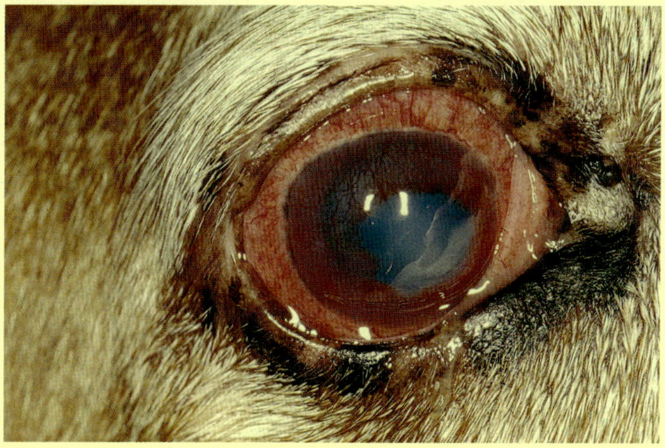

Figure 13-9
"Red eye"—corneal neovascularization and edema in an exophthalmic globe.

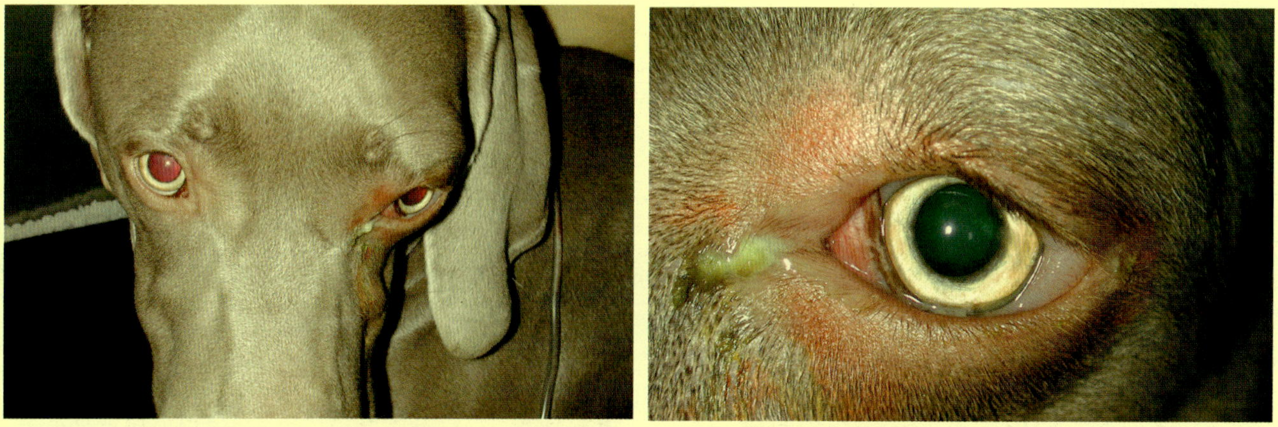

A

B

Figure 13-10 A-B
A, Weimaraner with exophthalmos of the left eye resulting from zygomatic sialocele. **B,** Close-up of left eye showing nictitans protrusion and chemosis.

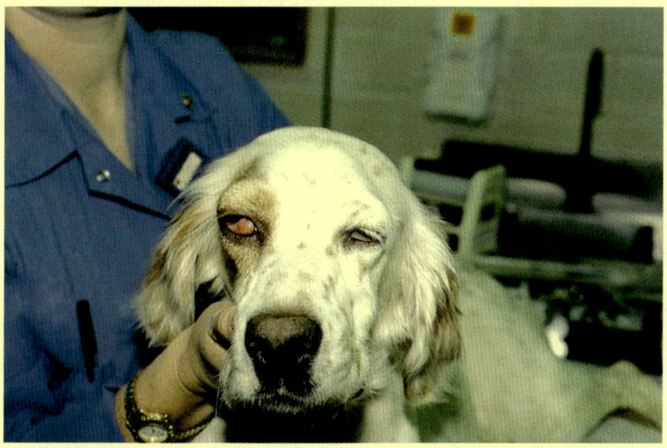

Figure 13-11
Exophthalmos of the left eye with protrusion of nictitans resulting from orbital squamous cell carcinoma.

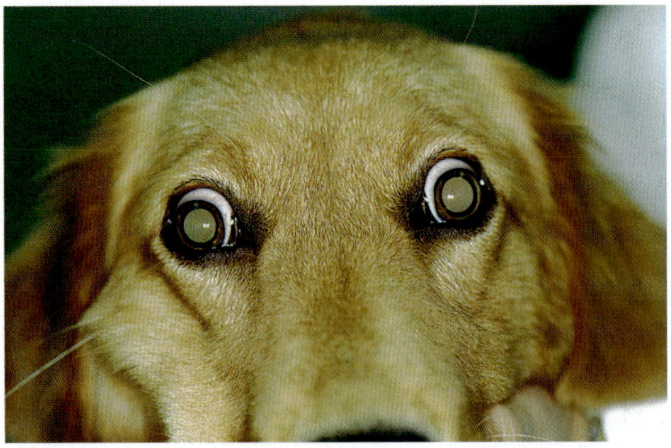

Figure 13-12
Exophthalmos in both eyes in a young golden retriever with extraocular myositis.

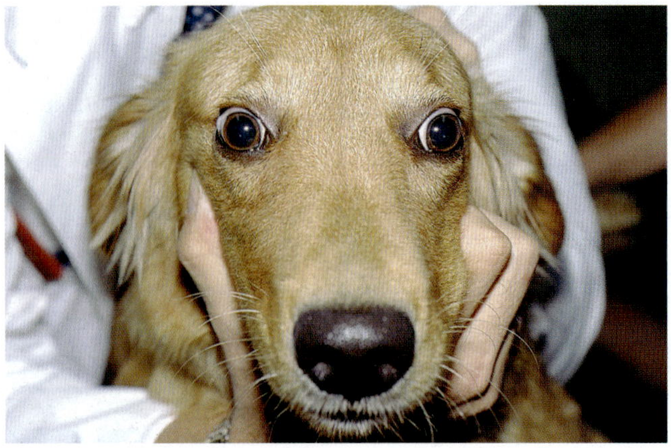

Figure 13-13
Exophthalmos in both eyes in a young golden retriever with extraocular myositis.

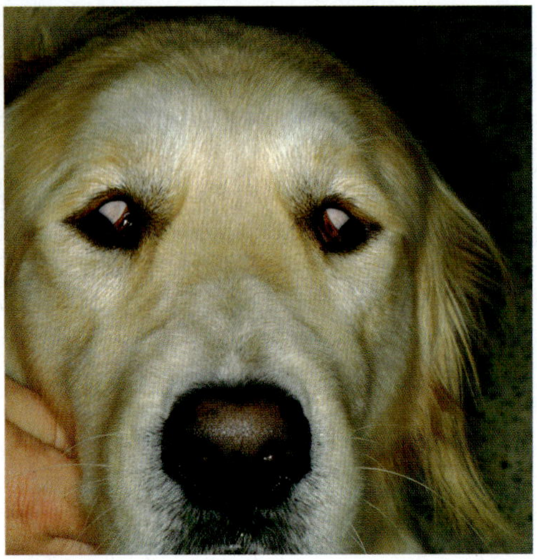

Figure 13-14
Muscle fibrosis secondary to retrobulbar extraocular myositis in a young golden retriever. Note the ventrolateral exotropia.

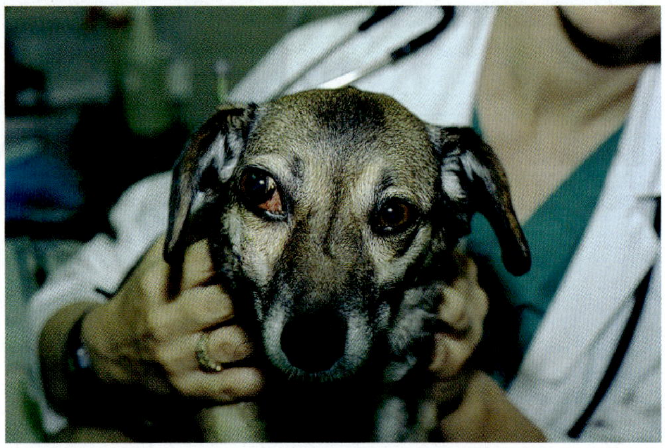

Figure 13-15
Exophthalmos of the right eye resulting from retrobulbar fibrosarcoma. Note the prolapsed nictitans.
(Courtesy Dr. Nancy Bromberg.)

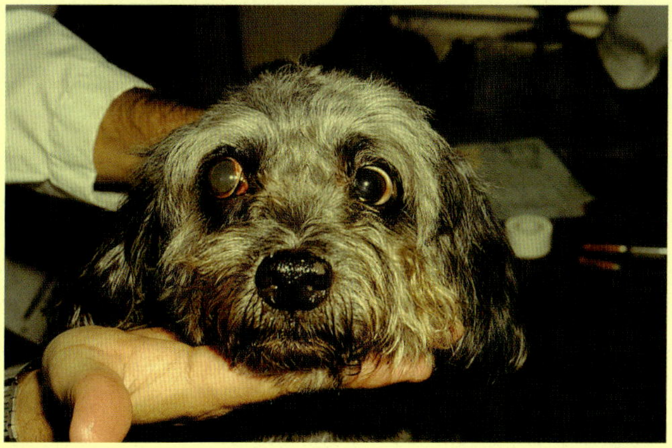

Figure 13-16
Exophthalmos of the right eye, lateral globe deviation, and mydriasis resulting from optic nerve meningioma.

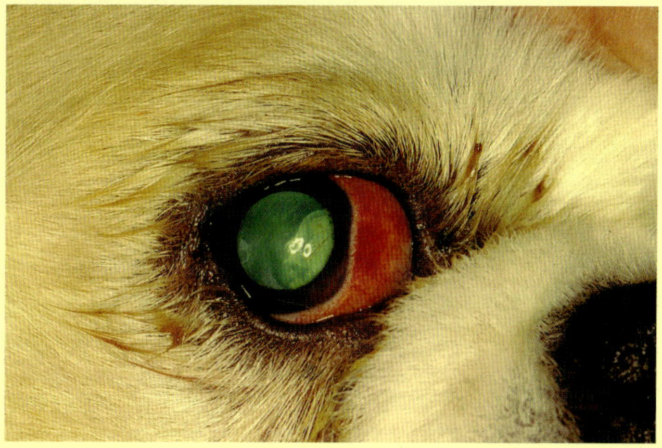

Figure 13-17
Traumatic proptosis (corrected) resulted in subconjunctival hemorrhage, lateral strabismus, and torn medial rectus muscle.

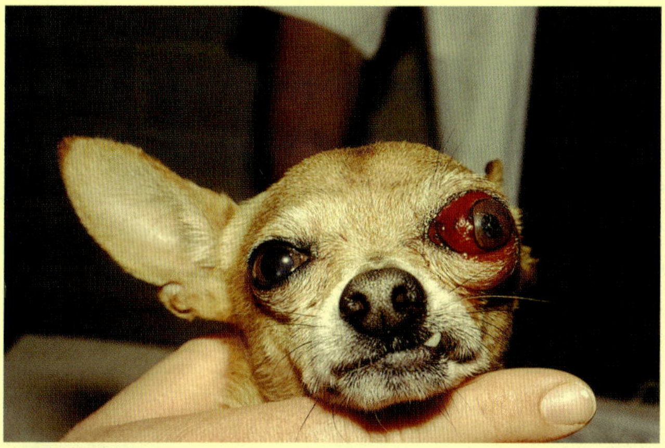

Figure 13-18
Traumatic proptosis with torn medial rectus muscle and subconjunctival hemorrhage.

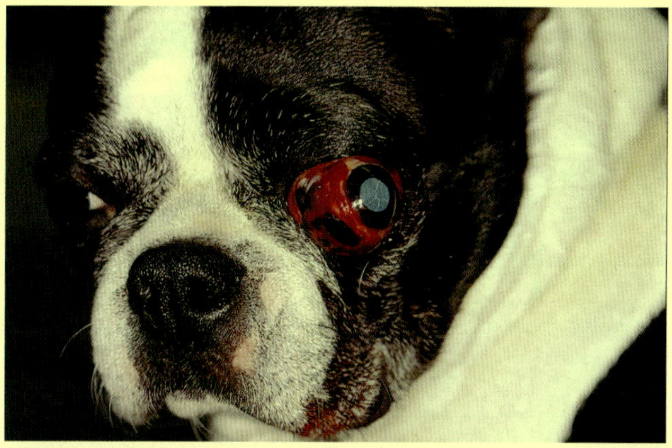

Figure 13-19
Proptosed globe in a Boston terrier, with avulsion of at least the medial rectus muscle.

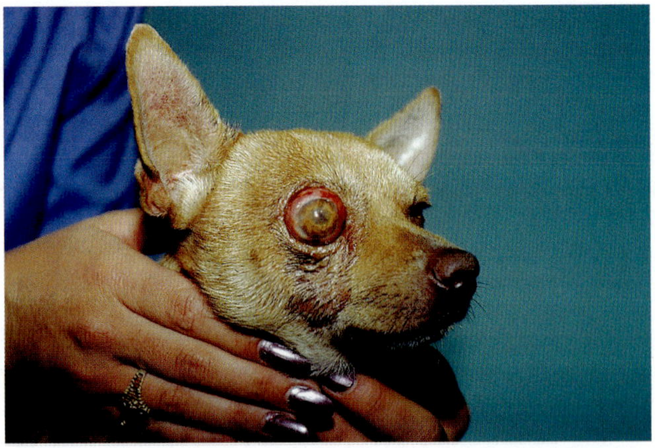

Figure 13-20
Traumatic proptosis. The animal was hit by a car door. Chemosis, subconjunctival hemorrhage, and miotic pupil are present.

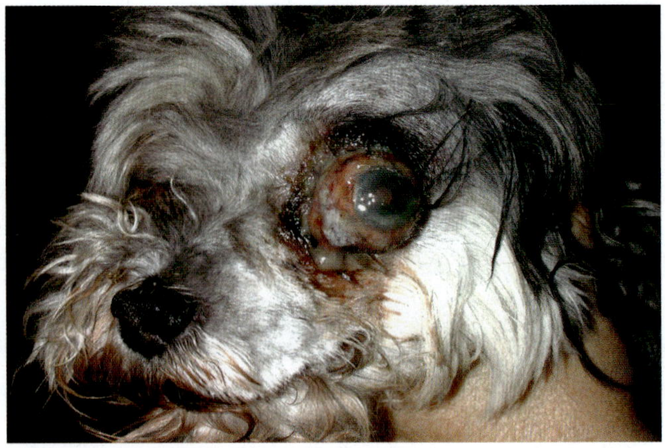

Figure 13-21
Severe and neglected ocular proptosis.

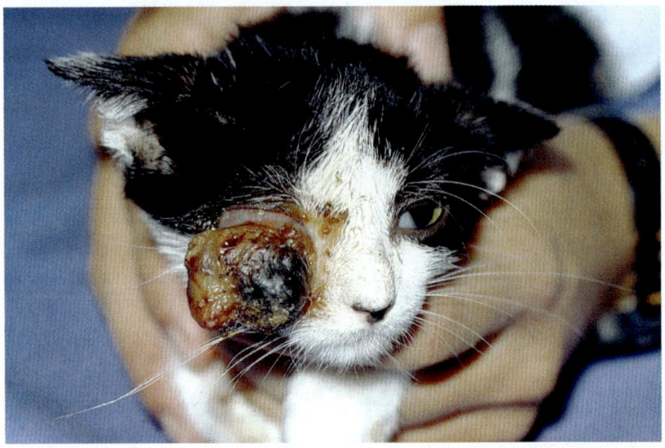

Figure 13-22
Neglected ocular proptosis in a kitten.

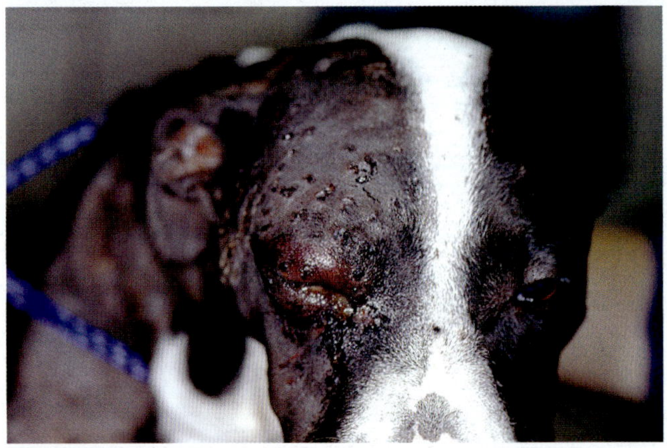

Figure 13-23
Accidental shotgun wounds of the face. The eye was enucleated because of uncorrectable damage to the eye.

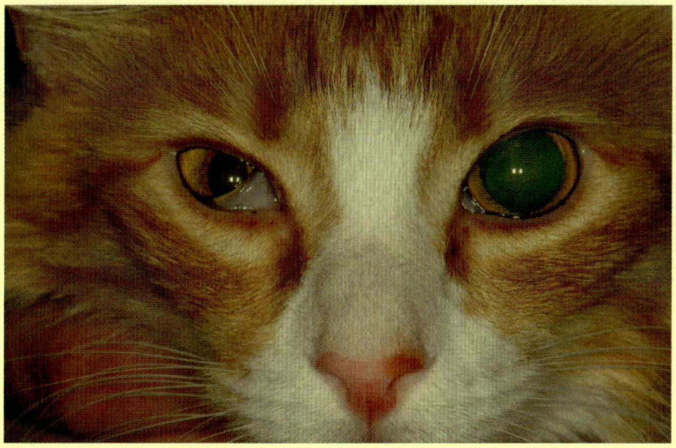

Figure 13-24
Presenting signs of Horner's syndrome (autonomic denervation) include a quadrad of ocular signs in small animals. In this cat with Horner's syndrome of the right eye the classic signs (MEPP) of miosis, enophthalmos, protrusion of the third eyelid, and ptosis are present.

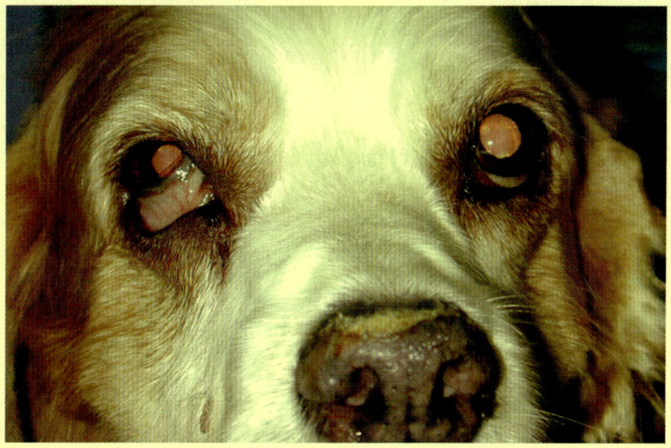

Figure 13-25
Spaniel with Horner's syndrome affecting the right eye. Ptosis, enophthalmos, miosis, and protrusion of the third eyelid are evident.

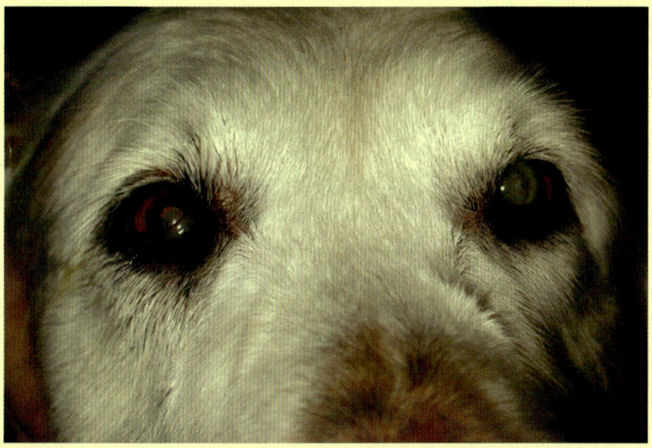

Figure 13-26
Horner's syndrome (idiopathic) in an elderly golden retriever. Miosis, enophthalmos, ptosis, and protrusion of the third eyelid (MEPP) of the right eye are present.

Index

A

Abyssinian
  hyperreflectivity, 171
  late PRA, 171
  optic atrophy, 171
  vascular attenuation, 171
Active chorioretinal lesions, *Ehrlichia* infection, 193
Active chorioretinitis, 187-198. *See also* Rottweiler
  aspergillosis, impact. *See* German shepherd
  focal areas, 187
Acute experimental chlamydiosis. *See* Cats
Acute glaucoma. *See* American cocker spaniel; Dogs
Acute perivascular cuffing (vasculitis), 191
Acute retinitis, 189
Acute uveitis, 82
Adenocarcinoma. *See* Dog upper eyelid
Adenoma. *See* Dog irises; Dogs
Advanced optic nerve cupping, 125
Afghan hound, immature cataract, 103
Ahmed valve implantation. *See* Basset hound
Akita
  corneal edema, 89
  tapetal retinal folds, 179
  uveitis, 89
Alopecia, 88
American cocker spaniel
  acute closed-angle glaucoma, 120
  acute glaucoma, 120
  cherry eye, 25
  congenitally imperforate lower nasolacrimal punctum, 31
  conjunctivitis, 30
  corneal edema, 30, 120
  dilated pupil, 120
  ectropion uveae, 86
  episcleritis, 62
  injected conjunctival vessels, 120
  KCS, 30
  mucopurulent discharge, 30
  myelinated nerve fibers, 145
  neovascularization, 30
  nontapetal fundus, retinal folds, 179
  peripheral corneal neovascularization, 120
  purulent material, release, 31
  red eye, 86, 120
  retinal folds, 178
  uveitis, 86
American water spaniel
  PRA, 161
  tapetal hyperreflectivity, 161
Aniridia. *See* Dogs
Ankyloblepharon, 10
  bacterial infection. *See* Eyelids
Anterior cataract, focused, 99
Anterior chamber
  chronic granulomatous infiltrates, 64
  fibrin clot, inferior position, 92
  free-floating iris cyst. *See* Boston terrier; Dogs
  haziness, 86
  iris cysts. *See* Irish wolfhound
  red blood cells, presence (hyphema), 83
  vitreous, slit lamp photograph, 112
Anterior lens capsule
  iris, swelling, 89
  pigment
    deposits, 68, 91
    presence, 89. *See also* Keeshound
  posterior synechiae, 89
  rubeosis iridis, 91
  smooth contour, change, 109
  vascularization, 94
Anterior lens luxation, 114. *See also* Fox terrier
Anterior luxation, 112
Anteriorly luxated lens, 113-114, 116. *See also* Golden retriever
Anterior sutures. *See* Immature cataract
Anterior uveitis, 89. *See also* Cats
Aphakic crescent
  superior position, 122
  visibility, 115-116
Aqueous, white cells (presence), 87
Aqueous flare, presence, 89
Aqueous humor, dark particulate matter, 86

Arcus lipoides. *See* Cocker spaniel; German shepherd
Area centralis hyperreflectivity, 173
Aspergillosis, impact. *See* German shepherd
Associated central cataract. *See* Cats
Asteroid hyalosis, 126, 127. *See also* Golden retriever
  stars, appearance, 98
Atrophy, 125, 208
Australian heeler
  corneal descemetocele, 44
  corneal neovascularization, 29
  KCS, 29
  mucopurulent discharge, 29
Australian shepherd
  buphthalmic right eye, 122
  central anterior stromal lipid deposits, 54
  choroidal dysplasia, 221
  choroidal vessels
    formation, 221
    visibility, 142, 148, 150, 152
  chronic glaucoma, 122
  conjunctiva, eyelid agensis, 1
  corneal dystrophy, 54
  corneal edema, 122
  dermoid, 1
  dyscoria, 66
  end-on-vessels, presence, 139
  hereditary multiple ocular anomalies, 221
  heterochromia iridis, 66, 70
  iris coloboma, 66, 221
    nasal extension, 66, 67
  lateral lower eyelid, eyelid agenesis, 1
  long posterior ciliary artery, 221
  microphakia, 97
  microphthalmia, 221
  normal nontapetum, 147, 148, 150, 152
  normal retina, 143
    light-colored tapetum, 136
    tapetal cells, presence, 139
  optic nerve, focal coloboma, 216
  peripheral fundus, staphyloma (presence), 221
  retinal dysplasia, 176
  retinal folds, 176
  RPE, pigmentation, 152
  staphyloma, presence, 221
  tapetum, development, 147
  tigroid fundus, 149
  vascularization, 122
  VKH, 89
Autoimmune cause, 13
Autonomic denervation, 227

B

Bacterial blepharitis. *See* Dogs
Basement membrane defects, 36
Basset hound
  advanced optic nerve cupping, 219
  buphthalmos, 122
  chronic glaucoma, 122, 219
  corneal edema, 55
  corneal endothelial dystrophy, 55
  corneal erosions, 55
  Descemet's membrane, tears, 122
  dilated pupil, 122
  glaucoma
    buphthalmos, 123
  glaucoma, Ahmed valve implantation, 121
  puppy, retina, 137
  red eye, 122
  secondary lens subluxation, 123
  vascularization, 55
Beagle
  corneal edema, 121
  dilated pupil, 121
  open iridocorneal angle, 119
  primary open-angle glaucoma, 119, 121
  red eye, 121
Belgian shepherd
  color change, 183
  degenerative retinopathy, 183
  hyperpigmentation, 183
  inherited degenerative retinopathy, 183
  tapetal fundus, circular dysplastic foci, 183
  tapetal hyperreflectivity, 183
Bichon frise
  bilateral depigmentation, 185
  cataract surgery, 60
  Descemet's membrane, inclusion cyst, 60
Bilateral cherry eye. *See* English bulldog
Bilateral combined eyelid agenesis, 8. *See also* Cats
Bilateral eosinophilic keratoconjunctivitis. *See* Cats
Bilateral eyelid agenesis. *See* Shorthair cat
Bilateral FCRD. *See* Siamese cats
Bilateral glaucoma. *See* Cats
Bilateral hypopyon. *See* Dogs
Bilateral lower eyelid ectropion. *See* Dogs; Dogue de Bordeaux
Bilateral macropalpebral fissure. *See* Pug
Bilateral severe entropion. *See* Shar-Pei
Bilateral superficial ulcers. *See* Yorkshire terrier
Bilateral upper eyelid agenesis. *See* Cats
Bilateral uveitis, 88, 124. *See also* Left eye
Bleeding disorders. *See* Systemic bleeding disorders
Blepharitis, 11, 12. *See also* Cats; Puppies
Blinking, 9
Blue-eyed cat, thinned iris stroma, 73
Border collie
  normal tapetum, 140
  red tapetal islets, 140
Borrelia burgdorferi, 86
Boston terrier
  anterior chamber, free-floating iris cyst, 74
  corneal dystrophy, 53
  corneal edema, 55
  corneal ulcer, perforation, 45
  diffused corneal edema, 55
  endothelial dystrophy, 55

Boston terrier *(Continued)*
immature cataract, 102, 103
incipient anterior cortical cataract, 55
iris sphincter atrophy, 55
lipid deposition, 53
medial canthus, erosive squamous cell carcinoma, 14
medial rectus muscle, 225
nasal limbal hemangiosarcoma, 61
proptosed globe, 225
Boxcar lesions, 206
Boxcarring. *See* Golden retriever
Brachycephalic breeds, facial folds (presence), 9
Brain tumors, 216
Briard
CPRA, 165
Brucella canis. *See* Dogs
Bulbar conjunctiva, lymphoid follicles, 20
Bulbar surface, lymphoid follicles. *See* Nictitans
Bullous retinal detachment. *See* Hypertensive cat
Buphthalmia. *See* Weimaraner
Buphthalmos, 122-124. *See also* Eyes; Shetland sheepdog
inclusion. *See* Basset hound

C

Cairn terrier
corneal edema, 123
limbus, pigment (presence), 123
pigmentary glaucoma, 123
sclera, pigment (presence), 123
Candida species, impact, 42
Canine adenovirus infection, 85
Canine herpesvirus, 176
Canine progressive retinal atrophy, 156-170
Canine SARD, 172-173
Canthus. *See* Lateral canthus
Capsule, wrinkling, 108. *See also* Poodle
Cartilage growth, abnormalities, 24
Cataract. *See* Focal anterior cortical cataracts; Immature cataract; Incipient cataracts; Peripheral vacuolar cataracts
association. *See* High enzyme-linked immunosorbent assay titer
poodle trauma uveitis, 86
surgery. *See* Dogs
Cataractous lens, 113-114
Cat corneas
cellular infiltrate, 41
dendritic ulcer, 38
foreign body, 47
neovascularization, 41
perforation, 45
sequestrum, 52-53
ulceration, 46
Cat irises
cyst, 75
feline leukemia virus (positive test), 90
major arterial circle, 65
prolapse, 46
Cat left eyes
bilateral eyelid agenesis. *See* Shorthair cat
conjunctival lymphosarcoma, 23
epiphora, 31
Cat nictitans
cellular infiltrate, 41
eosinophilic infiltrate, 26
lymphocytic infiltrate, 26
neovascularization, 41
Cats
active chorioretinitis, 196-197
acute experimental chlamydiosis, 19
advanced taurine deficiency, 175
area centralis
hyperreflective zone, 174
hyperreflectivity, 173
attenuated retinal vessels, presence, 170
bilateral combined eyelid agenesis, 8
bilateral eosinophilic keratoconjunctivitis, 40
bilateral glaucoma, 124
blepharitis, 41
blood vessels
diameter, decrease, 171
disappearance, 170, 171
chorioretinitis, 195-198
chronic low-grade anterior uveitis, 91
chronic perforated descemetocele, 46
chronic uveitis, 91
ciliary adenoma, 80
ciliary body cyst, 75
corneal scarring, 40
corneal ulcer, 36
diffuse iris melanoma, 79, 80, 119
dilated pupils, 124
drainage angle pigmentation, goniophotograph, 80
entropion, 8
eosinophilic conjunctivitis, 20
eosinophilic keratitis, 41
epithelium, loose edges, 36
equatorial vacuoles, 110
exposure keratitis, 124
focal idiopathic uveitis, 91
herpesvirus. *See* Feline herpesvirus
hyperreflective tapetum, presence, 170, 173
hypertension, 206-208
incipient cataracts, 110, 116
incipient suture line cataract, 110
iridocorneal angle, diffuse iris melanoma (extension), 79
iris-to-cornea PPM, 69
iris-to-lens PPM, associated central cataract, 69
keratic precipitates, 83, 92
lower eyelid
entropion, 7, 53
trichiasis, 7
lymphosarcoma, 92

Cats *(Continued)*
  medial canthus, mast cell tumor, 16
  multifocal granulomatous lesions, 195
  multifocal hyperpigmented chorioretinal scars, 213
  multifocal hyperreflective scars, 213
  nevus, 76
  normal fundus, 153-156
  ophthalmomyiasis, 213
  optic nerve
    active chorioretinitis, 194
    oval hyperreflective chorioretinal scar, 175
    tapetum, surrounding, 153
  optic neuritis, 195, 198
  pigmented iridocorneal angle, 119
  PPMs, 70
  PRA, 170
  preretinal hemorrhage, 205
  pupillary margin, thinned iris, 73
  pupil margin, iris cysts, 75
  retinal degeneration, 170-171
  retinal folds, 205
  retinal hemorrhage, 197, 205
  retinal thinning, 173
  right eye, bilateral upper eyelid agenesis, 2
    postoperative view, 2
  sequestrum, 52
  subluxated lens, 116
  subretinal hemorrhage, 205
  superficial corneal ulcer, 35
  superficial nonhealing corneal ulcer, 36
  superior bullous retinal detachment, 201
  tapetal color, 153
  tapetal hyperreflectivity, presence, 170, 171
  taurine deficiency, 174
  trichiasis, 8
  uveitis, 89-93
Cat ulcers
  corneal neovascularization, impact, 46
CEA. *See* Collie eye anomaly
Cellular infiltrates, 193. *See also* Cat corneas; Cat nictitans; Pembroke Welsh corgi
Central nervous system (CNS)
  neoplasia, 216
  tumors, 214
Central PRA (CPRA), 165. *See also* Briard
Cephalexin, treatment, 14. *See also* Oral cephalexin
Chemosis, 18, 20, 222, 226. *See also* Conjunctivitis
Cherry eye. *See* American cocker spaniel; Dogs; English bulldog; Third eyelid
Chihuahua
  corneal endothelial dystrophy, slit lamp photograph, 56
  corneal epithelium, fluid-filled lacunae, 56
  left eye, optic neuritis (retrobulbar optic neuritis), 218
  right eye, optic nerve (retrobulbar optic neuririts), 218
Chlamydial infection, 20
Choriocapillaris layer. *See* Retinal pigment epithelium
Chorioretinal scarring, 209
Chorioretinitis, 91, 211, 218. *See also* Active chorioretinitis; Chronic chorioretinitis; Inactive chorioretinitis
  visibility, 188
Choroid, black dots, 130
Choroidal depigmentation. *See* Springer spaniel
Choroidal hypoplasia, 183. *See also* Collie eye anomaly; Right eye; Shetland sheepdog
Choroidal pigment, 132
Choroidal vessels, 136
  presence. *See* Poodle
  tiger stripes, 150
  visibility, 151, 153. *See also* Australian shepherd; Fundus; Miniature longhaired dachshund; Siberian husky
Chow chow
  bilateral lower eyelid entropion, 7
  bilateral upper eyelid entropion, 7
  lower eyelid entropion, 6
  secondary pigmentary keratitis, 6
  upper eyelid entropion, 6
Chronic chorioretinitis, 192. *See also* Dachshund
Chronic corneal ulcer
  granulation, 5
  neovascularization, 5
Chronic glaucoma, 123, 125
Chronic granulomatous infiltrates. *See* Collies
Chronic KCS, 28, 44. *See also* Lhasa apso
  close-up. *See* Pug
Chronic superficial keratitis. *See* Pannus
Chronic ulceration, 52
Chronic uveitis, 94. *See also* Cats; Golden retriever
Ciliary adenoma. *See* Cats
Ciliary body adenoma. *See* Dogs
Ciliary body cyst. *See* Cats
Ciliary cleft, 95
Ciliary epithelium, nonpigmented cyst. *See* Dogs
Ciliary processes. *See* Stretched ciliary processes
Cilium, stoutness, 3
Closed iridocorneal angle, 119
Coagulaopathies, 203
Coccidioidmycosis, impact, 194. *See also* Dogs
  optic neuritis, 217
Cocker spaniel
  arcus lipoides, 57
  early PRA, 160
  ectropion uveae. *See* American cocker spaniel
  hypothyroidism, 57
  incipient cortical opacity, 103
  peripapillary edema, 217
  peripheral tapetal hyperreflectivity, 160
  pigment proliferation, focal areas, 166
  posterior cortical opacities, 103
  PRA, 166
  red eye. *See* American cocker spaniel

Cocker spaniel *(Continued)*
- retinal hyperpigmentation, 217
- RPE depigmentation, 166
- uveitis. *See* American cocker spaniel
- vascular attenuation, 160

Collie eye anomaly (CEA), 183-187
- choroidal hypoplasia, 184-186
- impact. *See* Shetland sheepdog
- nontapetum, retinal folds, 185
- optic nerve coloboma, 186-187
- peripapillary depigmentation, 186
- retinal folds, 185
- retinal nonattachment, 187

Collies
- iris, obscuration, 78
- NGE, 64
- normal nontapetum. *See* Merle collie
- normal tapetum. *See* Border collie
- sclera/eyelids/cornea, chronic granulomatous infiltrates, 64

Coloboma, 66, 185, 214. *See also* Australian shepherd; Lens; Optic disc
- iris dilator muscle, involvement, 67

Color dilute coat, 145

Commensals, 11

Congenitally imperforate lower nasolacrimal punctum. *See* American cocker spaniel

Congenital tortuous venules, 202

Conjunctiva, 17. *See also* Edematous conjunctiva; Injected conjunctiva
- dermoids, 17
- eyelid agenesis. *See* Australian shepherd
- pygmy rattlesnake bite. *See* Dogs
- redness/swelling, 44

Conjunctival cyst. *See* Dogs

Conjunctival dermoid. *See* Young dog

Conjunctival edema. *See* Springer spaniel

Conjunctival hemangioma. *See* Dogs

Conjunctival hemorrhage, 225

Conjunctival infiltrates, 92

Conjunctival lymphosarcoma. *See* Cat left eyes

Conjunctival melanocytoma. *See* Labrador retriever

Conjunctival papilloma. *See* Lhasa apso

Conjunctival sac, thelazia. *See* Dogs

Conjunctival surface, pigmented papilla. *See* Golden retriever

Conjunctival swelling, 18

Conjunctivitis, 20. *See also* Mucoid conjunctivitis
- chemosis, 18
- petechia, 18

Cornea, 34
- deep laceration, penetration, 48
- dendritic ulcer. *See* Cat corneas
- endothelial surface, 83
- facial folds, impact. *See* Pekingese
- hair
  - contact, 2
  - existence, 68
- inferior aspect, 83
- infiltration, 40
- laceration. *See* Perforating corneal laceration
- linear opacity, 86
- lower eyelid hair, contact, 6
- mucopurulent discharge, adherence, 28
- pigment, presence, 2
- PPM. *See* Cats

Corneal degeneration. *See* Dogs; Mixed-breed dog
- slit lamp photograph
  - lipid infiltrates, 57
  - neovascularization, 57

Corneal dermoids, 17. *See also* Dachshund
- hairs, inclusion, 35

Corneal descemetocele. *See* Australian heeler; Pointer

Corneal drying, impact, 35

Corneal dystrophy, 3. *See also* Boston terrier
- bilateral diseases, 53

Corneal edema, 85, 87, 89, 105. *See also* Akita; Boston terrier; Diffuse corneal edema; Focal corneal edema; Greyhound; Secondary corneal edema; Shih Tzu; Springer spaniel
- association. *See* Episcleritis
- inferonasal extension, 91
- presence, 42, 44-45, 123

Corneal endothelial dystrophy. *See* Chihuahua

Corneal endothelial pump, inflammation (interference), 86

Corneal endothelium, keratic precipitates. *See* German shepherd

Corneal injury, 61

Corneal lipid infiltrate. *See* Dogs

Corneal lubrication, absence, 35

Corneal neovascularization, 8, 85, 89, 121. *See also* Australian heeler; Dogs; Shetland sheepdog
- foreign body, impact, 47
- impact. *See* Cat ulcers
- presence, 29, 45, 123

Corneal pathologic problems, 3

Corneal perforation. *See* Cat corneas; Dogs

Corneal pigmentation. *See* Pug

Corneal scar
- anterior synechiae, 48
- cataract, 48

Corneal scarring, 28, 51. *See also* Cats

Corneal stroma, 43. *See also* Siberian husky
- lipid infiltration, 57

Corneal surface, mucopurulent discharge (adherence), 29

Corneal ulceration, 5, 39

Corneal ulcers, 3, 4. *See also* Cats; Deep corneal ulcer; Melting corneal ulcer; Nonhealing corneal ulcer
- granulation. *See* Chronic corneal ulcer
- neovascularization. *See* Chronic corneal ulcer
- perforation. *See* Boston terrier
  - healing, 46
  - uvea protrusion, 44

Corneal vascularization, absence, 37

Corneoconjunctival transposition. *See* Half-thickness corneoconjunctival grafts
healing, 48-49
Cortex, liquefaction, 108. *See also* Keeshound
nucleus, visibility, 108
Corticosteroids
preparation, 21
response, 213
treatment, 41
CPRA. *See* Central PRA
Cryosurgery, usage, 3
Cryptococcosis, 195, 197
Cyst. *See* Boston terrier; Dogs
tapetal reflex, transillumination, 74

D

Dachshund
chronic chorioretinitis, 210
corneal degeneration, slit lamp photograph, 57
corneal dermoid, 35
depigmented lesions, 210
lipemia retinalis, 202
nontapetum, chronic chorioretinitis, 213
normal retina. *See* Miniature longhaired dachshund
toxoplasmosis, 202
Dacryocystitis. *See* Weimaraner
Dalmatian, normal tapetal-nontapetal junction, 139
Deep corneal ulcer, 42
Degenerative retinopathies, 135
Dendritic ulcer. *See* Cats
Depigmentation. *See* Skin
areas, 192
Dermatitis. *See* German shorthaired crossbreed
Dermoid, 1, 17. *See also* Australian shepherd
hairs, inclusion. *See* Corneal dermoid
Descemetocele. *See* Cats; Dogs; Pointer
Descemet's membrane, 42
tears, 123
Diabetes mellitus. *See* Dogs
Diffuse corneal edema, 59, 86
Diffuse iris melanoma. *See* Cats; Siamese cats
Diffuse posterior cataracts, 100
Dilated pupil, 123. *See also* American cocker spaniel; Cats
presence, 120
Dirofilaria. *See* Eyes
Distemper
impact, 189
infection, 192
virus, 212
Distichia. *See also* Dog upper eyelid; Eyelids; Pekingese; Saint Bernard
emergence. *See* Meibomian gland
Distichiasis, 3
Doberman pinscher
GME, 190, 217
iris-to-lens PPM, 68
PHPV, 126
PHTVL, 126
sulfonamide-induced retinitis, 188
Dog irises
adenoma, 79
dark-colored iris, 143
nevus, 72, 76
tumor, 79
Dog lower eyelid
entropion, 7
imperforate punctum, 31
Dog nontapetum, 143-152, 191
chocolate-brown color, 145
multifocal white opacities, 211
reddish-brown color, 146
schematic diagram, 143
Dogs
acute glaucoma, 120
acute optic nerve edema, 125
aniridia, 65
anterior chamber, free-floating iris cyst, 74
anterior corneal stromal spicules, 59
bacterial blepharitis, 11, 13
bilateral hypopyon, 87
bilateral lower eyelid ectropion, 8
Brucella canis, 83
cardiac anomaly, engorged vessels, 203
cataract, post-surgery patients, 111
cataract surgery, 84
hypopyon, 87
cherry eye, 26
chest, compressive injury, 204
ciliary body adenoma, 77
ciliary epithelium, nonpigmented cyst, 73
color change, 210
conjunctiva, pygmy rattlesnake bite, 20
conjunctival cyst, 22
conjunctival hemangioma, 22
conjunctival sac, thelazia, 21
corneal degeneration, 58-59
corneal edema, 120
corneal lipid infiltrate, 64
corneal neovascularization, 59
dark-brown nontapetum, 144
descemetocele, 42-43
diabetes mellitus, 100
distemper, 190, 209
virus infection, 191
distichia, 3
engorged venules, 204
episcleritis, 64
extinguished electroretinogram, 172
eyelid, papilloma, 15
flat retinal detachment, 200
focal retinal detachment, 200
follicular conjunctivitis, 26
hair loss, 13
hemorrhage, 194, 204

Dogs *(Continued)*
hypermature cataract, 109
hypertensive retinopathy, 100
hyperviscosity syndrome, 204
hyphema, 84
inflammatory disease, recovery, 208
internal ophthalmomyiasis, 211-212
intrastromal corneal hemorrhage, 59
iridal swelling, 84
leukemia, 87
limbal melanoma, 61
lipid-laden opacities, 127
lymphosarcoma, 87
multifocal depigmentation, 211
multiple myeloma, 222
nevus, 76
nontapetal retina
depigmentation, 213
infiltrates, 191
normal fundus, 129
normal iridocorneal angle, 118-119
normal nontapetum, 143-152
normal tapetum, 129
optic neuritis, 188
peripapillary edema, 125
pupil
distortion, 77
margin, multifocal iris cysts, 74
red eye, 77
retinal dialysis, 198
retinal edema
focal areas, 190
multifocal areas, 189
retinal hemorrhage, 204
coccidioidmycosis, impact, 188
retinal infiltrates, focal areas, 194
retinal patchier, 204
right eye, corneal performation, 45
sclera, vascular tumor, 63
secondary pigmentation, 210
superior nontapetum, diffuse mottling, 144
swelling, 13
tapetum hyperreflectivity, focal areas, 210
tortuous retinal venules, 144
uveal melanoma, 78
uveitis, 83
V-shaped upper eyelid, 6
Dogue de Bordeaux, bilateral lower eyelid ectropion, 8
Dog upper eyelid
adenocarcinoma, 15
distichia, 3
meibomian gland adenoma, 15
Dorsal conjunctiva, dermoid. *See* Siamese cats
Dot and blot-shaped focal hemorrhages, 203
Drainage angle, 78, 94
pigmentation, goniophotograph. *See* Cats
Dyscoria, 66. *See also* Australian shepherd
posterior synechiae, impact, 93

E

Ectopic cilium
impact, 5
presence, 4
Ectropion, 8. *See also* Dogue de Bordeaux; Saint Bernard
uveae, 77, 85. *See also* American cocker spaniel
Edema, 39, 121. *See also* Corneal edema
Edematous conjunctiva, 19
Ehrlichia canis (E. canis), 191, 193
Ehrlichia infection. *See* Active chorioretinal lesions
Ehrlichiosis, 193
Electroepilation, usage, 3
End-on capillaries. *See* Normal retina
End-on vessels, presence. *See* Australian shepherd
Endothelial keratic precipitates, 90, 91
Endothelial pigmentation. *See* English pointer
End-stage PRA, 172, 173
English bulldog
adult, cherry eye, 25
facial fold, 26
lymphoid follicular enlargement, 26
medial entropion, 26
puppy, bilateral cherry eye, 25
English cocker spaniel
icterus, 22
immune-mediated hemolytic anemia, 22
English pointer
atrophic disc, 169
endothelial pigmentation, 60
PRA, 169
subalbionotic fundus, attenuated retinal vessels, 169
Enophthalmos, 220. *See also* German shepherd; Great Dane
Entropion, 5. *See also* Cats; Dog lower eyelid
absence, 8
Enucleated eye, histopathology, 79
Eosinophil, high numbers, 40
Eosinophilic conjunctivitis. *See* Cats
Eosinophilic infiltrate. *See* Cat nictitans
Eosinophilic keratitis. *See* Cats
Epiphora, 19. *See also* Cat left eyes; Golden retriever
Episcleritis, 63. *See also* American cocker spaniel; Dogs; Rottweiler
corneal edema, association, 62
impact. *See* Red eye
neovascularization, association, 63
Epithelial defect, arborizing, 38
Epithelial inclusion cyst, 61
Epithelium
loose lip, indolent ulcer, 38
loose tags, 38
tags, 37
Erosive squamous cell carcinoma. *See* Boston terrier
Erythema. *See* External nares; Eyelids
Exophthalmia, 222
Exophthalmic cat, retinal photograph, 201
Exophthalmic globe, edema, 223

Exophthalmos, 220
Exposure keratitis, 222. *See also* Cats; Shetland sheepdog
External nares, erythema, 89
Exudate, 187, 198
Eyelid, 1
agenesis. *See* Australian shepherd; Cats; Upper eyelids
ankyloblepharon, bacterial infection, 10
conjunctiva, lymphoid follicles, 20
distichia. *See* Upper eyelids
erythema, 89
malformations, 8
margins, 5
dermoid, 17
distichia, 3
melanoma, 16
mucocutaneous junction, thickening/erythema/erosion, 11
mucopurulent discharge, adherence, 28, 29
papilloma. *See* Dogs
protrusion, 5
Eyes
anomaly. *See* Collie eye anomaly
antibiotic, application, 10
bilateral uveitis. *See* Left eye
bleeding, causes, 128
buphthalmos, 89
poliosis. *See* Left eye
secondary glaucoma. *See* Left eye
subadult *Dirofilaria* organism, 87
uveitis. *See* Left eye

F

Face, shotgun wounds, 226
Facial folds. *See* English bulldog
impact. *See* Pekingese
presence. *See* Brachycephalic breeds
FCRD. *See* Feline central retinal degeneration
Feline central retinal degeneration (FCRD), 173-175. *See also* Siamese cats
lesions, 173
Feline herpesvirus
conjunctivitis, 18
infection, 18, 38
keratitis, multifocal areas, 40
keratitis, 39, 46
keratoconjunctivitis, 40
polymerase chain reaction testing, positive result, 41
Feline infectious peritonitis (FIP), 93, 196
uveitis, 93
Feline leukemia virus, 205
infection, 92
positive test, 92, 93. *See also* Cat irises
Feline panleukopenia virus, 176
Feline PRA, 170-171
Fibrils. *See* White fibrils
Fibrin clot, inferior position. *See* Anterior chamber
Fibrin clot, staining, 45
Fibrin plug, visibility, 45
Fibrovascular iridal membranes, 94
Fibrovascular membranes, 94
Field-trial Labrador retriever, retinal dysplasia, 180
FIP. *See* Feline infectious peritonitis
Flash reflection, 127
Fluorescein dye
staining, 35-38, 43-45
uptake, 51
usage, 31
Focal anterior cortical cataracts, 98
Focal chorioretinal scar, 209
Focal corneal edema, 113
Focal gray keratic precipitates, 95
Focal idiopathic uveitis. *See* Cats
Focal posterior synechia. *See* Fox terrier
Focal retinal detachment, 201
Focal retinal folds, 177
Focal tapetal hyperreflectivity. *See* Poodle
Follicular conjunctivitis. *See* Dogs
Fox terrier
anterior lens luxation, 115
attenuated vessels, 173
focal posterior synechia, 112
lens subluxation, 112
optic atrophy, 173
retinal dysplasia, 178
SARD, 173
Freckle. *See* Nevus
Free-floating iris cyst. *See* Boston terrier; Dogs
Frosted glass appearance. *See* Nuclear sclerosis
Fundus. *See* Dogs; German shorthaired pointer; Juvenile fundus; Red fundus; Subalbinotic fundus; Tapetal fundus
choroidal vessels, visibility, 151
normally pigmented tapetal area, cross-section, 130
visibility, 115

G

German shepherd
active chorioretinitis, aspergillosis (impact), 188
arcus lipoides, 56
atypical pannus, 26, 27
cataract, 110
cellular infiltrate, 26
corneal edema, 222
corneal endothelium, keratic precipitates, 110
corneal pigmentation, 50
enophthalmos, 222
granulation tissue, presence, 49
hypothyroidism, 56
lens-induced uveitis, 110
lesions, asymmetry, 50
mature cataract, 110
neovascularization, presence, 49

German shepherd *(Continued)*
nictitans
anterior surface, melanoma, 27
gland, cyst, 27
palpebral surface, plant seed foreign body, 27
pannus, 49-51
perilimbal arcus lipoides, 56
phthisis bulbi, 222
posterior synechiae, 110
traumatic uveitis, 222
German shorthaired crossbreed
dermatitis, 13
staphylococcal blepharitis, 13
German shorthaired pointer
fundus, 146
lower eyelids, lateral entropion, 5
nasolacrimal duct cyst, 32
nontapetum, RPE, 146
normal fundus, 132
optic nerve myelination, 132
upper eyelids, lateral entropion, 5
Ghost vessels. *See* Miniature longhaired dachshund
presence. *See* Pug
Giant retinal dialysis, 199
Giant schnauzer, preretinal arteriolar loops, 202
Glaucoma, 79, 220. *See also* Golden retriever; Left eye; Poodle; Secondary glaucoma
buphthalmos, inclusion. *See* Basset hound
Gliosis, 158
Globe, retraction, 5
GME. *See* Granulomatous meningoencephalitis
Golden retriever
anteriorly luxated lens, 114
asteroid hyalosis, 127
central corneal edema, 114
chronic uveitis, 89
epiphora, 31
exophthalmos, 224
extinguished electroretinogram, 172
extraocular myositis, 224
Horner's syndrome, 227
imperforate lower nasolacrimal punctum, 31
interpalpebral fissure, superficial corneal opacification, 34
nictitans gland adenocarcinoma, 33
normal retina, yellow-orange tapetum, 132
optic nerve atrophy, 219
posterior Y-suture cataract, 99
PRA, 159
puppy, bilateral blepharitis, 11
retinal atrophy, 219
retinal dysplasia, 178
retinal vessels, boxcarring, 159
retrobulbar extraocular muscle myositis, 224
SARD, 172-173
secondary glaucoma, 89
tapetal hyperreflectivity, 159
tapetum, multifocal circular areas, 178
upper eyelid
conjunctival surface, pigmented papilla, 4
trichiasis, 10
ventrolateral exotropia, 224
vessel attenuation, 159
VKH-like syndrome, 219
Gordon setter
PRA, 158
retinal blood vessels, attenuation, 158
tapetal hyperreflectivity, 158
Granulation, 5. *See also* Chronic corneal ulcer
Granulomatous meningoencephalitis (GME), 190. *See also* Doberman pinscher
Great Dane, enophthalmos, 222
Greyhound
corneal edema, 86
normal nontapetum, 146
pannus, 51
RPE, pigment (absence), 146
uveitis, 86

H

Hair loss. *See* Dogs
Half-thickness corneoconjunctival grafts, 48
Hematoxylin-eosin [H&E] stain, 176
Hemorrhage, presence, 203
Herpesvirus
conjunctivitis. *See* Feline herpesvirus
infection. *See* Feline herpesvirus
keratitis. *See* Feline herpesvirus
Heterochromia, 153. *See also* Siberian husky
iridis, 66, 70, 71. *See also* Australian shepherd
High enzyme-linked immunosorbent assay titer, cataract (association), 86
Histoplasmosis, 195, 213
Horner's syndrome, 81. *See also* Golden retriever; Spaniel
signs, 227
Husky
posterior Y-suture cataract. *See* Siberian husky
trauma-induced uveitis, 82
Hyaloid artery, 126
Hyaloid remnants, 202
attachment. *See* Posterior lens capsule
Hypermature cataract, 59, 106, 108. *See also* Dogs; Poodle
lens liquefaction, 106
slit lamp photograph. *See* Liquefied hypermature cataract
Hyperpigmentation, areas, 192
Hyperplasia, 165
Hyperreflective tapetal lesions, 189
Hyperreflective tracks, 210
Hypertensive cat
aneurysms, 206
bullous retinal detachment, 206, 207
external photograph, 207
optic atrophy, 206
retinal degeneration, 206

Hypertensive cat *(Continued)*
retinal detachment, 207
retinal folds, 206
retinal hemorrhage, 206-208
small petechiae, 206
total bullous detachment, 208
Hypertensive retinopathy. *See* Dogs
cases, 203
Hyperviscosity syndrome. *See* Dogs
Hyphema, 83, 128. *See also* Anterior chamber; Dogs
presence, 48
Hypopyon, 87. *See also* Dogs
presence, 42
Hyporeflective tapetal lesions, 189

I

Icterus. *See* English cocker spaniel
Immature cataract, 74, 102, 104. *See also* Afghan hound; Boston terrier; Miniature poodle; Miniature schnauzer; Siberian husky
anterior sutures, 91
anterior Y-shaped sutures, prominence, 105
Immune-mediated hemolytic anemia. *See* English cocker spaniel
Immune-mediated thrombocytopenia, 21
Imperforate lower nasolacrimal punctum. *See* Golden retriever
Imperforate punctum. *See* Dog lower eyelid
Imuran, treatment, 64
Inactive chorioretinitis, 208-213
Incipient anterior cataracts. *See* Standard poodle
Incipient anterior cortical cataracts. *See* Boston terrier
Incipient anterior opacities. *See* Cocker spaniel
Incipient cataracts, 98
vacuoles, 100
Incipient cortical cataract. *See* Labrador retriever
Incipient posterior polar Y-suture cataract. *See* Rottweiler
Incipient suture line cataracts. *See* Cats
Incipient-to-immature cataract. *See* Miniature poodle
Indirect ophthalmoscopy, 189
Inherited cataract, dilation, 82
Inherited retinal degeneration, 208
Injected conjunctiva, 19, 122
Internal ophthalmomyiasis. *See* Dogs
Interpalpebral fissure, superficial corneal opacification. *See* Golden retriever; Puppies
Intraocular lens (IOL), 112
haptics, 111
usage, 111
Intraocular neoplasia. *See* Rottweiler
Intraocular pressure
chronic insidious rise, 79
60 mm Hg, 121
Intraocular tumor, 128
Intrastromal corneal hemorrhage. *See* Dogs
Intumescent diabetic cataract, 106
Iridal blood vessel, dilation, 82
Iridal swelling. *See* Dogs
Iridocorneal angle, 117. *See also* Beagle; Closed iridocorneal angle; Dogs
diffuse iris melanoma, extension. *See* Cats
Iriododialysis, 95
Irises. *See* Subalbinotic iris
atrophy, 39
bombé, 86, 94
coloboma, 66. *See also* Australian shepherd
color change, 90. *See also* Left eye; Right eye
cyst. *See* Cat irises; Dog irises; Irish wolfhound
dilator muscle
atrophy, 72, 73
involvement. *See* Coloboma
distortion, 77
major arterial circle. *See* Cats
melanomas, 74, 77. *See also* Cats
visibility, gonioscopy (usage), 78
nevus. *See* Dog irises
obscuration. *See* Collies
pigmentation, 59
sphincter atrophy. *See* Boston terrier; Shetland sheepdog
sphincter muscle atrophy, 72
stroma. *See* Blue-eyed cat
surface, 76
swelling (iritis), 82, 85. *See also* Anterior lens capsule; Pit bull
traumatic separation, 95
tumor. *See* Dog irises
Irish setter
glial proliferations, 158
optic atrophy, 158
peripheral tapetum, 157
rod-cone dysplasia type 1, 157-158
tapetal hyperreflectivity, 157-158
vessel
attenuation, 157
thinning, 158
Irish wolfhound
anterior chamber, iris cysts, 74
pupillary margin, iris cysts, 74
Iris-to-cornea PPM. *See* Cats
Iris-to-iris capsule, 68
Iris-to-iris PPM, 68
Iris-to-lens PPM, 67, 68. *See also* Doberman pinscher
associated central cataract. *See* Cats
Itraconazole, treatment, 188, 194

J

Juvenile fundus, 137, 143, 147
presence, 157

K

KCS. *See* Keratoconjunctivitis sicca
Keeshound
  anterior lens capsule, pigment (presence), 107
  cortex, liquefaction, 107
  morgagnian cataract, 107
Keratic precipitates, 83, 93. *See also* Cats; Endothelial keratic precipitates; Focal gray keratic precipitates
Keratitis, 9. *See also* Feline herpesvirus
  multifocal areas. *See* Feline herpesvirus
Keratoconjunctivitis sicca (KCS), 25, 28-29. *See also* American cocker spaniel; Australian heeler; Chronic KCS; Shih Tzu; Siberian husky; Springer spaniel
Keratopathy. *See* Lipid keratopathy
Kittens
  lipemia, 69
  lipemic iridal vessels, 69
  lipoprotein lipase deficiency, 69
  patent PPMs, 69

L

Labrador retriever
  cataract, 96, 158
  ciliary adenocarcinoma, 78
  conjunctival melanocytoma, 23
  geographic retinal dysplasia, 180, 181
    vascular loops, 181
  hyperreflective tapetum, 158
  incipient cortical cataract, 104
  limbal melanoma, 61
  microphakia, 96
  nontapetum, 145
    depigmentation, 166
    hyperpigmentation, 166
    retinal dysplasia, circular area, 181
  normal retina, 131
  optic nerve hypoplasia, 215
  peripheral retinal tear, post intracapsular lens removal, 200
  peripheral tapetum, hyperreflectivity, 159
  posterior polar Y-suture cataract, 99
  PRA, 158-159, 166
  puppy
    inherited chondrodysplasia, 180
    multiple ocular anomalies, 180
  retinal dysplasia, 181. *See also* Field-trial Labrador retriever
    circular area, 181
    superior, 180
  tapetal reflection, 158
  upper eyelid distichium, 4
  vessel attenuation, 159
  zonules, nasal extension, 96
Lacrimal system, 28
Lacrimal tissue removal, surgery failure, 32
Lacrimation, 4
  increase, 11
Lateral canthus, involvement, 2
Lateral lower eyelid, eyelid agenesis. *See* Australian shepherd
Lateral strabismus, 225
Left eye
  bilateral eyelid agenesis. *See* Shorthair cat
  bilateral uveitis, 88
  exophthalmia, 223
  exophthalmos, 225
  iris color change, 90
  lateral globe deviation, 225
  midriasis, 225
  poliosis, 88
  secondary glaucoma, 88, 89
  uveitis, 89
Lens. *See* Luxated lens
  coloboma, 97
  displacement, 116
  equator, broken zonules, 115
  fibers
    meeting, 105
    separation, anterior Y-shaped sutures, 106
  introduction, 96
  luxation. *See* Anterior lens luxation; Mixed-breed dog
  protein, leakage, 105, 109
  subluxation, 78. *See also* Fox terrier
Lens capsule
  pigment deposits. *See* Anterior lens capsule
  PPM remnants, 68
Lens-induced uveitis, 59, 105, 109. *See also* German shepherd
Lesions, red-stained, 39
Leukemia. *See* Dogs
Lhasa apso
  chronic KCS, 29
  conjunctival papilloma, 22
  optic atrophy, 219
  periocular dermatitis, 29
  proptosis, 219
  retinal atrophy, 219
  upper eyelid, sebaceous adenoma, 14
Limbal melanoma. *See* Dogs; Labrador retriever
Limbal (scleral) staphyloma, 95
Linear opacity, 68
Lipemia. *See* Kittens
  retinalis. *See* Dachshund
Lipemic iridal vessels, 69
Lipid degeneration, 56
Lipid infiltrates. *See* Shetland sheepdog
Lipid keratopathy, 74. *See also* Siamese cats
Lipids, corneal deposit, 51
Lipofuscin, foci, 165
Lipoprotein lipase deficiency. *See* Kittens
Liquefied hypermature cataract, slit lamp photograph, 108

Lower eyelids
  distichia, 4
  ectropion. *See also* Saint Bernard
  entropion, 6. *See also* Cats; Chow chow; Dogs; German shorthaired pointer; Shar-Pei; Shorthair cat
  erosion, squamous cell carcinoma impact. *See* White cat
  hair, contact. *See* Cornea
  trichiasis. *See* Cats
Luxated lens, 112. *See also* Anteriorly luxated lens
Lymphocytic infiltrate. *See* Cat nictitans
Lymphocytic-plasmacytic corneal infiltrate, 49
Lymphoid follicles. *See* Bulbar conjunctiva; Eyelids; Nictitans
Lymphoid follicular enlargement. *See* English bulldog
Lymphosarcoma, 91, 195. *See also* Cats; Dogs
Lysine, treatment. *See* Oral lysine

M

Major arterial circle. *See* Cat iris
Maldeveloped retina, geographic areas, 176
Mastiff
  bullous retinal detachments, 182
  hemorrhage, 182
    ventral gravitation, 182
  multifocal retinal detachment, 182
  nontapetum, retinal dysplasia, 182
  retinal dysplasia, 182
Mature cataract, 105. *See also* German shepherd; Saint Bernard
  presence, 2
Medial canthus
  cartilage, T-piece, 24
  erosive squamous cell carcinoma. *See* Boston terrier
  malignant melanoma, 15
  mast cell tumor. *See* Cats
  nasolacrimal duct cyst. *See* Terrier
Medial entropion. *See* English bulldog; Pug
Medial rectus muscle. *See* Boston terrier
Medial trichiasis, 59
Meibomian gland
  abscess, 12
  adenoma. *See* Dog upper eyelid
  distichium, emergence, 4
Meibomianitis, 12
Melanoma, 201. *See also* German shepherd; Iris; Standard poodle
  diagnosis, 76
  distention, 78
Melting corneal ulcer, 42
Membrana nictitans. *See* Third eyelid
MEPP. *See* Miosis enophthalmos protrusion of the third eyelid ptosis
Merle collie, normal nontapetum, 149
Microphakia. *See* Australian shepherd; Labrador retriever
Microphthalmos, 220
Migrating epithelium, adherence, 36
Milk supplement, impact. *See* Nuclear cataract
Miniature longhaired dachshund
  advanced PRA, 161, 167
  choroidal vessels, visibility, 142
  disc, myelin loss, 161
  ghost vessel, 167
  normal retinas, 142
  pigment clumping, 167
  PRA, 161
  retinal vascular attenuation, 161
  RPE depigmentation, 167
  tapetal hyperreflectivity, presence, 161
  tapetum, development, 142
  vessel attenuation, 161
Miniature poodle
  immature cataract, 102
  incipient-to-immature cataract, 104
  retinal edema, focal area, 191
Miniature schnauzer
  equatorial fundus, PRA, 162
  immature cataract, 103
  PRA, 162
  vascular attenuation, visibility, 162
Miosis, 81
  presence, 89
Miosis enophthalmos protrusion of the third eyelid ptosis (MEPP), 227
Miotic pupil, 226
Mixed-breed dog
  corneal degeneration, 58
  depigmentation, 167
  hyperpigmentation, 167
  lens luxation, 114
  lipemia retinalis, 217
  mineralization, occurrence, 58
  nontapetum
    depigmentation, 169, 170
    hyperpigmentation, 170
  papilledema, 217
  PRA, 167, 169, 170
  retinal arterioles, caliber variations, 164
  retinal degeneration, 164
  retrobulbar meningioma, 217
  secondary glaucoma, 114
  staphylococcal blepharitis, 14
  tapetum, yellow color (patchy variability), 164
Morgagnian cataract, 107. *See also* Keeshound
  slit lamp photograph, 107
Mucocutaneous junction
  thickening/erythema/erosion. *See* Eyelids
Mucocutaneous junction depigmentation (vitiligo), 89
Mucoid conjunctivitis, 20
Mucoid discharge, 11, 19
Mucopurulent discharge. *See* Australian heeler; Shih Tzu; Springer spaniel

adherence. *See* Cornea; Corneal surface; Eyelids; Pekingese
Mucopurulent ocular discharge, 18
Mucous discharge, increase, 28
Multifocal chorioretinal scars, 209. *See also* Nontapetum
Multifocal conjunctival petechiae, 21
Multifocal cutaneous draining tracts. *See* Weimaraner
Multifocal hyperreflective areas, 208
Multifocal iris cysts. *See* Dogs
Multifocal retinal hemorrhage. *See* Poodle
Myelinated nerve fibers. *See* American cocker spaniel

N

Nasal keratitis. *See* Pug
Nasal limbal hemangiosarcoma. *See* Boston terrier
Nasolacrimal duct
- cyst. *See* German shorthaired pointer; Terrier
- scarring. *See* Young cats

Necrotic stroma, 52
Neovascularization, 5, 28, 85. *See also* Chronic corneal ulcer; Corneal neovascularization
- association. *See* Episcleritis
- 360 degrees, presence, 46
- presence, 89

Nevus (freckle), 76. *See also* Cats; Dog irises; Dogs
- ectropion uveae, 77

NGE. *See* Nodular granulomatous episclerokeratitis
Nictitans. *See* Cats; Scrolled nictitans
- anterior surface
  - follicular conjunctivitis, 20
  - plaque, 26
- bulbar surface, lymphoid follicles, 19
- elevation, 27
- glands
  - adenocarcinoma. *See* Golden retriever
  - cyst. *See* German shepherd

Night blindness, 156
Nodular granulomatous episclerokeratitis (NGE), 64. *See also* Collie
Nonhealing corneal ulcer, 36, 39
Nonhealing superficial corneal ulcer, 37
Nonhealing superficial ulcer, 37
Nonhealing ulcer, 4, 38
Nonpigmented cyst. *See* Dogs
Nontapetal fundus, 165. *See also* Tigroid nontapetal fundus
- linear gray opacities, 192
- RPE, reaction, 209
- vitreal hemorrhage, 193

Nontapetum. *See* Dog nontapetum
- depigmentation. *See* Mixed-breed dog
- multifocal chorioretinal scars, 212
- multifocal white opacities. *See* Dogs
- retina, choroidal vessels (visibility), 149
- tracks, 211

Normal fundus, 202. *See also* Cats; Dogs; German shorthaired pointer
Normal nontapetum. *See* Australian shepherd; Dogs; Greyhound; Siberian husky
Normal retina, 130-143. *See also* Australian shepherd; Labrador retriever; Springer spaniel
- arterioles, 134
- disc, pigmented conus, 133
- end-on capillaries, 134
- gray tapetal color, 136
- nontapetal junction, 133
- optic disk, odd myelination, 133
- optic nerve vessels, prominence, 134
- physiologic cup, visibility, 133
- pigmented conus, presence, 135
- schematic, 157
- speckled tapetum, 131
- superior fundus, tapetum islets (presence), 141
- tapetal islets, presence, 141
- tapetal junction, 133
- tapetal-nontapetal junction, 135
- tapetum
  - variable color, 134
  - visibility, 140
- white tapetum, 140
- yellow-orange tapetum. *See* Golden retriever
- yellow-red tapetum, 132

Nuclear cataract, milk supplement (impact), 100
Nuclear sclerosis, 72, 97-98, 104. *See also* Poodle
- frosted glass appearance, 97

O

Ocular anomalies, 66
Ocular irritation, 5
Ocular proptosis, neglect, 226
Ocular tumors, 83
Old English sheepdog, persistent hyaloid remnant, 126
Ophthalmia neonatorum, 10
Ophthalmomyiasis, 210. *See also* Cats; Dogs
Optic atrophy, 209, 215. *See also* Abyssinian; Fox terrier; Hypertensive cat; Irish setter; Springer spaniel; Tibetan terrier
Optic disc
- colobomas, 183
- myellination, 130

Optic nerve, 214, 217
- atrophy, 125
- choroidal hypoplasia. *See* Right eye
- coloboma. *See* Collie eye anomaly
- cupping. *See* Advanced optic nerve cupping; Basset hound
- hemorrhage, 197
- hypoplasia. *See* Labrador retriever; Poodle; Russian wolfhound; Samoyed
- meningioma, 225
- obscuring, 199
- retinal edema, 190
- tapetum, nerve (surrounding). *See* Cats
- vessels, prominence. *See* Normal retina

Optic neuritis, 215, 218. *See also* Cats
Optic papilla, 214
Ora ciliaris retinae, 198
Oral cephalexin, treatment, 12
Oral lysine, treatment, 40
Orbit, 220. *See also* Pug

P

Pannus (chronic superficial keratitis), 26. *See also* German shepherd; Greyhound; Pembroke Welsh corgi
  occurrence, 51
Papilledema, 216-217
Patent PPMs. *See* Kittens
Pekingese
  cornea
    facial folds, impact, 9
    mucopurulent discharge, adherence, 60
  corneal epithelium, superficial pigment (infiltration), 60
  KCS, 60
  nasal fold trichiasis, 60
  pigmentary keratitis, 9
Pekingese, distichiasis, 3
Pembroke Welsh corgi
  cellular infiltrates, 52
  neovascularization, temporal quadrant, 52
  pannus, 52
Perforating corneal laceration
  cat scratch, impact, 48
  slit lamp photograph, 48
Perilimbal arcus lipoides. *See* German shepherd
Periocular dermatitis. *See* Lhasa apso
Periocular erythema, 20
Peripapillary edema, 218
Peripheral corneal neovascularization. *See* American cocker spaniel
Peripheral equatorial vacuoles, 100
Peripheral retina, thinning, 135
Peripheral retinal tear. *See* Labrador retriever
Peripheral tapetal hyperreflectivity. *See* Cocker spaniel
Peripheral vacuolar cataracts, 98
Persistent hyaloid remnant. *See* Old English sheepdog
Persistent hyperplastic primary vitreous (PHPV), 126-127. *See also* Doberman pinscher; Pointer
Persistent hyperplastic tunica vasculosa lentis (PHTVL), 126-127. *See also* Doberman; Pointer
Persistent pupillary membrane (PPM), 67, 68. *See also* Cats; Iris-to-iris PPM; Iris-to-lens PPM; Kittens
  decrease, 69
  remnants. *See* Lens capsule
Petechia(e). *See* Conjunctivitis; Hypertensive cat; Multifocal conjunctival petechiae
Phacoemulsification, usage, 111
Photoreceptor dysplasias, 176
PHPV. *See* Persistent hyperplastic primary vitreous
Phthisis bulbi, 220
PHTVL. *See* Persistent hyperplastic tunica vasculosa lentis
Pigmentary keratitis, 59. *See also* Pekingese
Pigmentation, 9
  increase, 39, 77
  reduction, 70
Pigment deposits. *See* Anterior lens capsule
Pigmented iridocorneal angle. *See* Cats
Pigment spots, 210
Pit bull
  iris, swelling, 82
  uveitis, 82
Planum nasale, 88
PMMA. *See* Polymethymethacrylate
Pointer
  cataracts, 127
  corneal descemetocele, 43
  endothelial pigmentation. *See* English pointer
  intralenticular hemorrhage, 127
  normal fundus. *See* German shorthaired pointer
  PHPV, 127
  PHTVL, 127
Poliosis. *See* Left eye
Polymerase chain reaction testing, positive result. *See* Feline herpesvirus
Polymethymethacrylate (PMMA), 111
Poodle
  anterior suture lines, prominence, 104
  atrophic optic nerve, 163
  capsule, wrinkling, 107
  choroidal vessels, presence, 168
  depigmentation, 167
    foci, attenuation, 168
  focal depigmentation, 168
  focal tapetal hyperreflectivity, 163
  glaucoma, 109
  hypermature cataract, 107, 109
  hyperpigmentation, 167, 168
  hyperreflective tapetum, 162
  immature cataract, 104. *See also* Miniature poodle
  multifocal retinal hemorrhage, 167
  nontapetum RPE, depigmentation, 168
  nuclear sclerosis, 104
  optic nerve
    head, myelin loss, 163
    hypoplasia, 216
  papilledema, 216
  peripapillary depigmentation, 162
  peripheral tapetum, segmental hyperreflectivity, 163
  PRA, 104, 162-163, 167-168
  PRCD-1, 163
  retinal arterioles, loss, 162
  retinal detachment, 109
  retinal veins, attenuation, 162
  tapetal fundus

Poodle *(Continued)*
central hyperreflectivity (presence), 162
peripapillary hyperreflectivity (presence), 162
trauma uveitis. *See* Cataract
uveal melanoma. *See* Standard poodle
vascular attenuation, 163
vascular loss, 168
white foci, presence, 168
Portuguese water spaniel
choroidal vessels, presence, 169
diffuse hyperreflectivity, presence, 164
hyperpigmentation, small foci, 169
PRA, 164, 169
Posterior capsular opacity, 127
Posterior cataracts. *See* Diffuse posterior cataracts
Posterior cortical cataracts. *See* Standard poodle
Posterior cortical opacity, 127. *See also* Cocker spaniel
Posterior lens capsule
gray retina, 201
hyaloid remnant, attachment, 126
Posteriorly luxated lens, 115, 116. *See also* Shar-Pei
Posteriorly subluxated lenses, 124
Posterior polar Y-suture cataract. *See* Labrador retriever
Posterior synechiae, 86, 89. *See also* Anterior lens capsule
360-degree, 94
impact. *See* Dyscoria
trauma, secondary, 93
Posterior Y-suture cataract. *See* Siberian husky
feathering, 99
Postnucleation lacrimal cyst, 32
PRA. *See* Progressive retinal atrophy
PRCD-1. *See* Progressive rod-cone degeneration-1
Prednisone, treatment, 12, 14, 64
Preretinal arteriolar loops. *See* Giant schnauzer
Preretinal hemorrhage. *See* Cats; Sheltie
Preretinal venous loops, 202
Progressive retinal atrophy (PRA), 135, 156, 208. *See also* American water spaniel; Cocker spaniel; Feline PRA; Golder retriever; Gordon setter; Labrador retriever; Poodle; Portuguese water spaniel; Pug
advanced. *See* Miniature longhaired dachshund; Springer spaniel; Tibetan terrier
equatorial fundus. *See* Miniature schnauzer
impact. *See* Retinas
Progressive rod-cone degeneration-1 (PRCD 1), 163. *See also* Poodle
Proptosis, 220. *See also* Lhasa apso
Pseudodiphtheritic membrane formation, 18
Ptosis. *See* Miosis enophthalmos protrusion of the third eyelid ptosis
Pug
attenuated retinal vessels, visibility, 159
bilateral macropalpebral fissure, 9
chronic KCS, close-up, 30
corneal pigmentation, 30
ghost vessels, presence, 166
medial entropion, 8
nasal keratitis, 8
nontapetum
depigmentation, 166
hyperpigmentation, 166
pigmentation, 8
PRA, 159, 166
scarring, 30
shallow orbit, 9
trichiasis, 8
Pupil
dilation, 91
distortion, 77. *See also* Dogs
margin, 115
iris cysts. *See* Cats
multifocal iris cysts. *See* Dogs
Pupillary margin
iris cysts, 106. *See also* Irish wolfhound
thinned iris. *See* Cats
Puppies
bilateral blepharitis. *See* Golden retriever
eyelids
fusing, 10
opening, 11
interpalpebral fissure, superficial corneal opacification, 34
upper eyelid, blepharitis (focal area), 11
Pus, drainage, 10

R

Red cells, settling, 84
Red eye, 82, 105, 114, 121-123. *See also* American cocker spaniel; Dogs
corneal neovascularization, 223
episcleritis, impact, 62
presence, 42, 89, 120, 222
Red fundus, 146
Red reflex, 110
Retinal atrophy, 209. *See also* Canine progressive retinal atrophy
Retinal blood vessels, blood, 125
Retinal degeneration, 170, 175, 208. *See also* Hypertensive cat; Mixed-breed dog
schematic, 165
Retinal detachment, 83, 109, 128, 198-201, 218. *See also* Poodle
area, 196
Waldstrom's macroglobulinemia, impact, 205
Retinal dialysis. *See* Dogs; Giant retinal dialysis
Retinal dysplasia, 176-183. *See also* Australian shepherd; Fox terrier; Mastiff; Springer spaniel
histopathologic specimen, 176
superior. *See* Labrador retriever
Retinal edema
focal areas, 192
linear areas, 197
Retinal effusion. *See* Rottweiler

Retinal folds, 176-179, 193, 201. *See also* Akita; American cocker spaniel; Australian shepherd; Focal retinal folds; Golden retriever; Springer spaniel
Retinal hemorrhage, 190-191, 203, 217. *See also* Cats
  coccidioidmycosis (impact). *See* Dogs
Retinal holes, 199
Retinal hyperpigmentation. *See* Cocker spaniel
Retinal infiltrate, 194
Retinal nonattachments/detachments, 176, 183
Retinal pigment epithelium (RPE), 129-130, 198
  cell hypertrophy, 165
  choriocapillaris layer, 136
  depigmentation, 212. *See also* Cocker spaniel; Miniature longhaired dachshund; Rottweiler
  dystrophy, 165
  pigment, 139
    absence, 138
    sparseness, 139
  pigmentation, 139, 142. *See also* Superior fundus
  response, 165
Retinal tears, 109, 199
Retinal thinning, 104
Retinal vascular attenuation. *See* Miniature longhaired dachshund
Retinal vessels, 203
  boxcarring. *See* Golden retriever
  presence, 198
Retinas, 129. *See also* Normal retina
  inflammation, 187
  inner limiting membrane, 140
  PRA, impact, 157
Retinopathies, 165
Retinoschisis, 200
Retrobulbar abscess, 190
Right eye
  exophthalmia, 223
  exophthalmos, 224
  iris color change, 90
  optic nerve, choroidal hypoplasia, 184
  prolapse nictitans, 224
  secondary glaucoma, 124
Rod-cone dysplasia type 1. *See* Irish setter
Rose bengal, staining, 39
Rottweiler
  active choroiditis, 190
  chorioretinitis, 190
  episcleritis, 190
  incipient posterior polar Y-suture cataract, 100
  intraocular neoplasia, 84
  nontapetum, pigmentation (increase), 167
  PRA, 167
  retinal effusion, 190
  RPE depigmentation, 167
Rough collie, CEA, 183
RPE. *See* Retinal pigment epithelium
Rubeosis iridis. *See* Anterior lens capsule
Russian wolfhound, optic nerve hypoplasia, 215

S

Saint Bernard
  distichia, 110
  ectropion, 110
  mature cataract, 110
Saint Bernard, lower eyelid (ectropion), 9
Samoyed, optic nerve hypoplasia, 215
Sarcoma. *See* Lymphosarcoma; Traumatic sarcoma
Sclera, 62
  nodular swelling, 63
  vascular tumor. *See* Dogs
Scleral staphyloma. *See* Limbal staphyloma
Scleral vessels, 122
Scrolled nictitans, 24-25
Secondary corneal edema, 92
Secondary glaucoma, 94, 109. *See also* Golden retriever; Left eye; Mixed-breed dog; Right eye
  presence, 116
Secondary lens subluxation. *See* Basset hound
Secondary pigmentary keratitis. *See* Chow chow
Shar-Pei
  bilateral severe entropion, 6
  lower eyelid entropion, 7
  posteriorly luxated lens, 115
  upper eyelid entropion, 7
Sheltie, preretinal hemorrhage, 204
Shetland sheepdog. *See also* Lipid degeneration
  buphthalmos, 123
  CEA, impact, 183
  choroidal hypoplasia, 184
  corneal neovascularization, 54
  crossbreed
    hypothyroidism, 58
    perilimbal corneal degeneration, 58
  exposure keratitis, 123
  inherited corneal dystrophy, 54
  iris sphincter atrophy, 56
  lipid degeneration, 56
  lipid infiltrates, 54
  multiple myeloma, ocular involvement, 123
  stromal lipid dystrophy, 54
Shih Tzu
  corneal edema, 29
  KCS, 29
  mucopurulent discharge, 29
  vascularization, 29
Shorthair cat
  left eye, bilateral eyelid agenesis, 2
  lower eyelid entropion, 36
  neovascularization, 36
Siamese cats
  bilateral FCRD, 174
  diffuse iris melanoma, 80
  dorsal conjunctiva, dermoid, 17
  hyperreflectivity, symmetric bands, 174
  lipid keratopathy, 56
Siamese-type fundus, 155
  tapetal cells, 155

Siberian husky
  choroidal vessels, visibility, 151
  cornea
    mucoid discharge, adherence, 30
    plant material foreign body, 46
  corneal stroma, 53
  corneal vascularization, 30
  eyelids, mucoid discharge (adherence), 30
  fundic reflex, 147
  immature cataract, 102
  KCS, 30
  normal nontapetum, 147
  subalbinotic iris, 150
Skin
  depigmentation (vitiligo), 88
  grafting, 2
Spaniel, Horner's syndrome, 227
Speckled tapetal cells, 140
Sphincter muscle atrophy. *See* Iris
Springer spaniel
  advanced PRA, 160
  choroidal depigmentation, 182
  conjunctival injection, 30
  corneal edema, 30
  KCS, 30
  mucopurulent discharge, 30
  nontapetal fundus, retinal folds, 177
  normal retina, 131
  optic atrophy, 160
  retinal dysplasia, 182
  superficial neovascularization, 30
  tapetal fundus, retinal folds, 177
  tapetal hyperreflectivity, 160
  tapetum
    absence, 182
    changes, 160
  vessel attenuation, 160
Squamous cell carcinoma, impact, 223. *See* White cat
Standard poodle
  incipient anterior cataracts, 99
  posterior cortical cataracts, 99
  uveal melanoma, 78
Staphylococcal blepharitis. *See* German shorthaired crossbreed; Mixed-breed dog
Stretched ciliary processes, 97
Striate retinopathy, 192
Stroma. *See* Corneal stroma; Necrotic stroma
  presence, 42
Stromal dystrophies, 53
Stromal lipid dystrophies. *See* Shetland sheepdog
Stromal lipid dystrophy. *See* Shetland sheepdog
Subadult *Dirofilaria* organism. *See* Eyes
Subalbinotic fundus, 110, 149
  choroidal vessels, 155
Subalbinotic iris, 70, 71
Subconjunctival hemorrhage, 225, 226. *See also* Traumatic subconjunctival hemorrhage
Subconjunctival plaque, 21
Subluxated lens. *See* Cats
Subretinal serous exudate, impact, 206
Sudden acquired retinal degeneration (SARD), 172. *See also* Canine SARD; Fox terrier; Golden retriever
Superficial corneal opacification. *See* Golden retriever; Puppies
Superficial corneal ulcer. *See* Cats
  healing, 36
Superficial neovascularization. *See* Springer spaniel
Superior fundus, RPE pigmentation, 139
Superior nontapetum, diffuse mottling. *See* Dogs
Superior tapetum, 187
Suture lines, formation, 105
Symblepharon, 19. *See also* Young cats
Synchysis scintillans, 126
Syneresis, 126
Systemic bleeding disorders, 83
Systemic clotting disorders, 128
Systemic hypertension, 206

T

Tapetal cells. *See* Speckled tapetal cells
  islets, 151
Tapetal color, 140
Tapetal fundus, 147
  inflammation, multifocal small foci, 198
  pigmentary abnormalities, 198
  reflectance, reduction, 176
Tapetal hyperreflectivity. *See* American water spaniel; Belgian shepherd; Cocker spaniel; Golden retriever; Gordon setter; Springer spaniel; Tibetan terrier
  presence. *See* Miniature longhaired dachshund
Tapetal hypoplasia, 138
Tapetal hyporeflectivity, 187
Tapetal islets, 147
Tapetal-nontapetal junction, 139. *See also* Dalmatian; Normal retina
  scalloping, 139
Tapetal reflex, 42
  brightness, 104
  transillumination. *See* Cyst
Tapetum, 131. *See also* Dogs
  destruction, 196
  linear tracks, 197
  multifocal circular areas, 178
  presence, 142
  retinal folds, 178-179
  sparseness, 153
  thinning, 138
Tapetum hyperreflectivity, focal areas. *See* Dogs
Taurine deficiency. *See* Cats
Tear porphyrins, 52
Tear staining, 20. *See also* Young cats
Terrier. *See* Boston terrier; Yorkshire terrier
  lens subluxation. *See* Fox terrier
  pigmentary glaucoma. *See* Cairn terrier
  PRA. *See* Tibetan terrier
  right medial canthus, nasolacrimal duct cyst, 32

Thelazia. *See* Dogs
Thinned iris. *See* Cats
  stroma. *See* Blue-eyed cat
Third eyelid (membrana nictitans)
  cherry eye (scrolled cartilage/prolapsed gland), 24. *See also* American cocker spaniel; English bulldog
  conjunctiva, bulbar surface, 25
  manual repositioning, 25
Thrombocytopenia. *See* Immune-mediated thrombocytopenia
Tibetan terrier
  advanced PRA, 164, 165
  arteriolar attenuation, 169
  choroid, depigmentation, 169
  optic atrophy, 164
  PRA, 164, 169
  ridging (striping), choroidal vessels (impact), 165
  tapetal hyperreflectivity, 164, 165
  thinned retina, 165
  vascular attenuation, 164
  vessel attenuation, 164
Tigroid fundus. *See* Australian shepherd
Tigroid nontapetal fundus, 148
Topical dexamethasone, response, 41, 51
Topical trifluridine, response, 41
Torn medial rectus muscle, 225
Toxoplasmosis, 196. *See also* Dachshund
Trauma, 83, 192
  bleeding, 203
Trauma-induced uveitis. *See* Husky
Traumatic proptosis, 225, 226
Traumatic sarcoma, 94
Traumatic subconjunctival hemorrhage, 21
Trichiasis, 8. *See also* Cats; Golden retriever; Medial trichiasis; Pug
Trifluridine, treatment, 40

U

Ulceration. *See* Chronic ulceration
Ulcer stains, 42-43
Upper eyelids
  agenesis, 2
  copperhead snake bite, 42
  distichia, 4. *See also* Dog upper eyelid; Labrador retriever
  entropion. *See* Chow chow; German shorthaired pointer; Shar-Pei
  poor conformation, 6
  sebaceous adenoma. *See* Lhasa apso
Upper respiratory tract infection, 18
Uvea, introduction, 65
Uveal melanoma. *See* Dogs; Standard poodle
Uveitis, 77, 81, 85. *See also* Acute uveitis; Akita; American cocker spaniel; Dogs; Greyhound; Husky; Left eye; Pit bull
  presence, 89

V

Vacuoles. *See* Incipient cataracts; Peripheral equatorial vacuoles
Vascular anomalies, 202
Vascular disease, 202-208
Vascularization, 39. *See also* Anterior lens capsule; Neovascularization; Shih Tzu
Vasculitis, 83, 128. *See also* Acute perivascular cuffing
Vitamin E deficiencies, 165
Vitiligo. *See* Mucocutaneous junction depigmentation; Skin
Vitreal exudate, 91
Vitreal fibrosis, 212
Vitreal hemorrhage, 128
Vitreous, 126
VKH. *See* Vogt-Koyanagi-Harada
Vogt-Koyanagi-Harada (VKH) syndrome, 88, 125. *See also* Australian shepherd
  VKH-like syndrome. *See* Golden retriever

W

Waldstrom's macroglobulinemia, impact. *See* Retinal detachment
Weimaraner
  buphthalmia, presence, 122
  chronic glaucoma, 122
  dacryocystitis, 32
  exophthalmos, 223
  lacrimal puncta, pus drainage, 33
  multifocal cutaneous draining tracts, 32
  tapetal reflex, 136
White cat, lower eyelid erosion (squamous cell carcinoma impact), 16
White fibrils, 112
White foci, presence. *See* Poodle

Y

Yorkshire terrier, bilateral superficial ulcers, 35
Young cats
  feline herpesvirus infection, 19
  nasolacrimal duct, scarring, 19
  symblepharon, 19
  tear staining, 19
Young dog, conjunctival dermoid, 17

Z

Zonules, 96. *See also* Lens
  nasal extension. *See* Labrador retriever
Zygomatic sialocele, impact, 223